Good Research Practices

Good Research Practices

A practical guide to the implementation of the G*x*Ps

Edited by

Nigel J. Dent

Scientific Consultant,
Country Consultancy, UK

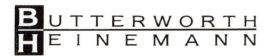

Butterworth-Heinemann
Linacre House, Jordan Hill, Oxford OX2 8DP
A division of Reed Educational and Professional Publishing Ltd

ℜ A member of the Reed Elsevier plc group

OXFORD   BOSTON   JOHANNESBURG
MELBOURNE   NEW DELHI   SINGAPORE

First published 1997

© Reed Educational and Professional Publishing Ltd 1997

British Library Cataloguing in Publication Data
A catalogue record for this book is available from the British Library

Library of Congress Cataloguing in Publication Data
A catalogue record for this book is available from the Library of Congress

ISBN 0 7506 2266 0

Typesetting and artwork origination by David Gregson Associates, Beccles, Suffolk
Printed and bound by Hartnolls Ltd., Bodmin, Cornwall

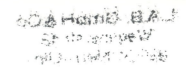

Contents

Part Three   Clinical trials and good clinical practice

Part Four   Multinational studies – pitfalls and benefits

Part Five   Animal health industries and good clinical practice

Part Six   Biotechnology

Contributors

Professor D Bobilewicz, MD, PhD
Head of Department of Laboratory Diagnostics, Postgraduate Medical Centre, Central Hospital, Warsaw, Poland

Dr R Brase
Central Hospital 'Links der Weser', Bremen, Germany

Mr E Brown
QA Manager, GMP, UK

A. Brzeziński, MD, PhD
Head, Department of Laboratory Diagnostics, Medical University, Łódź, Poland

Ms R A Corrigan
International Head of QA, Innovex (UK) Ltd, UK

Dr S W Cummings, PhD
Merck Sharpe and Dohme (Europe) Inc., Brussels, Belgium

Mrs C N Dent
Clinical Development, Hoechst Roussel Vet, UK

Mr N J Dent
Scientific Consultant, Country Consultancy, UK

Dr V G Edy
Head of Quality, British Biotech Pharmaceuticals Ltd, UK

Dr D S Freestone, FFPM
Retired. Formerly Director of Medical and Applied Research, Wellcome Research Laboratories and Part Time Senior Medical Officer, MCA, UK.

G M Gawlik, Bsc
Associate Director, Worldwide Quality Assurance Resources, Animal Health and Agricultural Development, Merck & Co., Inc., Rahway, NJ, USA.

Ms S Hughes, BSc
Lilly Research Centre Ltd, UK

Mr R L Hutchison
Director, Regulatory Compliance, SmithKline Beecham Pharmaceuticals, UK

Dr R W James, BVetMed, PhD, FRCPath, MRCVS, MIBiol, CBiol
Soteros Consultants Ltd, UK

Dr D L Jefferys
Director of Licensing, Medicines Control Agency, UK

Mr C Jenkins
GCP Auditor, Ashdown Clinical Research, UK

Dr R Kaplan
Group Director, QA, Ortho Biotech, USA

Mr G J Marsat
Director, Regulatory Compliance GCP, SmithKline Beecham Pharmaceuticals, UK

Mrs B Moore, MSc
Kesteven Statistical Services, UK

Mrs S Ollier, BSc
Clinical Research Consultant, QED Partnership, UK

Mr T Ott
Director, Worldwide Regulatory Compliance, Bristol-Myers Squibb Corporation, USA

Professor T L Paál
National Institute of Pharmacy and Imre Haynal University of Health Sciences, Budapest, Hungary

Dr H Plettenberg
LAB Europe, Germany

Mr G Prout
Technical Director, Kennet Bioservices Ltd, UK

Professor B Rozman, MD, PhD
University Medical Centre, Ljubljana, Slovenia

Ms S H Segalstad
Segalstad Consulting, Oslo, Norway

Mrs P M Squibb
QA Manager, British Biotech Pharmaceuticals Ltd, UK

Dr O Svendsen, DVM, PhD, DSc
Scientific Director, Scantox, Denmark

Dr M ten Ham
Chief, Drug Safety Unit, WHO, Geneva, Switzerland

Dr R H Visanji, MSc
QA, Hoechst Roussel Vet, UK

Dr J Walters, PhD
Elanco Animal Health, UK

Mr B C Warren
Research Quality Assurance, Pfizer Ltd, UK

Dr P L Worthington
PRISM Europe Ltd, UK

Preface

Over the past two decades the arrival of good practices has been of paramount importance to the bioscience industries.

The first arrival, which could be called the grandparent, was the good manufacturing practice (GMP) regulations governing the manufacture of medicinal and allied products.

Later the good laboratory practice (GLP), introduced by the Food and Drug Administration (FDA) of the USA, gave rise to consternation in many parts of the world because of the possibilities of a bureaucratic straitjacket on scientific research. Since 1976 this has proven not to be the situation; in contrast, it has increased the standard of science and people's awareness of the topic of preclinical and clinical research. This set of regulations or guidelines, as they are in some countries, could certainly be called the parent of the GxPs.

The most recent innovation is the good clininal practices (GCPs), the infant of them all. Although already established for some time in the USA, more formal introductions have recently been seen throughout Europe and Japan, culminating in the tripartite harmonization of the International Conference on Harmonization (ICH) document on GCP.

The term GxP has now been coined for many of these good practices. In addition to the main ones mentioned, GMP, GLP and GCP, we are seeing an evolution of similar guidelines throughout the industry.

In 1995 we saw the birth of GCP for the conduct of clinical trials for veterinary medicinal products (GCPV) in a European Union note for guidance.

There has been talk of good statistical practice, good computer practice, good warehouse practice and good scientific practice in university and similar establishments.

The whole industry is becoming aware of the need to promote a professional front and the guidelines over the next decade will proliferate.

The prime concern of the GMPs is still with the production of the finished product. This, however, has been extended through several

European Community directives and regulatory statutes into the provision of medicinal products for clinical trials in human pharmaceutical medicine.

GLP still remains as a regulatory requirement for the development of preclinical work covering safety and efficacy. However, within the industry, there is some divergence of opinion and the classic absorption, distribution, metabolism and excretion (ADME) and safety pharmacology (a topic yet to be clearly defined) remain open to interpretation by several regulatory agencies as to the need for their compliance with GLP.

In the GCP arena, there are again several differences of opinion as regards informed consent, ethics committee or institutional review body (IRB) composition and source data verification. Throughout the world we see a variance in the standards of inspectorate: some countries already have a very active group while others are beginning to set up such a unit. The International Conference on Harmonization 3 (ICH 3) was active in producing universal acceptance of documentation to further these areas of research and development.

At the time of publication, the animal health industry is coming to terms with GCPV and the provision of an independent quality assurance unit (QAU). Working to a set of guidelines which, again, has no formal inspectorate.

Following on from the ICH conferences relating to human pharmaceuticals and chemicals, April 1996 saw the first meeting of the International Cooperation on Harmonization of Technical Requirements for Registration of Veterinary Medicinal Products (VICH), take place. Of the key topics a mandate has been given to develop a tripartite guideline on the basis of existing guidelines to harmonize good clinical practice.

The programme is scheduled to run into 1998 with the GCP document expected at the end of 1997.

The GCPs, therefore, unlike the other good practices, suffer somewhat from the interpretative needs of companies and lack of formal inspection.

Again, over the next decade, it is the editor's impression that we will see some rationalization of inspection to cover these good practices and it is hoped that this book will help readers to make as smooth a transition as possible from their current situation to one of a compliant state.

This book has been designed to be a *practical guide*. All the authors have been chosen by the editor for their specific in-depth knowledge of the subject on which they have written. They are all practical persons who are active in their field and known to be up-to-date in the subject.

The section on GLP indicates how the QAU should move into the 21st century and covers particular problems in the production of drug substance, animal health studies and areas where biological vaccines will be reviewed in the GLP vein.

The next section, covering GCP, is really to be seen from the investigator's viewpoint. It is always very clear from the sponsor's point of view what needs to be done but this section deals with particular problems and overcoming such problems as are seen by the investigator when asked by a sponsor to carry out a clinical trial. The aspect of dealing with, and operating, contract research organizations (CROs) is also addressed in this section and gives both the sponsor and the CRO valuable information on what is required from both parties.

As clinical trials and GCP become more complex, the next section has chosen to outline preparing for an FDA inspection, submitting an investigational new drug application and bringing total quality management into clinical trials. A particular problem area in harmonization is that of ethics committees and here a chapter sets out to guide the reader along this particular stony path.

The section is followed by a chapter covering the practical problems of auditing multinational studies – again a very practical application, identifying the pitfalls and how to avoid them.

Within the animal health industry the book has taken great pains to cover the regulatory aspect, the practical aspect of setting up and monitoring clinical trials, along with assuring quality in these. The studies themselves cover companion animals through to large animal studies.

Biotechnology has been addressed in both the production of materials from GMP through to compliance with GLP and the implementation of the G*x*Ps has been looked at in the light of other current accreditation standards, such as EN 29 000.

The latter part of the book has set out to introduce the reader to the regulatory agencies and a review of the World Health Organization (WHO) and the Medicines Control Agency (MCA) leads the reader into what is often a grey area, extending outside that of preclinical and clinical testing.

The situation in Central and Eastern Europe is rapidly changing politically, and equally complex with regard to the G*x*Ps. A thorough review of all good practice has been undertaken and provides the reader with an up-to-date situation in this area.

An area that is often overlooked in producing a good scientific study is the final report and here three authors have undertaken to cover the expert report and the production of meaningful statistics.

No book would be complete without the overall review of computers and here the prime concern has been the validation of the computer database, to comply with GLP and GCP specifically.

Nigel J. Dent

Acknowledgements

As the editor, I would sincerely like to thank all the authors who have spent so much time producing excellent chapters and have been at the receiving end of my constant nagging, reminding them of fast-approaching deadlines.

Their excellent chapters left me needing to make little editorial comment, as each had stuck to the brief exactly, giving little overlap needing correction. As all were professionals, either in the quality assurance area or their relevant professions, the initial manuscripts were received with the minimal number of typographical errors which, again, made editorial review much easier.

Also thanks must go to Butterworth-Heinemann and Tim Brown for having faith, once again, in producing a second book covering good practices.

In preparation of the final manuscript I acknowledge the help of my wife in transcribing the individual authors' editorial comments and the patience of Ben and Saxon who missed out on many Sunday afternoon walks.

PART ONE

Good laboratory practice

1   The practical quality assurance unit: observations for the 21st century

R L Hutchison

Introduction

Opinions of what constitutes quality, and how to control it, have changed over the years, and will undoubtedly change again. Mostly these ideas have originated in manufacturing industry, particularly engineering. They have been adapted for other purposes. Thus, there has been a progression from inspection of the final product simply using accept/reject criteria, to component and final product inspection, then came the addition of statistical control with the use of Sherwart charts, and the Dodge and Romig tables. Eventually, in Japan, the line workers were taught the necessary measuring skills and statistics and an era of self-control of quality began. This form of quality control was something of a reversion to a pre-industrial-revolution self-control of quality by craftsmen, especially when focused on customer requirements. At the same time the definition of quality passed from 'fitness for purpose' (which in practice meant no better than it needed to be) to customer satisfaction.

The Japanese concepts of quality also grew out of the need to eliminate waste. Thus, foremen in car factories worked on the line as team leaders, and workers did their own quality control. At the same time there was a return to small batch component production and just-in-time delivery to eliminate inventory and warehouse costs.

The movement from one phase of quality theory to the next was caused by the realization either that the current methods were not working properly, or that that particular method did not fit a particular culture. Therefore, while statistical quality control was largely developed in the Bell Telephone laboratories, before the Second World War, and taken by Americans to Japan after the war, it was the mores and culture of Japanese society and in particular industrial organization which determined its use and transition to what is now known as total quality control, or total quality management (TQM). When, because of the success of Japanese industry worldwide, western governments and industrialists started to examine what could be the probable causes of that success, costs, delivery and quality were fixed upon as major factors. Then the question became: how can these control processes be transferred to western industry? Maybe what was seen first was the pressure on costs and delivery, and the quality processes came as part of the package. Whatever the reason, at that time, Dr Ishikawa (1985), the Japanese thinker and teacher on quality processes, expressed the view that someone who did not read Chinese script and had not been brought up in a Confucian and Buddhist culture could not successfully operate total quality control systems. In other words, a system of thought is directly related to the language and culture in which it is expressed. Change either the language or the culture, and the thought processes also change. Dr Ishikawa subsequently changed his opinion. Nevertheless there are powerful differences of culture, employment practices and attitude which do not make for an easy transfer of ideas of quality from Japan to the west, particularly North America. Japan is a society which generally proceeds by consensus; that is not true of some western countries where individualism, individual rights and expression are ideals.

There are therefore difficulties in introducing TQM into some western countries. Partially these are caused by company structures and partially by employment practices. For instance, in the UK and USA the executive officers of manufacturing companies often originate largely from sales or accounting backgrounds. They therefore have had only peripheral interest or involvement in problems associated with product quality. TQM demands their involvement.

However, despite the differences in company practices and structures, TQM has been successfully introduced in 30% of the US companies which have tried to use it. This shows that it can be done, but the introduction of TQM may not be easy. In Europe quality management systems have often been introduced through ISO 9000 registration. While there have been successes with the introduction of quality systems through this route, there have also been complaints from smaller companies about the expense and bureaucracy associated with ISO 9000 registration.

If TQM systems are to be introduced into those industries controlled by the good practice regulations, what is needed to ensure their success?

First, there must be clear and unequivocal top management support for the introduction of TQM throughout the company. Managements, not unnaturally, show a high commitment to costs and delivery, but often pass responsibility to the quality assurance group or the quality control department for all aspects of product or performance quality until something goes wrong. In a TQM environment this is not a feasible attitude. Quality of product, service or performance must be treated by management with equal seriousness and commitment to the way they treat costs and delivery. Quality standards and improvement on those standards are after all as much a market advantage as low costs and prompt short delivery times. To gain such an awareness of quality standards involves continuing formal and informal education and training, as well as applicable work experience, for both management and staff.

Externally there are forces which mitigate against the successful introduction of TQM. The pharmaceutical industry is highly regulated, particularly for drug development and manufacture. The three sets of regulations which govern preclinical development (good laboratory practice; GLP), clinical development (good clinical practice; GCP) and manufacturing (good manufacturing practice; GMP), particularly in the European Union, have distinctive requirements for quality assurance (QA), but each description of QA is different. It is therefore possible, even within the pharmaceutical industry, for QA practitioners to describe activities which are clearly different, but which each calls QA. Thus it becomes necessary to define which type of QA is being practised. If an organization is also attempting to gain ISO 9000 registration, it will also have to follow another concept of quality management.

Of the three regulated descriptions of QA within the European Union, by far the widest and most comprehensive is that for GMP:

> The basis concepts of Quality Assurance, Good Manufacturing Practice and Quality Control are inter-related. They are described here in order to emphasise their relationships and their fundamental importance to the production and control of medicinal products ...

> Quality Assurance is a wide ranging concept which covers all matters which individually or collectively influence the quality of a product. It is the sum total of the organised arrangements made with the object of ensuring that medicinal products are of the quality required for their intended use. Quality Assurance therefore incorporates Good Manufacturing Practice plus other factors outside the scope of this guide.

By contrast, the GLP definition of QA is limited in both its conception of what constitutes quality and how to achieve it:

Quality assurance programme

General

1 The test facility should have a documented quality assurance programme to ensure that studies performed are in compliance with these Principles of Good Laboratory Practice.

2   The quality assurance programme should be carried out by an individual or by individuals designated by and directly responsible to management and who are familiar with the test procedures.
3   This individual(s) should not be involved in the conduct of study being assured.
4   This individual(s) should report any findings in writing directly to management and to the Study Director.

Responsibilities of the Quality Assurance personnel

1   The responsibilities of the quality assurance personnel should include, but not be limited to, the following functions:
   a)   ascertain that the study plan and Standard Operating Procedures are available to personnel conducting the study;
   b)   ensure that the study plan and Standard Operating Procedures are followed by periodic inspections of the test facility and/or by auditing the study in progress. Records of such procedures should be retained;
   c)   promptly report to management and the Study Director unauthorised deviations from the study plan and from Standard Operating Procedures;
   d)   review the final reports to confirm that the methods, procedures, and observations are accurately described, and that the reported results accurately reflect the raw data of the study;
   e)   prepare and sign a statement, to be included with the final report, which specifies the dates inspections were made and the dates any findings were reported to management and to the Study Director (Ishikawa, 1985).

This is the description of QA from the Organization of Economic Co-operation and Development's *Principles of Good Laboratory Practice (OECD, 1992)*, which is now the system of GLP formally adopted by the European Union. It is by far the loosest description of QA in any of the GLP principles or regulations. All demand final product testing, in the form of a review of each final study report; all demand that each study shall be regularly inspected. None of the regulations makes a formal distinction between QA and quality control. In fact, the GLP description of QA conforms more to any other description of quality control than most other descriptions of QA.

This description of QA suffers from all the faults of the old system of quality control. First, quality is divorced from the work being done. The QA unit is responsible for quality and the scientists are responsible for science. Second, the measure of quality is compliance with GLP, nothing more. Third, the insistence on reviewing each report on every study creates a situation where, at best, the job of the QA unit is to ensure the accuracy and validity of each report; at worst they are proof-readers. This creates a situation in which the report is examined to discover errors, rather than to show that the process by which data are collected and the report produced is in control. As the QA unit is responsible for the accuracy of the report and therefore for discovering errors, errors are actually created or not properly addressed prior to a QA examination, because it can safely be left to QA to find those errors. While most QA groups adopt various stratagems to limit the number of errors in reports being received, such as to reject whole or part reports with an unacceptable error rate, this still remains a quality control process. This responsibility for the accuracy and validity of a study report must reside in the study team and its study director. To remove that responsibility to another group actually diminishes the quality of the report.

If the processes by which a study is performed and the report written are demonstrably in control, and if those processes have good quality control procedures, which are regularly reviewed and improved, why should it be necessary for another group to review the accuracy of the report? The quality of a product is defined by the people who produce it, not by the quantity of external inspection. Of course it may be necessary for QA personnel to review final reports and data, but this is to show that the processes by which data are generated and the report produced are what they should and could be, rather than to ensure the accuracy of the report. That should already be assured.

It is true that companies have introduced total quality techniques into various aspects of safety testing, and where these introductions have been successful there is a great deal of enthusiasm for the results. However, if every study report is audited to discover data and reporting inaccuracies, rather than to confirm or improve the process by which the report is produced, a tension is produced between two conceptions of quality control, which makes the introduction of TQM more difficult than is necessary.

If the various GLP principles and regulations were altered to a description of quality management similar to the European Union GMP guidelines and included a paragraph such as:

> There shall be a formal system of quality assurance which, among other matters, will ensure compliance with these principles of GLP

such a definition would allow a variety of QA systems to be practised. Provided the regulatory objective of GLP compliance is met, how it is met is a matter for each individual company, not the government regulatory inspection teams.

How the theory and practice of quality management will develop will largely be determined by the organization of individual companies within the pharmaceutical and chemical industries, management practices, increasing use of computers, and the training and work practices of scientific staff.

Company organization

Many companies in all industries are examining company organization and structures. They are shedding management staff and putting many tasks and indeed whole departments out to contract, because those activities are no longer considered core to the company's main functions. Even core projects are being undertaken by teams of contractors or temporary staff who are only employed for the duration of that project. Other companies are making extensive use of homeworkers who are linked only by computer and telephone to the company.

Pharmaceutical companies, in particular, are under increasing pressure from governments to reduce the costs of medicines, particularly where the government is the sole buyer. Similar pressures are being exerted in other countries by insurance companies or Pharmacy Benefit Management (PBM)companies. At the same time costs are increased by more stringent and more frequent application of regulations. Internal cost reduction has therefore become imperative and ways are being sought to reduce the time taken to do various tasks, to reduce the costs involved in doing those tasks, or both simultaneously. Alternatively, work which until recently would always have been done in-house is being passed to specialist contractors. Indeed, it is entirely possible that one piece of work could be spread or passed between several different contractors depending on their particular expertise. How far companies are prepared to follow such a path in drug development is open to speculation. Would they be able to exert sufficient control over development, or to anticipate particular problems, if more than a certain percentage of work were put out to contract?

In any event, it is entirely possible that each contractor may have its own quality standard which may or may not be congruent with those of the contracting company. It is a given fact that all these companies should conform to GLP, but is that a measure of quality, or a tool with which to achieve quality? If it is a measure, then it is only a minimum standard. If it is a tool, what is the best way to use it, and what other tools need to be used in order to achieve an acceptable quality standard? These are not new problems, but in the environment which has existed since 1979 all that was necessary was for the contracting company to ensure compliance to GLP. In today's concepts of quality, the quality of work, the delivery of that work and its economy are all intertwined. The quality control and other factors reside within the workgroup; therefore these are issues which must be resolved between the two companies as the contract is negotiated. This means that those people negotiating a contract must be prepared to discuss openly what the quality expectations and quality control systems are. It will not be sufficient to enquire about GLP compliance and if that meets requirements to assume that the quality standards are adequate. It is quite possible to meet all the requirements of GLP and to perform poor studies, all of which are beautifully documented. Therefore there has to be extensive training of negotiators in quality control. Something beyond who can do the job quickest and cheapest is required. Of course these are important factors, but any gains made by aiming solely at economy and delivery can easily be lost through unsatisfactory quality, which could cause delays through partial or complete rework of a project.

Inside producing companies there is considerable pressure to reduce both the costs and the time taken to produce work. Much of this can be achieved by introducing more efficient equipment of one form or another. To be successful, companies have to exert equal pressure at least to maintain quality, if not to improve it. In turn this means that the work teams have to be aware of what constitutes good quality and to build work processes which automatically ensure it. Certainly quality cannot be assured by routine inspections, except to confirm that the processes by which quality is controlled are in place and working properly. However, in a rapidly changing work environment it must be the QA unit's responsibility that the changes and improvements in delivery and cost not only do not compromise quality, but that gains in quality standards are also made.

Management practices

It is interesting that several writers on quality control, notably Ishikawa (1985) and Juran (1988), strongly express the view that the company president should take more than a passing interest in quality control. Not only should he or she chair the company quality council, but also should conduct his or her own periodic quality audits. This has some advantages, the most obvious of which is to emphasize total company commitment to quality. However, while an inspection by the company president or chief executive officer may be easily feasible in a small or middle-sized company with few sites in a limited area, the problems posed to a company president of a large multinational company with factories and research sites around the world are formidable. But no company president does not pay particular attention to production and sales figures and the problems associated with prompt and economic delivery. It ought not be too difficult, therefore, to find a way of both encouraging the development and enforcement of quality standards. Without a clear and active participation in quality activities by senior management, quality control and assurance work can easily be shunted to a suitably named department without any real power to change much.

Many companies offer prizes for outstanding process improvement projects and organize celebrations annually to give credit to project teams. Fewer celebrate achievements which are related purely to quality improvement projects.

Perhaps the presidential quality audit and the quality improvement celebrations could be organized in the following way. The company president chooses one site to audit a particular function, similarly each successive line manager will also audit a particular aspect of their own areas. The audit should be aimed at the quality control procedures of the group being audited. The results of the audit should then be discussed with all members of the team in an unaggressive way, and where necessary commitments for improvements made or to offer congratulations on good work. Of course at the same time there may be quality circles meeting to seek improvements in quality systems. These groups will also report their activities through line management. The reports of all audits and the quality circles could be then be passed to a reviewing committe who would choose the best to celebrate.

Such a system commits all management to quality activity and emphasizes to staff that they also must make an equal commitment. Not only have management to commit to quality, they have to learn about and how to solve quality problems. Staff also have to go through the same learning process.

Traditionally managers have concentrated on costs and delivery. This concentration has been reinforced in scientific groups by the way the GLP regulations have been written since 1979, where science appears to be divorced from considerations of quality. If management has appointed a QA unit which reports regularly on quality issues, then scientists can concentrate on science and managers can manage. Of course, this is a caricature of the situation in most laboratories. However it is not that uncommon; as Imai (1986) points out, all managers' jobs are concerned with quality, costs and delivery. He has redrawn the Deming circle with these three words at the centre.

The message is clear. If managers leave considerations of quality to quality professionals, their staff will follow suit. Science and quality are not separate entities, but totally interconnected. The one is not possible without the other.

Computers

The increasing use of computers has had a dramatic effect on laboratory work and the quality of data and reports scientists are producing. When

GLP was first introduced, computers were used as sophisticated calculators and some companies were beginning to collect some data by direct entry to the computer. Now it is possible for protocols to be written, data collected, reports to be written and transferred to regulatory affairs, compiled into a dossier and a disk prepared for onward transmission to a health ministry, all on the same system.

In addition, standard operating procedures (SOPs) have been transferred from paper to computer. The technology exists already, and is being sold, for sound and video film to be incorporated into SOPs. This raises the possibility that similar graphics and spoken comment could also be used in study reports.

Clearly the computer has been and will continue to be a potent force for standardization and accuracy of data, and hence for its quality. As computer technology continues to change and becomes more powerful, and similar changes are taking place with scientific equipment, what are the implications for quality management?

The computerization of SOPs, if the most modern techniques are used, could cause regulatory problems. All the regulations or principles of GLP call for 'written standard operating procedures'. Of course most of them were written in the middle to late 1970s, and what was envisaged were bound volumes of SOPs with pages of text, and presumably some illustration. Today most people receive information either through spoken word or by television. Therefore SOPs which could be presented graphically, by still photographs or by video, with spoken commentary would probably be more easily accepted than many pages of text. Of course some matters may have to be presented through text, but there is no reason why more than one method of presentation should be be used.

Such a set of SOPs will present new problems of control, but they should not be any more difficult than ensuring that everyone is working to the same text. The definitive SOP is that on the computer, and if copies are made these can be clearly dated to show a very short expiry period. There will be different problems of archiving such SOPs, but these are no more difficult than storing standard computer tapes, videodisks or microfilm, which is now being done.

As computing technology quickly becomes central to running and reporting safety studies, all staff associated with servicing the computer or writing software will also move from the periphery of regulated activities towards the core of those activities. This means that the awareness of quality of all computing staff will have to be raised. Of course in those companies introducing TQM or seeking ISO 9000 accreditation this should already be happening. However as computer control of studies is extended from study protocol to final submission disk, everyone connected with or actively involved with that line which information passes along must be more than aware of what controls must be applied to information and what can and cannot be done to it. Quality control, QA and validation of that information line are therefore imperative.

The big problem for QA groups will be the pace of change of both computer and equipment technology. Already most people are working with on- or off-line personal or portable computers and have the power to execute their bright ideas very quickly – if company discipline is not properly maintained.

There is therefore a requirement for a big regulatory and quality input to those members of the computer group who, until recently, have considered themselves outside regulatory control, and into areas such as regulatory affairs who may find they have powers of access to data of which they had not even dreamed.

Scientific and technical staff

All the quality control of studies will be undertaken by the scientific and technical staffs. In fact the biggest influence on good practices and good data in most large safety studies is technicians. They will spend more time with the study than anyone else. The study director or a principal scientist will spend time with the study, but their role is coordination, ensuring satisfactory progress and the resolution of problems. In the main the study is progressed by technicians. Yet the GLP regulations consider them least of anyone; essentially they should have appropriate documentation, come to work, keep clean, wear correct clothing for the job and not work if they are sick.

As pressures to work smarter increase, the pressures on technicians to produce higher-quality work will also increase. There is therefore a need for continuing education and training of technicians in the techniques of quality control, and quality improvement. Much of this training will come from specialist facilitators in total quality control techniques or from QA personnel. In most companies technicians are the 'poor bloody infantry' of the scientific world, and yet these are the people who see the study most of every day and therefore can contribute most to improving both processes and quality. This is probably where, in future years, the QA group will spend most of its time in training activities.

Senior scientists and study directors will already have a sense of customer satisfaction. This of course will heighten as they either work with technicians or among their peers on process improvements. Already they are responsible for the application of GLP to studies. In practice the expertise lies with the QA unit. This ought not to be the case. If in-process quality control from protocol to report is to be a reality, those responsible for the application of GLP must develop an equal expertise and awareness, to that which the QA group possesses. Without knowing thoroughly what are the minimum standards, improving on them is not a possibility.

Scientists at this level are most likely to be leaders of process or quality improvement teams and be responsible for in-process quality control of all study activities. It is therefore imperative that they have strong conceptions of quality control and improvement, and are properly trained and educated to fulfil that function.

Quality assurance

If the GLP regulations and guidelines are changed to give a more flexible approach to quality management, and if the trends in quality management continue to develop as they are at the moment, then there will be a change in the nature of the work of the QA unit from that presently practised.

As laboratories become more dependent on analytical equipment of greater power, and this equipment is linked to computer network, the development processes are becoming less dependent on people, except for the interpretation of results. Theoretically, provided the equipment and computer systems are properly set up and validated, the raw data content of study reports should be more accurate than it has ever been. If at the same time better and validated quality control systems are introduced into data and report production, there should be no need for the routine examination of every study and its report by the QA unit. When then will the work of the QA unit lie?

The trends that have been identified in this essay have been:

1   More diverse ways of working – outworking, more use of specialist contractors, as well as existing contract houses.
2   Greater involvement of management in the quality control processes.
3   Increasing use of linked computer systems.
4   Increasing use of quality control methods by study staff.

Where will this leave the work of the QA unit? Obviously it is unlikely to remain as it is. The emphasis is likely to change away from audits based around studies, to investigating the processes by which data, reports and submissions are generated. It is entirely possible that specific studies or study reports will be audited, but as the purpose of the audits may be different, to ensure that the processes by which the data and reports are produced are in control and satisfactory, the nature of the review will change.

By far the biggest impact on the QA unit will come from the diverse way all industries are tending to employ people. If a team of experts, many of whom may not be employees of a company, is put together for a particular project and disbanded when the project is complete, what input should QA personnel have on that team? Should it always be part of the team, or act as a consultant to the team? Obviously the answers to such questions depend on the nature of the project. But it is clear that if expertise is being purchased temporarily from outside a company, it is unlikely that personnel so employed are likely to have any feel for the quality management procedures inside the company. They may suggest alternatives or they may be opposed to those that already exist. In either event there must be a role for the QA unit to play in ensuring that any such systems produce satisfactory quality and are workable, economic and practical. There is also a strong need for them to train outside experts in the quality management procedures which already exist.

It is also possible that more company personnel could also work from home, with only a computer or telephone link to the company site. Pharmacokinetic analysis, some pathology work and even some aspects of QA could already be undertaken in this way. The problem then will be to control the drift away from a common standard of working methods and quality. There is a tendency for people working apart to drift apart and behind in their working methods, unless they are brought together periodically for retraining and further training. If people are working away from the main group, how does the QA unit assure their work practices? Are frequent visits to them necessarily the best solution? Should the QA emphasis be on ensuring the processes by which they work, and to push them into working in an accepted and acceptable manner? Should home-workers always be involved in process improvement teams to ensure they are aware of the current company policies?

The most difficult problem will arise when a contracting company which is downsizing and using outworkers makes a contract for work with a company using similar management techniques. In this case the personnel handling the contract and the QA unit from the contracting company will have to be very sure of the complete chain in the contract, and will need to know the capacity and quality of each link in the chain. What happens if one facet of the study is not satisfactory to the contracting company? This may not now be a new problem, but the push by companies to put even parts of their core operations to contractors, consultants and sundry homeworkers increases the probability of someone in the chain misinterpreting the scientific or quality criteria which are driving a particular study. It emphasizes the need to plan the contract very carefully, particularly the quality control and QA aspects of the study.

The involvement of management in the inspection of the quality control systems of their own department may prove something of a culture shock to many scientific managers. Many managers have been happy to leave quality problems to QA personnel while they looked after science, budgets and deadlines. QA personnel will be required to educate, train, persuade and cajole managers to accept their responsibilities for quality control and quality management. The direct involvement of management is crucial to the spread and revision of better-quality techniques among scientists and technicians. It has to be emphasized to managers that often the techniques of quality control or assurance are involving them in cycles of work and rework, inspection and reinspection, all of which adds to the cycle time for particular projects. If they wish to reduce project costs and cycle times, managers must involve themselves in inspection and discussion of their own quality control systems.

The task of QA personnel in guiding and coaching managers is both vital and delicate. It is clear that they are responsible for training managers in inspection techniques, the most recent concepts of quality control and quality problem-solving. It is equally clear that they must not be seen as overtly pointing managers at problems. Of course, as now, QA personnel will discover problems and suggest solutions to systems and processes, some of which will cross functional boundaries, but the staff working those systems are responsible for resolving those problems and seeking management assistance.

The increasing power of computers will pose equally exquisite problems for QA personnel. As the power of the components of computers is expanding exponentially, and the uses of the same or linked systems also grow, the traditional techniques of validation also needed to be re-examined. As companies expand internationally their computer systems expand with them to encompass national and international telephone systems. This in turn means the use of telephone cable and satellite systems. Work can be progressed round the clock round the globe. Already some companies in Europe where work costs say £50 an hour are transferring it via computer and satellite to Asia where the same work costs £7 an hour. Some others have adopted 24 hours-a-day working practices, by moving work through a worldwide network every 6–8 hours. In this way they can obtain 3 days' work in 24 hours.

In a sense the way work is transferred through computer networks mirrors the fragmented way either individual projects or whole development programmes are being conducted. Already small companies contract to develop a compound through a series of subcontractors. As more countries in Eastern Europe and Asia adopt the good practice regulations, work will be transferred to those areas, provided they can show good scientific and good regulatory practices, for cost savings alone. This will mean that very careful track will need to be kept of the flow of work through contractors and subcontractors.

The problem this presents to QA personnel is not only that the various contractors and subcontractors are compliant, but also that they have in place good-quality management systems and that those systems work. In turn this means that not only should they have an expertise in the regulations as they exist worldwide, or in a particular country, and their interpretation, but also they need a deep knowledge of evolving quality management systems. As the work processes become more fragmented between developing and contracting companies, and as computer systems turn development and registration into a continuous process, quality management will need to be at the centre of the planning process.

In this brave new world of product development it is obvious that the theory and practice of quality assurance will change. There will be an increasing need for the QA unit to be educated and trained in new quality management techniques, and in turn for them to educate people practising quality control. The emphasis must be on ensuring that the processes by which data are collected, reported and their onward transmission are satisfactory and have proper quality control systems built into them. These challenges will be solved differently by each QA team, as their own company evolves different work practices.

Conclusion

With time, systems of quality management have changed and will change again. This has been an attempt to project those changes which are happening now in both general industrial management and quality management and guess what the future may bring. However the fashions and trends may change and the future management styles may lead in a totally different direction. Only one thing is certain – it will not remain as it is now.

References

Commission of European Communities (1992) *The Rules Governing Medicinal Products in the European Community. Volume IV: Good Manufacturing Practice for Medicinal Products.*

Imai, M. (1986) *Kaizen – The Key to Japan's Competitive Success.* New York: McGraw Hill.

Ishikawa, K. (1985) *What is Total Quality Management? The Japanese Way.* Englewood Cliffs, NJ: Prentice Hall.

Juran, J. M. (1988) *Juran's Quality Control Handbook* 4th edn. New York: McGraw Hill.

2 Good manufacturing practices in the manufacture of drug products for clinical trials

E Brown

Introduction

It seems natural, and indeed, almost to be expected, that anyone who manufactures drug products for clinical evaluation would want to apply appropriate Good Manufacturing Practices (GMPs), not just to the manufacturing operation itself, but also to the packaging, labelling and assembly activities. But which GMPs should be applied, and to what extent? This chapter will attempt to identify the principal areas where GMPs should be applied, in the manufacture of drug products for clinical trials.

At first sight, available rules and regulations appear to be contradictory. In the UK, the *Rules and Guidance for Pharmaceutical Manufacturers 1993* (the so-called *Orange Guide*) includes the EC's *Guide to Good Manufacturing Practice for Medicinal Products*. This section of the *Orange Guide* has several annexes, including *Annex 13. Good Manufacturing Practice for Investigational Medicinal Products*. The introduction to this *Annex* states: 'Medicinal products intended for research and development trials are not at present subject to either marketing or manufacturing Community legislation'. However, it then goes on, quite rightly, to suggest that it is illogical for experimental products not to be subject to the controls which would apply to the formulations of which they are the prototypes. On the other hand, the EC *Good Clinical Practice Guidelines* (i.e. *Good Clinical Practice for Trials on Medicinal Products in the European Community*) under the section on the responsibilities of the sponsor requires the provision of 'fully characterized investigational medicinal products prepared in accordance with Good Manufacturing Practice (GMP), suitably packaged and labelled in such a way that any blinding procedure is ensured'. So, the more that anyone considers the subject of GMPs as applied to the manufacture of clinical trials supplies, the more it is realized how essential it is to apply GMPs, in order that patients or volunteers receive investigational drug products of the desired quality. Indeed, it is essential that those involved or associated with clinical manufacture should have a thorough understanding of not just *Annex 13*, but the *Guide to Good Manufacturing Practice for Medicinal Products* itself. The note in *Annex 13* states: 'The principles and many detailed guidelines of *Good Manufacturing Practice for Medicinal Products* (Volume IV of the series *The Rules Governing Medicinal Products in the European Community*) are relevant to the preparation of products for use in clinical trials'. Their relevance will be explored in the following pages.

Quality Management

It was the Lakeland poet John Ruskin, in the 19th century, who penned the words 'Quality is never an accident, it is always the result of an intelligent effort. There must always be a will to produce a superior thing'. No one will disagree with this simple yet profound observation. Another way of expressing this truth is to say that quality has to be managed into a process to result in the end-product of the desired quality. For the manufacture of clinical trials materials, a quality management system is essential, if we are going to be able to guarantee the quality of the patient supplies. And it follows that the right patient will be provided with the correct dose form, properly manufactured, in the appropriate container, which is properly labelled, and has satisfied its quality control specification, by the use of relevant analytical methods. The quality management system will help in identifying the component parts which, when put together, will provide the assurance of the necessary quality. These component parts include:

1   Personnel.
2   Premises.
3   Equipment.
4   Production.
5   Packaging and Labelling.
6   Quality Control.
7   Documentation.
8   Quality Assurance.

Each of these subjects will receive due consideration in this chapter.

But first of all, some definitions of the often-used terms on the subject. *Quality Assurance* is a wide-ranging concept which covers all matters, which individually or collectively influence the quality of a product. It is the sum total of the organized arrangements made with the object of ensuring that medicinal products are of the quality required for their intended use.

Good Manufacturing Practice is that part of quality assurance which ensures that products are consistently produced and controlled to the quality standards appropriate to their intended use, as required by product specification or clinical trial certificate (or other regulatory requirement).

Quality Control is that part of GMP which is concerned with sampling, specifications and testing, and with the organization, documentation and release procedures which ensure that the necessary and relevant tests are actually carried out, and that materials are not released for use, nor products released for supply, until their quality has been judged as satisfactory.

Personnel

Any quality management system or system for quality assurance relies heavily on the people involved. Another perspective on this topic would draw the conclusion that quality assurance is the responsibility of *everyone*. It is, more often than not, the people who make the mistakes. It is the people who do not follow the procedures. It is the people who forget to record some data or information. It is the people who deviate from accepted practices, and take short cuts. It is thus patently obvious that special attention needs to be focused on the subject of the people who are involved in the manufacture of drug products intended for clinical valuation. It needs to be ensured, in simple terms, that the right people are doing the right job. Thus we need persons who have the necessary qualifications, who have the relevant experience, and who have received the training which is appropriate to their needs. To back up this requirement, it is sensible to maintain a curriculum vitae, and a job description, for everyone. The job description should not only define the main elements of the job, but set out a person's responsibilities and reporting lines. A record of all training that takes place, both internal – on-the-job – and external, should be maintained. All persons involved or associated with the manufacture of drug products should receive regular training in GMPs. There are specific responsibilities that individuals will have, dependent on the nature of the work that they are involved in. Those involved directly with manufacturing and those required to enter manufacturing areas need to pay special attention to personal hygiene, and the possibility of carrying infections into controlled areas. Manufacturing areas should only be entered when the appropriate garments are worn (usually clean overalls, hats, gloves and shoes). Eating, drinking, chewing and smoking must not be permitted in manufacturing or laboratory areas.

Those who are familiar with Good Laboratory Practices will be familiar with the term and responsibilities of the study director. Under the requirements of GMPs, there are two key personnel, namely the person responsible for manufacture (the head of production or production manager), and the person responsible for quality control (the quality control manager or the quality controller). Within a full manufacturing facility, each of these persons has clearly defined roles, many of which are directly applicable to clinical supply manufacture. The responsibilities of the head of production for clinical supplies will include:

1 ensuring that products are manufactured and stored according to appropriate documentation, in order to obtain the required quality;
2 approval of instructions relating to production operations, and ensuring their implementation;
3 ensuring that production records are evaluated and signed by an authorized person before they are sent to the quality control department;
4 ensuring that maintenance of equipment and premises is carried out; and
5 ensuring that appropriate training of department personnel is carried out.

The quality control manager's responsibilities include:

1 approval, or rejection, as he or she sees fit, of starting materials, packaging materials, intermediate, bulk and finished products;
2 evaluation of manufacturing and packaging records;
3 ensuring that all necessary testing is carried out;
4 approval of specifications, sampling instructions, test methods and other quality control procedures;
5 ensuring that maintenance and calibration of equipment and premises (as appropriate) are carried out
6 ensuring that training of department personnel is carried out.

It is imperative that the heads of production and quality control are independent of each other (neither reports to the other), otherwise some bias may be introduced.

There is a wide range of documentation which must be used and completed during manufacturing and quality control activities, and this will be considered in further detail in the section on documentation, below.

Premises

The premises used for the manufacture of clinical supplies may be on a production site, in which case the full range of GMPs will be accepted as normal, and routine. Alternatively they may be located on a site used for research and development activities where there may be many personnel who are not familiar with the requirements of the GMPs. If the latter is the case, then special attention needs to be given to the location of manufacturing facilities, as the risks of cross-contamination need to be kept to a minimum. All premises should be located, designed, constructed, adapted and maintained to suit the operations to be carried out. The layout and design must aim to minimize the risks of errors and permit effective cleaning and maintenance, in order to avoid cross-contamination, build-up of dust or dirt, and in general, any adverse effect on the quality of products manufactured and packaged therein. As far as possible, only those who need to enter manufacturing areas should be permitted to do so.

Premises where specialized manufacturing operations take place, such as those for the production of sterile products for injectable use, require specialized facilities for air handling and ventilation, to ensure that the air quality is maintained so that air-borne particles and bacterial levels are kept at a minimum. Similar standards need to be maintained for the manufacture of sterile products for clinical trials, as those applied to the manufacture of sterile products which are to be marketed.

All premises should be easy to clean. Manufacturing areas should have coving between walls and floors, to prevent recesses where dust can accumulate. When there are manufacturing rooms where dust-generating activities take place, which are adjacent to one other, the air-handling systems should be balanced so that air is not transferred from one manufacturing room to another.

Storage areas should be of sufficient capacity to allow orderly storage of starting and packaging materials, intermediate, bulk and finished products, materials in quarantine, or which have been released, rejected or returned. Good storage conditions must be maintained, and temperature and humidity may need to be controlled (as in manufacturing areas also). Quarantine status may be achieved by separation, in which case access into quarantine areas must be restricted. Any system which replaces physical quarantine must give equivalent security.

Quality Control laboratories should normally be separate from production areas, and separate rooms may be necessary for the housing of sensitive analytical equipment, to minimize vibration. Rest and refreshment rooms and toilets should be well-separated from manufacturing facilities.

If there are any animal houses on site, they should be well-separated from manufacturing areas, and have separate air-handling facilities.

Equipment

The range of equipment that is used in the manufacturing and analysis of drug products for clinical evaluation can be quite extensive. Manufacturing equipment could include mixers and granulators, tablet presses and capsule fillers, ampoule and vial-filling machines, ovens and autoclaves, to name just a few. With all of these, and other pieces of manufacturing equipment, the principles of GMP that are applied should be quite similar. The equipment should be reliable and reproducible in its operation and output. Its design, location and maintenance programme should suit its intended purpose. Repair and maintenance operations should not present any hazard to the quality of the products. Lubricants should not be introduced into the product. Manufacturing equipment should be easy to clean. There should be no surfaces which come into contact with the product, for which the cleanliness cannot easily be confirmed. It is unlikely that equipment which is dedicated to one product will be available for the manufacture of products for clinical trials. Cleaning is, therefore, particularly important, if it is to be demonstrated that no contamination has been introduced from inadequately cleaned equipment.

It is particularly important that balances, and other weighing and measuring devices used during manufacture, can be demonstrated as being reliable. A regular calibration programme is essential, and standardization should take place sufficiently frequently to provide confidence in the balances. It is also important to use a balance of the appropriate range for the material being weighed.

For the manufacture of sterile products, it is essential that autoclaves and ovens are fully validated, so that the sterility of the final product can be guaranteed. The validation exercises will need to involve temperature-mapping studies for various load configurations of each container size of the finished drug product.

Production

In this section, the scope of production is defined as beginning with receipt of starting materials, and ending with release of bulk drug product. Packaging and labelling are considered in the following section.

Upon receipt of the starting materials, which will include drug substances, excipients and packaging materials, a system for Quality Control should come into operation. None of the starting materials can be used until their quality is judged as being satisfactory. To determine this, a sample is taken, in accordance with procedures approved by the Quality Control Manager, and submitted for Quality Control assessment, whilst the bulk of the material is appropriately labelled, and placed under quarantine. (Quality Control will be considered in some detail later.) Upon release of the material, the bulk is re-labelled with a release label, and transferred to a released materials storage area.

Manufacture of a batch of drug product begins with the dispensing of the starting materials, using a batch manufacturing instruction, which includes the formulation and required quantities for the batch. (Refer to the section on documentation, below, for details of the requirements for batch manufacturing instructions.) The dispensing operation is carried out by one person, and checked by a second person (who checks that the material, the quantity and release number are all correct). This check is recorded by the signature of the checker against the dispensing record. The manufacturing area and equipment to be used must be inspected for cleanliness and the absence of materials or paperwork relating to previous manufacturing activities, and a record made of the inspection. Area and equipment log books can provide a history of usage, cleaning and inspections. The manufacture takes place in accordance with the batch manufacturing instructions, and records are taken of such items as mixing times, temperatures, pH and physical characteristics. All critical actions are checked by a second person, and documented by signature in the manufacturing records. At the end of distinct phases in the process, yields are calculated, and providing that they are within acceptable limits, the manufacture can proceed to the next phase. Any deviation from the defined processing instructions or any unexpected yields must be fully investigated, explained and documented before the product can be submitted to Quality Control. In-process testing, such as moisture content, tablet hardness and weights and disintegration times may be carried out by production personnel, and the records will form part of the manufacturing documentation.

For the manufacture of sterile products for parenteral use, special care needs to be taken. Environmental monitoring forms an essential part of the processing activities. Particulate and bacterial levels need to be monitored and demonstrated to be within acceptable limits. Charts and printouts from ovens and autoclaves are retained as evidence that the appropriate sterilizing conditions have been achieved.

At the end of the manufacturing process, samples for analysis are taken by Quality Control personnel, according to sampling procedures approved by the Quality Control Manager. A record of this sampling will be made in the manufacturing documents, and a full reconciliation using theoretical and actual yields will be made. Any discrepancies must be fully investigated and documented. The bulk product will then be stored under quarantine, pending availability of analytical data and release by the Quality Control Manager.

During the whole of the manufacturing process, the manufacturing area, the equipment and any receiving vessels and containers, including those for waste, must be properly labelled with product name and batch number. It is important to remember that labelling is the major cause of problems and mix-ups in the pharmaceutical industry as a whole, and the manufacture of materials for clinical trial use is not devoid of similar problems.

The area and equipment will then undergo a full cleaning programme, according to authorized procedures. Depending on the nature of the compound being manufactured, it may be necessary to carry out studies to demonstrate the validity of the cleaning programme, particularly if highly potent drug products are being manufactured. Area and equipment log books are used to record the fact that cleaning has taken place, together with necessary inspections after cleaning.

The manufacturing record should, at this point, be complete, having recorded all steps in the process, with signatures, times and dates of all significant stages. The record will include the in-process data with charts and printouts, and a completed record of reconciliation. Any calculations performed should be checked by a second person, and that check recorded. The completed records will then be audited, signed and dated by a supervisory person from the manufacturing department. The completed batch manufacturing record is then ready for audit by the Quality Control department.

Packaging and labelling

The packaging and labelling of supplies for clinical studies is a particularly critical phase in the whole manufacturing operation. Indeed, it is often a much more complex operation than the packaging and labelling of marketed products. One of the fundamentals of GMPs requires that only one product is permitted in an area at a time. But many packaging operations for clinical trials require that more than one product is assembled into the same pack. And as if that weren't enough, different products are made to match one another so that neither patient nor doctor is aware of which treatment is being administered at any one time. One trial which is brought to mind involved four tablets, which were made up of two placebos and two different active products being assembled into the same blister. This kind of situation demands that procedures are carefully drawn up which will minimize the risk of any mix-up, and Quality Control personnel have an important part to play in ensuring that the right product is supplied in the right container.

The label preparation process is also a critical part of the operation. The clinical study protocol will give details of the content of each label, but there may be variations, depending on the territory in which the study is to take place. Approval of a draft label would normally be sought from Drug Regulatory Affairs for the particular territory, and also from the medical department in the territory, who can confirm accuracy of the language used. Some regulatory agencies will require expiry dating of supplies, whilst others will not. Once approval has been received, then printing of the labels can take place. It must be ensured, however, before any printing takes place, that the printer and area are free from any other printed materials, and this inspection should be documented. The required number of labels, including those to be retained with the packaging records, can then be printed. Unless the printing system is properly validated, it will be necessary to carry out a 100% inspection of the labels. This check will include review of the text, against the approved draft, and the clarity and legibility of the labels, and of course, this check will be documented. The label text will normally include the name of the sponsor, the trial reference number (or protocol number), the batch number, the patient identity number (if applicable), the storage conditions, and the expiry or retest date.

The required quantity of drug products will be dispensed for the assembly of a particular order. An assembly room, which has been cleaned and inspected, will be labelled with the order number. For a trial involving, say treatment A, treatment B and treatment C in the same patient pack, it is usual that all of treatment A will be packed first in the area, and labelled, then treatment B, and finally treatment C. Only one bulk container and one set of labels will be permitted in the room at any one time. In addition to the required number of containers being packed, an additional container will be packed, for Quality Control examination and identity confirmation. Alternatively a person from the Quality Control department may be present during the entire assembly operation, and sign the packaging documentation to confirm that the right product has been packed into the right labelled container. The packaging records will receive an audit from the quality control or quality assurance department, and the assembled order will be packed into its shippers upon release from the Quality Control Department.

Quality Control

The term Quality Control may be misunderstood by those who are not familiar with the subject, because this function does not control the quality at all, but rather tests for the desired quality at various stages during the process. Staring materials, including packaging materials, intermediate, bulk and finished drug products, and the final packed and labelled product will all be subject to varying degrees of testing, but unless the release process also includes an audit of the manufacturing, packaging and labelling records, the value of the testing on its own will be limited. Specifications need to be drawn up for all starting materials, intermediate, bulk and finished drug products. These will be based upon the analytical methods which have been developed and validated for the particular drug substance and product under evaluation. It is important that the stability of the drug product is determined, usually under accelerated conditions, in order that an appropriate specification is drawn up. Excipient specifications, as far as is possible, will be based upon pharmacopoeial monographs. It is the responsibility of the Quality Control Manager to approve all specifications and related analytical methods. The Quality Control Manager will require to have appropriate analytical equipment under his or her management, which is properly maintained and calibrated, as appropriate, to carry out all of the necessary testing. The testing will be carried out on samples which have been taken by Quality Control personnel, following sampling methods which have been approved by the Quality Control Manager. Once all of the necessary testing has been completed (physical, chemical and microbiological, as necessary), and a check has been completed of all calculations, and all of the data conform with the requirements of the specification, and the manufacturing records have been audited by Quality Control personnel, the Quality Control Manager is in a position to be able to release or reject the material as he or she sees fit. It is beneficial, however, to have a non-conforming materials review committee whose function is to review any non-conforming materials, as during the development phase of medicinal products, it may be that it is the specification that should be changed, rather than the product rejected.

The role of quality control in the packaging and labelling operation is primarily to ensure that the right product is in the right container, which is properly labelled. This will be determined by carrying out an audit of the labelling and packaging records, and by carrying out a final identity check on the final packed product. If there is more than one dose level of product available, and especially if the products are matched in appearance, then the identity will need to be quantitative as well as qualitative. Orders which have been assembled, but are not released, require to be quarantined. This may be accomplished by the quarantine of the packaging area itself, until release is granted.

Providing that identity checks and the Quality Control audit of the packaging and labelling operation are satisfactory, then a Quality Control release can be granted for the particular order. However, before the shippers can be despatched, to the site of the trial, confirmation is needed that the particular trial is authorized by the appropriate regulatory agency to take place, and that a clinical trial certificate (or equivalent) has been granted. It is also often the case that orders will need to be despatched in parts, based upon storage availability at the site of the trial, patient recruitment, the duration of the study and the stability of the drug product. It is important, in this situation, to be able to reconcile the whole order with the parts which have been despatched, and with those awaiting despatch.

Documentation

It is essential, for any quality management system, that good documentation is available and used. The documentation roughly falls into two different types – those that provide instructions, and those that collect data and information. All documentation requires a distribution and retrieval system, which will ensure that only the current version is available for use. Outdated versions should be retained in historical files.

First, then, the main instructional documents.

Batch Manufacturing Instructions

By the time a drug product is ready to undergo clinical evaluation, a stable formulation will have been developed, and clear instructions should be able to be written which, when followed, will produce a batch of the drug product that is of the desired quality, in a consistent manner. The instructions will include the formulation, with the required quantities of all of the ingredients, both the drug substance and the excipients, and space to record the dispensing records and batch numbers (or release numbers) of all of the necessary materials, including packaging materials. All of the major equipment to be used will be defined. The document will include space to record the identity and cleanliness of the manufacturing area and the cleanliness of the manufacturing equipment before manufacture commences. Step-by-step instructions will follow, for the manufacture to take place. The instructions will require that all major steps in the manufacturing sequence will be signed by the person performing the activity, and countersigned by a second person who checks the operation. Wherever specific conditions are requested, such as temperatures, times, pHs and pressures, spaces will be provided to record the actual conditions. The instructions will require that batch quantities are recorded at significant phases during manufacture, enabling a full reconciliation to be made. They will also require that any deviation from the intended procedure is fully documented and justified. Any unexpected results from the reconciliation need also to be fully explained. The instructions will also specify the times and quantities of any samples to be taken during manufacture, and provide space to record the actual sample quantities removed.

Packaging Instructions

Because of the nature of clinical trials, it is very likely that individual packaging instructions will need to be prepared for each clinical trial, unlike the packaging of marketed products, which is often a totally repetitive operation. The clinical protocol will outline the packaging requirements, which may include the blinding of supplies, so that patient and physician are only aware of the different treatments by a code. It is important that these instructions are clear and unambiguous, and stipulate the requirement for clear separation, in time, if not in packaging area, of the different components in the trial. They will begin with an authorized requisition for all of the drug products and packaging components required for the packaging operation to take place. The packaging instructions will also include procedures for the preparation of the labelling required for the trial. As with the manufacturing instructions, space will be provided to record the fact that all necessary actions have taken place, with signatures and countersignatures as appropriate. Similarly, space will be provided to record all quantities used, to permit a full reconciliation of the packaging activity.

Specifications

A specification will normally include a range of tests, with acceptable limits, and the methods to be followed to derive the corresponding data. Specifications for starting materials will normally include the name of the supplier, together with sampling procedures. Those for bulk or finished products will include a similar range of tests with acceptance limits, and methods to be followed to derive the data. During the development phase of a new compound, it is to be expected that the specifications for drug substance and drug product will change in the light of new experience. The distribution and retrieval system is particularly significant in ensuring that only current versions are accessible to the Quality Control personnel who use these documents.

Standard Operating Procedures (SOPs)

There is a need for written instructions for the performance of operations which are not necessarily specific to one product or material, but which are standard procedures. These should be prepared for such activities as equipment operation, maintenance and cleaning, cleaning of premises, environmental control, sampling and inspection.

It may be found useful to define, in the SOP, the *objective* (what will be achieved by following this SOP), the *scope* to which the SOP applies, and to whom it is applicable. As SOPs are intended to be management instructions, it may be found useful to outline each step as an instruction, and, as such, to begin each sentence with a verb. SOPs should be approved or authorized by someone who has the managerial authority to do so. As with other documentation, a good distribution and retrieval system is essential, so that only current versions are available to the user.

And now, those documents which collect data and information.

Clinical Trial Order

The order for a clinical trial should give all of the information necessary to manufacture and assemble the products required in the trial. It should therefore stipulate, as a minimum, the dosage form, strength and formulation reference, the quantities per unit pack and the number of packs, the principal investigator and the protocol number for the study. Labelling requirements may also be specified. The order should be authorized, usually by the medical director and a responsible person in drug regulatory affairs.

Manufacturing Records

The aforementioned batch manufacturing instructions may be used to record data and information as the manufacture proceeds. Undoubtedly, other data and information will be collected during the process, such as temperature and pressure charts, balance printouts and such items as dispensing labels. The record should be complete in itself, permitting the reconstruction of all that happened in the process, at a later date.

Packaging Records

Similarly, packaging records, assembled at the time of the packaging operation, should permit a complete reconstruction of the packaging activity at a later date.

Analytical Data

All analytical data should be recorded at the time of analysis, and will usually include observations, and records of physical, chemical and micro-biological tests, as appropriate. Supplementary information will include balance printouts and chromatographic traces. The data should include a reference to the specification and analytical methods used. All supplementary data should be cross-referenced to the analyst's laboratory notebook, and other information, such as the lot numbers of reference materials and the identity of equipment used, should also be recorded. The name of the analyst should be identified on the laboratory notebook page and on any supplementary data, together with any persons who have checked or transcribed data.

Equipment and Area Log Books

Initially, the log books should be used to record evidence that acceptance testing and qualification and/or validation have been completed. Information such as cleaning, inspections, use, maintenance and calibration should be recorded in the appropriate log books, so that a chronological record is maintained for equipment and manufacturing areas. The log books should also record any failures or breakdowns, and the actions taken to rectify the situation and restore the equipment or area to its validated state.

Distribution and Shipping Records

These should permit easy review to determine the location of every batch of clinical product, so that prompt action can be taken if there is a need for recall of products.

Standard Forms

There is a likelihood that many standard forms will be needed for the collection of information and records, during the whole of the process, from receipt of an order, and the starting materials, through to despatch of assembled clinical supplies. It is important that all such forms are carefully designed, are unambiguous, and are easy to use. When updated versions are introduced, all available previous versions should be withdrawn from use.

Quality Assurance

There is a need for self-inspection of the whole clinical manufacturing, packaging, labelling, release and shipping process. Such inspections can be carried out by auditors from the quality assurance department, who can provide assurance to management that all of the necessary systems and procedures are in place, and also that the systems and procedures are being used and followed.

Conclusion

This chapter has not done much more than identify some of the main considerations in applying GMPs to the manufacture of drug products for use in clinical studies. Topics, such as qualification and validation, the use of computers, and archiving of data have received little or no mention. However, if anyone is to generate the confidence that a patient, who is taking part in a clinical trial, has received the intended product of the right quality, then it will involve the generation of detailed records of the series of actions that have been taken, in appropriate premises, with materials that have complied with their specifications, and where appropriately qualified and trained staff, using the appropriate equipment, have followed the relevant procedures. These are the fundamentals of the quality management system that is needed.

References

Good clinical practice for trials on medicinal products in the European Community. (1990) In *The Rules Governing Medicinal Products in the European Community*, Vol. III, Addendum July 1990. Luxembourg: Office for Official Publications of the European Communities.

Rules and Guidance for Pharmaceutical Manufacturers 1993 (1993) London: HMSO.

3 Good laboratory practice in animal health studies

B C Warren

Scope

The vast majority of good laboratory practice (GLP)-compliant studies are performed to examine test substances from human medicine for the purpose of obtaining information on their properties and especially safety with respect to human health or the environment.

A smaller but important sector of non-clinical investigation for regulatory review is the determination of the pharmacokinetics, metabolic fate, excretion and safety of a veterinary pharmaceutical compound in production (farm) and companion animals. These studies may involve calves, dairy cows, pigs, sheep, goats, horses, poultry (chicken, turkey), dogs, cats or even fish.

Studies demonstrating the systemic and local tolerance in the indicated animal species (target animal safety studies, TASS) are required to be carried out to GLP guidelines/regulations. The international debate which has been ongoing on whether or not absorption, distribution, biotransformation and excretion studies should be performed to GLP standards is somewhat easier to decide for tests involving food-producing animals as these studies are associated with the establishment of the safety of the test substance in humans.

Thus large (farm) animal, poultry and fish studies fall within the scope of GLPs if they investigate:

1 The determination of the target compound/metabolite (marker residue) in the target tissue for the establishment of the maximum residue limit (MRL) of a new active substance.
2 The depletion of residues in tissues and body fluids for determination of the withdrawal period for the formulated product.

Associated studies on assay method development and validation and any unit providing analytical, pathology or similar service to a GLP study should also adhere to GLP principles in working procedures.

Animal health companies have recognized and welcomed the benefits of GLP in raising the quality of safety data and some have decided to operate to GLP standards for all non-clinical work in full development, including pharmacodynamic studies. This decision has also be made to avoid dual standards where safety and pharmacology studies are performed by the same group within the same laboratory.

The application of GLP principles to animal health studies

There are many similarities in the organizational processes, technical aspects and conduct of farm animal compared to laboratory animal GLP studies. These similarities relate primarily to the required documentation, its structure and content.

However, it is recognized by regulatory authorities that farm animal test systems used in veterinary studies do not easily conform to the precise GLP requirements defined in the regulations.

The interpretation of GLP principles is discussed below with reference to animal health studies. Problems are identified which may be presented to management, scientific staff and the quality assurance (QA) unit, relating to the planning, performance and monitoring of such studies.

Facilities and organization of animal health studies

Following a management decision to perform a non-clinical veterinary investigation, the organization of the study by the appointed study director (sometimes called the study manager) may involve many groups at the experimental facility. The first action is likely to be requisition of the appropriate quantity of the test substance or test formulation. This action often occurs prior to completion of the study protocol. Early involvement of the QA unit in a GLP study is assured if QA has routine sign-off on these veterinary trial requisition forms for the inspection of the documentation relating to the test material formulation, manufacture, analysis, container labelling, clearance and supply. It is preferable that QA audit this documentation before release to the study director.

The supply of the test farm animals to a study, their accommodation, care and maintenance are described in detail in later sections of this chapter.

The other organizational processes required under GLP for the proper running of a study are not dealt with in detail here as they have been fully covered in a previous publication in this series (Carson and Dent, 1990).

For various reasons, sponsors may select to contract out the live phase of a farm animal pharmacokinetic/residue study but provide the laboratory expertise required to evaluate the test substance in the test system. One course of action to ensure GLP compliance is to arrange for two separate studies to be carried out. These are planned, performed and reported under the control of two study directors (sponsor and contractor).

The sponsor study director's responsibilities could cover the following activities:

1 Preparation of a generic protocol for the work contracted out, from which the contract facility study director generates the live-phase study plan.
2 Preparation of an overall study protocol detailing the arrangements agreed with the contractor, the in-house laboratory investigations and the procedures for reporting the study data.
3 Coordinating the despatch of the test material and relevant documentation to the contract site and receipt of the test animal samples for the sponsor analyses.
4 Supervising the in-house laboratory investigations.
5 Preparing an overall report for the two study phases with the contract house report included as an appendix.

Ideally, a study which is required to conform to GLP should be performed at a GLP-compliant site. However, difficulty will be encountered in finding GLP-compliant facilities to carry out animal health studies or parts of studies such as:

1 Long-term toxicity or residue investigations in certain farm animals.
2 Residue studies in fish, such as salmon (the salmon fish farms in the far reaches of Scotland and in Scandinavia are commercial enterprises).
3 Slaughter and disposal of farm animals in tissue residue or tolerance studies.

With the study control in the hands of the sponsors study director, the essential exercise to achieve compliance is to ensure that evidence of adherence to the sponsor study protocol together with all the required elements of GLP compliance are generated for each study and placed in each individual study file.

In these circumstances it is essential that the study director pays due attention to the preparation of the protocol. An example of the structure of a protocol for an animal health safety study is provided in Appendix 1 of this chapter. This covers the protocol elements required under GLP with particular emphasis on the sections dealing with the test animals.

Examples of the interactions that may occur between the study director and staff, the information sought for inclusion in the protocol and for the performance of the study are:

1   Farm manager and stockperson(s):
   (a)   Determination of the holding areas/pens for the study animals.
   (b)   Timing of the supply of animals and feed.
   (c)   Animal maintenance/husbandry details.
   (d)   Animal handling techniques required for carrying out the live-phase study procedures.
   (e)   Preparation of treatment sites (e.g injection sites).
   (f)   Availability of animal weighing crates, check weights and other equipment.
   (g)   Arrangements for the disposal of test animals.
2   Veterinary studies test substance supplies unit:
   (a)   Timing of the test substance supplies and associated documentation (see page 32 for details).
   (b)   Safety-in-use information.
3   Attending veterinary surgeon(s);
   (a)   These may be on the staff of the facility or from a local veterinary practice.
   (b)   Discussion of the required clinical procedures, record entry forms; timing of study visits.
4   Statistical unit (or contract statistician):
   (a)   Study group test animal randomization method.
   (b)   Method of collection and presentation of study results; timing of forwarding the results to the unit; analysis methods to be employed.
   (c)   Timing of statistical report.
5   Laboratory units servicing study:
   (a)   Number/volumes of blood samples; anticoagulants to be used.
   (b)   Specific requirements for the collection of other body fluids/samples during the study.
   (c)   Treatment of samples collected.
   (d)   Storage of samples and any particular precautions required during transit to the laboratory.
   (e)   Supply of the required postmortem sample collection vessels, fixatives.
   (f)   Timing of the attendance by the pathologist (who may be contracted in) and support staff.
   (g)   Issue of the pathology report.

The risk of committing recording and operational errors will be reduced by adapting standard record forms and procedures used by the sponsor to those routinely used at the contract facility, e.g. feeding regimes, cow milk yield records, the preferred sequence of treatment of udder quarters with an intramammary product, body weight and feed intake records.

The study director should discuss the details of the study plan with all relevant personnel, establish the required lines of communication between sites and ensure that personnel clearly understand their individual responsibilities (the latter may be presented as instructions in the appendices of the protocol).

Other essential actions are:

1   Provision of copies of all the study procedures to be performed at the site and explanation to relevant staff.
2   Provision by the sponsor of the required procedures for the operation and calibration of study equipment.
3   Addition to the study file of husbandry, feeding and other animal care procedures together with curricula vitae or management statements of competence for contract facility staff involved in the study.
4   Monitoring by the study director of all procedures at the site (alongside the sponsor QA inspection programme) and recording of these actions on the study record forms (e.g. pre-dose procedures, selection of test animals, treatment, sample collection, storage and despatch, post-mortem procedures).

The study director should, of course, declare the fact of the non-GLP-compliant site (and the activities performed there) on the study report compliance statement. Comments could also be included regarding the specialist scientific knowledge or expertise of the staff and the checks and monitoring carried out by the study director at the site.

A brief outline of the organization of a multisite study is presented below in the comments on studies involving fish (see page 39).

Experimental animals, accommodation, care and maintenance

Source

It is rare for experimental farm animals or poultry to be bred on site. By far the majority are purchased for a specific study or series of studies requiring, for example, mixed sexes, a certain weight range or age. In the UK, the requirement that experimental animals be obtained from a licensed supplier is waived for farm animals and horses. The source will be a specialist/local farm supplier or they may be market-derived stock. The source, date of receipt on site, age, sex and breed should be recorded. Additional information on the disease history, number of lactations and milk yield records may be available for dairy cows.

All new arrivals should be isolated until their clinical condition is established. Animals arriving from different sources at the same time should initially be separated until any latent disease has emerged and been treated, if required, and to minimize the risk of cross-contamination. Medication of animals should be recorded in detail and the information made available to the study director for consideration in the selection of the test animals.

The animals are acclimatized in the holding pens for a predetermined period or until specific pretreatment study criteria are met, e.g. disease antibody status. Animals are routinely subjected to a veterinary examination as part of the pre-dose procedures for selection of the study animals.

Identification

All farm animals which are moved between sites in the UK must be identifiable by means which meet the Ministry of Agriculture, Fisheries and Food standards, under the Diseases of Animals Act. In the case of cattle this will be by uniquely numbered ear tags and/or breeding records.

Individual identification for experimental purposes can be by various methods:

1   Cattle: metal or plastic ear tags, coloured and/or numbered neck collars, freeze-brand numbers, numbered tail bands. It is an advantage for the dairy cow to have a numbered tail band or a freeze-brand number on the rump to allow identification in the parlour at milking.
2   Calves: ear tags.
3   Pigs: ear tags, ear tattoos, slap marker (tattoo) on the body.
4   Sheep: ear tags.
5   Horses: name associated with markings.
6   Poultry: wing bands or tags.
7   Fish: fin tags.

Individual study groups may also be identified by different colour markings, for example, on the backs of pigs and sheep and coloured tape around the tails of cattle. This colour coding can also be extended to cover the plastic ear tags, feed sacks (if treatment is administered as medicated feed) and the group pen labels.

Accommodation

This will vary considerably, ranging from environmentally controlled buildings with set air-change patterns, temperature control and incorporating purpose-built rooms, pens, metabolism units, water and feeding systems, to animal housing and holding units on commercial farms, with outside seasonal grazing of stock. Protocol demands for pasture trials may set criteria for helminth burden status, stocking density, sward type, availability of water and other parameters.

In the normal farm situation, excessive protocol claims should be avoided for the environmental conditions under which test animals are housed.

Dairy units may have the facility to measure individual-quarter milk yields and automated systems for recording yields. A computer-based system for calculating and recording cow milk yields should be validated to ensure data integrity.

Quarantine facilities are essential. Adequate separation of individual or groups of animals should be ensured, particularly where there is a risk of cross-contamination of biological agent or the applied topical treatment.

Diet and bedding

A feed batch record for a compound feeding stuff to be offered to study animals is required for GLP purposes. This identifies the supplier, batch number, ration ingredients, nutrient analysis, storage recommendations and precautions in use. The expiry date for the diet is determined by the vitamin content and the batch record usually refers to a 'best before' date stamp on individual feed bags. This latter information should also be added to the study file.

The compound feed batch (and drinking water) should be tested for contaminants that may be capable of affecting any study procedure. An example is the test for the presence of inhibitory substances that will interfere in the microbiological assay of an antibiotic in animal body fluids or tissues.

The standard farm practices for the bulk storage of bedding (straw bales, polythene-bagged wood shavings or shredded paper/cellulose waste) and animal feed (in multiple layered paper sacks on wooden pallets), with short-term supplies in the area where the test animals are housed, are acceptable for GLP compliance.

Sources of wood shavings and paper waste should be checked to ensure the product has not been treated with chemicals that might interfere with the outcome of the experimental work.

Husbandry and feeding

The overriding considerations governing the husbandry of farm animals are the welfare of the farm animal and its health and the health and safety of the farm staff and others handling the animals.

Points to consider when developing the procedures for the maintenance and feeding of study farm animals are:

1 The buildings and accommodation should be identified and described, including penning arrangements for individual animals or as groups,

bedding areas, dunging/feeding areas. Consideration should be given to the separation of animals and staff to avoid injury.

2   Bedding for the individual animal species to be identified; the frequency of adding the bedding to the pen/holding area.

3   Draught-free ventilation, ambient temperature; requirement for supplementary ventilation and/or heating. The monitoring of temperature, air flow and humidity should be considered.

4   Natural lighting, supplemented as necessary by artificial lighting; light/dark cycles.

5   Feeding a daily diet which is adequate to maintain full health and vigour; feeding method, frequency, timing.

6   Details of storage of limited supplies in feed preparation area: storage of bulk supplies elsewhere.

7   The UK Home Office demands continuous access of stock to a clean water supply unless the project licence issued stipulates alternatives. The type of drinkers should be specified where relevant.

8   Daily routine for cleaning out animal holding areas; procedure for cleaning accommodation between studies.

Weighing farm stock

The portable walk-in calf/sheep etc. weighing crate is standard equipment on an experimental farm. Care should be taken to ensure that the animal-retaining cage is clear of any obstruction, the equipment is correctly zeroed and check-weighed prior to use.

Multiple 25 kg check weights are convenient to handle and two or three will cover the weight range of most experimental animals. The weighing bridge is often utilized for adult cattle; a calibration check is performed at each service interval.

Standard operating procedures

An indication of the range of procedures associated with farm activities and study animals is shown in the list below. It is advisable that each procedure, in the set of standard operating procedures sited in the farm area, is covered with plastic laminate.

1   Handling systems (examples to aid animal treatment and examination): use of yoke stalls, race and crush or other facility with quick-release devices for cattle; race and handling pens with adjustable gates for sheep; V-shaped troughs for restraint of small pigs.

2   Clinical examination: ophthalmic, skin, intrauterine/intravaginal; pre-/posttreatment and terminal examinations.

3 Farm animal husbandry and management: as described above in the section on husbandry and feeding. General procedures for milking dairy cows and the use and cleaning of the dairy parlour.
4 Animal feeding: covers various species and ages of stock.
5 Treatment: by parenteral, oral, intramammary or topical routes of administration.
6 Sample collection: examples are milk, blood, urine, faeces, lacrimal fluid, interstitial fluid.
7 Sacrifice and disposal: methods, postmortem techniques.
8 Vermin/pest control: often performed on-site by a specialist contractor at prescribed intervals.
9 Miscellaneous: weighing animals, identification methods.
10 Administration: receipt of animals, criteria for acceptance into a study, completion of veterinary report.

Many of these procedures are routinely performed by the farm staff at a facility. One of the main contributory factors to a well-run farm animal study is the trained, experienced (and caring) stockperson whose skill in handling and restraining animals, observing and recording changes in the health and behaviour of study animals is a great asset to the study director.

Comments on studies involving fish

To illustrate the various GLP compliance issues relating to studies in fish, components of a tissue depletion study are described. In this study the test substance is administered via the feed.

Most probably the experimental work would be shared between a commercial fish farm (live phase) and the sponsor laboratory, with the sponsor study director providing the overall study supervision.

Responsibilities

The sponsor study director should be responsible for:

1 Setting up the lines of communication with the contract site.
2 The study plan and all record forms.
3 Test drug handling and preparation of the medicated feed.
4 Performance of the laboratory assays for residue determination in tissues and other samples.
5 The final report and archiving of all study raw data at the sponsor site.

The scientific manager (site investigator) at the commercial fish farm would be responsible for the husbandry, treatment and sampling of the fish:

all study-related site procedures should be documented and made available to the sponsor study director.

Specific requirements and details of the various components of the live phase of the study are:

Test system

1   The species of fish and source, e.g. Atlantic Salmon (*Salmo salar*) derived from the common stock at the fish farm.
2   Method of housing the fish, e.g. in sea-water tanks with known flow rates.
3   Procedure for monitoring the water temperature.
4   Numbers of fish per tank and method of identification of individual fish or groups housed in multiple tanks; tank labelling.
5   Details of the fish diet (e.g. standard salmon feed pellets), batch source, analysis and expiry date: the diet should be checked for any contaminants that may interfere in the residue analysis.
6   Acclimatization period to adjust to the tank water and to establish a regular feeding pattern.
7   Monitoring of the fish by the responsible scientist to establish their clinical condition and suitability for experimental purposes.

Pre-dose procedures

1   Determination of the amount of feed that is readily consumed to calculate the daily intake per tank.
2   Pretreatment sampling of fish (control tissues) for the purpose of validation of the residue analytical method.

Treatment

1   Preparation of the individual tank doses by coating/mixing the required quantity of feed pellets with the pre-weighed aliquots of test drug (the latter preferably prepared at the sponsor site) to achieve the study treatment regime: attention should be paid to the appropriate labelling of the treatments.
2   Feeding the fish (by the stockperson) and recording the proportion of each dose consumed (surface feeding).

Post treatment procedures

1   Sampling of fish at the intervals specified in the protocol.
2   Weighing (check-weighed balance), preparation, bagging, labelling and storage of the sampled fish (if the fish are stored frozen, the temperature of the deep freeze should be recorded at regular intervals).
3   Transportation procedures for transfer of the samples to the sponsor facility (the condition of the samples to be recorded on arrival).

Study monitoring
The study director should monitor the following live-phase procedures:

1   Pre-dose; treatment; sampling, preparation, weighing and storage of the sampled fish.
2   Audit of all study record sheets and other documentation at the site.
3   Transport of all samples.

Sponsor quality assurance inspections (before and during the live phase)

1   Examination of the draft and final protocols; the procedures established to ensure the live-phase site personnel are fully aware of the protocol requirements.
2   Pre-dose procedures.
3   Treatment and subsequent fish sampling, preparation, weighing, labelling and storage at the fish farm.
4   Live-phase study records.

Quality assurance activities

In addition to the various activities described above, a major QA function is to advise and guide management and staff concerning regulatory compliance issues relating to safety-oriented studies. A member of the QA unit at an animal health research and development facility is usually an integral part of the project team for the development of a veterinary product and he or she provides valuable input to the proper planning and running of the non-clinical GLP studies, particularly where these involve more than one experimental site (for example, the fish residue study outlined above).

Are there then differences between the QA activities in animal health studies compared to laboratory animal studies?

The answer, of course, is that there are no fundamental differences in any of the QA responsibilities or tasks to assure management that animal health studies (or laboratory animal studies) are conducted in accordance with GLP principles. The veterinary investigations do demand, though, a somewhat different approach to the QA monitoring of the operational phases.

Protective clothing

The laboratory white coat is not the protective clothing of choice when inspecting a farm animal study. It may well unsettle the study animals and the standard laboratory coat will not provide full protection against unforeseen happenings. For example, it must be remembered that what goes into a cow at one end, usually at a leisurely pace, comes out the other end with considerable force. Also the timing of the often-heard comment from the stockperson for the QA assessor to 'Step aside!' always appears to come a little late. The recommended attire is a dark-coloured boiler suit and rubber boots with steel toe caps (cattle are heavy). Full kit, including an airstream helmet, would be advisable under some conditions such as floor pen houses in poultry units.

Study inspections

For reasons of safety, QA staff should ensure they are familiar with all farm activities that they may encounter during inspections.

The following procedures may be observed by QA staff in an animal health non-clinical study, together with the associated documentation:

1 Pre-dose sample collection and analyses; clinical examination, selection and randomization of the test animals, weighing, treatment site preparations and any surgical procedures.
2 Preparation of test compound for dosing, including individual animal doses.
3 Treatment.
4 Penning/caging of animals.
5 Collection of post treatment body fluids and other samples.
6 Postmortem; tissue collection and storage.
7 Laboratory procedures.

Examples of QA checklists for monitoring critical study phases are presented in Appendix 2.

Particular attention is paid to observing compliance with the protocol details and/or relevant standard operating procedures for:

1 Animal identification method (was due care taken to identify animals in the live-phase work?).
2 Animal handling (was there adequate restraint of animals to perform the procedure as intended?).
3 Pen-labelling method and details (permanent for the period of the study and sufficiently specific and clear?).
4 Identification of the correct udder quarter for treatment and the treatment dose labelling (sufficient to cope with a study which may involve a comparison of up to four different formulations in each dairy cow, with eight animals in a study?).
5 Dairy cow udder/quarter cleaning prior to milk sampling (effective teat disinfection prior to collection of samples for bacteriological examination?).
6 Collection of milk samples (was the type of sample collected as indicated in the protocol: strip milk, fore-milk or total bulk quarter sample?).

7 Storage conditions for milk and other samples (sufficient to ensure stability?).
8 Preparation of animals at postmortem for collection of tissue samples in a residue study (was the animal thoroughly washed/brushed prior to sample collection and were proper precautions taken to avoid cross-contamination? Were tissue samples adequately labelled?).
9 Feeding of fish with the medicated feed (was sufficient care taken to avoid disturbing the fish during feeding?).

The farm environment, unfortunately, can provide the opportunity for possible extraneous influences on the performance of a study and the QA inspector should take care to observe, note and report any such site activities in and around the study animal-holding area. Examples are: drift of chemicals from field spraying, use of noxious substances near the study animals, unauthorized changes to cleaning procedures in the study pens.

Other activities

The animal health QA inspection activities will also include assessment of the compliance of in-house laboratory and animal facilities, concentrating on the procedures and systems not observed during study inspections.

Routine periodic inspections of contract laboratories that provide analytical, pathological or diagnostic support to veterinary GLP studies are included in the work programme of the QA unit. Sponsor QA inspection visits are also made to facilities contracted to carry out complete studies.

Training is another important function of the QA unit. Typically, training of scientific staff progresses through:

1 A short introduction to GLP for new personnel covering the essential elements of the GLP principles including those related to the site archive.
2 More detailed training on the application of GLP to specialized areas of work (laboratory and animal care staff).
3 The responsibilities of the study director.
4 Refresher courses.

It is recommended that due attention is paid to imparting knowledge of GLP on a one-to-one basis or in small group sessions with staff during (or soon after) study or laboratory inspections where examples of typical compliance problems arise and can be explained.

Postscript

Farm animal studies provide QA staff with a wide range of very interesting live-phase inspection experience but some of the working conditions can be a little uncomfortable. Consider the following scenario. It is mid-winter, the temperature is well below zero and you arrive by car at the farm to inspect the early-morning milking, sample collection and subsequent treatment of the dairy cows. The time is 5.30 a.m. (you were up at 4.30 a.m. at the local hotel); by torch light you retrieve your cold protective clothing, solid-looking rubber boots and study file from the car and with a somewhat forced cheerful and friendly disposition enter the dairy unit to change and spend the next hour looking as though you really are enjoying the inspection.

Your saviour, of course, is the stockperson who saw you arrive and welcomes you into the dairy office with a steaming hot mug of tea!

Reference

Carson, P. A. and Dent, N. J. (1990) *Good Laboratory and Clinical Practices: Techniques for the Quality Assurance Professional.* Oxford: Heinemann Newnes.

Appendix 1: Typical protocol structure for a veterinary target animal tolerance study

Study number and study title

Study background

Purpose
Selection of test species
Route of administration
Duration:
        Acclimatization period
        Treatment period
        Post treatment period

Study monitor(s)

Study site(s) – (full address, telephone/fax numbers provided)

Animal phase
Laboratory phase(s):
        Various analyses/tests
        Pathology/histopathology

Personnel

Study director
(Assistant study director)
(Study supervisor)
QA department
Animal phase:
        Veterinary surgeon(s)
        Stockperson(s)
        Day-to-day animal care responsibility

Laboratory phase(s):
>   Responsible contacts at each laboratory

Proposed dates (and study day numbers)

Start of acclimatization period
First day of treatment
Last day of treatment
Termination

Test system

Species and type
Number and sex
Body weight (range, approximate weight)
Age (range, approximate age)
Supplier (source: stock, purchased in)

Test substance

Identification
>   Source
>   Name/description
>   Reference number
>   Batch number
>   Date of manufacture

Purity
>   Nominal content/analysis result from certificate of analysis

Stability/expiry date
Storage recommendations
Dose preparation:
>   Dose calculation
>   Method of preparation

Control substance(s) e.g. test substance vehicle or formulation base; positive control

As itemized above for the test substance

Animal treatment and maintenance

Location:
>   Site, building, holding area reference

Housing:

> Pretreatment/posttreatment accommodation, details of pens/ housing, water supply and feeding methods, bedding, environmental conditions and monitoring

Feeding:

> Roughage, concentrates (supplier, batch number), water (supplier)
>
> Frequency, period (daily) intake rate
>
> Statement on possible feed contaminants and their effects on the integrity of the study; pre-study contaminant analyses; feed sample retention for subsequent analyses, if required

Veterinary care:

> Pre-study immunizations/medication/worming; clinical examination(s)
>
> Study inclusion/exclusion criteria
>
> Study veterinary examination(s), frequency
>
> Use of therapeutic treatments – effect on the aims and integrity of the study

Animal identification

Experimental design:

> Randomization method
>
> Treatment site preparation (if relevant)
>
> Feeding regime during treatment period
>
> Study groups, e.g. ×0, ×1, ×3, ×5 recommended dose rate
>
> Dose levels; mg active substance per kg body weight per day
>
> Treatment method

Observations and sampling

Animal health:

> Frequency of clinical observations
>
> Parameters monitored
>
> Details of clinical scoring systems

Bodyweight:

> Recording frequency

Feed and water intake:

> Subjective assessments or quantified observations

Blood, urine/faeces samples:

> Collection methods and sampling frequency (pre-, posttreatment)
>
> Tests to be performed

Terminal procedures:

> Procedure in the event of treatment-related adverse effects

leading to death of animal (postmortem examination, macroscopic/microscopic procedures)

Procedure for handling animals surviving to the study end (method of slaughter, postmortem procedure, tissue/body fluid sampling, preservation and processing details)

Statistical analyses

Parameters to be tested, methods employed; handling of data for males, females, combined results

Further information

Records:
> Storage of records during the performance of the study
> Storage of records and samples on completion of the study report

Safety:
> Precautions to be followed with regard to handling animals and test materials

Quality assurance:
> GLP compliance standards under which the study will be performed
> Proposed QA study inspection programme

Reporting:
> Procedures for issue of the draft/final versions of the study report

Schedule of study events

A comprehensive list of study events with specified dates/study days

Protocol approval

Dated signatures for study director (line management, QA).

Protocol distribution list

Appendices

Record forms:
> Animal housing environmental monitoring
> Feed issue and weigh-back
> Treatment
> Veterinary inspection and diary sheets

      Clinical procedures (pre-, posttreatment observations)

      Adverse event reports

      Body weights

      Tissue/body fluid sampling, storage (and despatch, if relevant)

Clinical pathology observations:

      Haematology, biochemistry

Tissue list for gross and microscopic pathology

Individual study personnel responsibilities

      Details of who does what and when

Appendix 2: Quality assurance monitoring of study critical phases
(examples of checklist items)

General items

Study number
Name of person performing procedure
Name of person(s) assisting
Date/timing of monitoring
Animal identification method
Method of labelling pen/holding area

Animal weighing

General items (see above)
Does the timing of animal weighing comply with the protocol?
Type of weighing scales/weighing machine used?
Has the weighing equipment been zeroed and check-weighed?
Were kg check weight(s) employed?
Procedure employed to identify animals (before, during or after weighing)?
Method of handling/weighing animals? Does this comply with the relevant standard operating procedure (SOP) for the animal species?

Animal dosing

General items (see above)

Preliminary documentation audits

Has the treatment formulation documentation been audited?
Does the treatment form dosing schedule (treatment quantity per body weight, unit dose per animal, frequency of treatment) comply with the protocol?
Does the labelling on the unit dose dispensers comply with the dosing schedule for each animal?

Labelling on the multidose treatment containers: does this comply with the protocol details?

Dosing

Does the dose quantity comply with the calculated quantity for each animal?
Was each animal correctly restrained?
Was each animal identified prior to treatment?
Is the syringe and hypodermic needle size as specified in the protocol or relevant SOP?
Route of administration: as stated in the protocol?
Was the animal number, dose and time administered recorded promptly and correctly?

Collection of body fluids

General items (see above)

Documentation audits

Does the timing of collection comply with the protocol?
Collecting/sample container labelling: does this identify the study, animal and time of collection?

Blood samples

Sample container: with additives? without additives?
Does this comply with the protocol?
Is the syringe size and needle gauge as specified in the protocol or relevant SOP?
Was each animal correctly restrained?
Was due care taken to identify the animal and labelled sample container?

Milk samples

Udder/quarter: were they cleaned before collection of sample?
Were the teats treated with a disinfectant wipe prior to collection of samples for bacteriology?
Was due care taken to identify animal, quarter and labelled sample container?
Type of milk sample collected: as stated in the protocol (strip milk, fore-milk or bulk quarter sample)?
Was the quarter milker thoroughly washed out before milking each animal?
Was the individual animal milk discarded as indicated in the protocol?

Other

Were the samples stored under the conditions specified in the protocol or SOP?

Collection of tissues and body fluids at portmortem

General items (see above)

Sacrifice interval (time of last dose to time of sacrifice)

Weights prior to sacrifice if specified in protocol: have the scales been check-weighed?

Type of euthanasia/means of sacrifice

Were animals adequately restrained at sacrifice?

Were animals cleaned prior to collection of tissue samples?

Were tissue samples collected as per SOP?

Collection of blood/tissue samples: does the collecting vessel labelling identify study, animal, tissue/body fluid, withdrawal period, date of sacrifice, species, radioactive identification (if applicable)?

Has the relevant postmortem documentation been completed, signed and dated?

4 Good laboratory practice in animal vaccine

R H Visanji

Introduction

It is in the interest of all companies to provide the highest possible standards and professionalism in recording and providing data for research and registration of veterinary products: implementing good laboratory practice (GLP) is a way of achieving this.

The veterinary manufacturers have lagged behind the pharmaceutical industries in the implementation of GLP. This is partly due to the nature of the economics. The use of vaccine for animals is dependent on cost. Many farm animals have a short life span and are slaughtered within 6–12 months of being born. If the manufactured vaccines are expensive then there is a possibility that farmers will risk not vaccinating animals.

Introduction of new legislation and the creation of the single market is forcing companies to produce vaccines of high quality. The use of new technology like genetic engineering to produce better and cheaper vaccines has brought about additional pressures from environmentalists. This has encouraged rigorous scrutiny of data from health and safety, regulatory and licensing agencies and has forced companies to seek accreditation to quality systems, the major ones being GLP, ISO 9000 and National Accreditation of Measurement and Sampling (NAMAS).

Recently a new service has been created called United Kingdom Accreditation Service (UKAS, 1995) merging from the two organizations NAMAS and National Accreditation Council for Certification Bodies (NACCB) and this is now recognized as a sole national body for accreditation of conformity assessment. UKAS Mission Statement is 'To generate confidence in the UK's conformity assessment process so as to enhance the competitiveness of UK business and reassure public'. Agreements are in place now where there is cooperation between NAMAS, GLP and ISO900 authorities to conduct joint inspections when requested in companies which have two or more of the above accreditations.

Each of these quality systems has its own distinct objectives and sphere of influence. For example, GLP was originally set up to prevent falsification of data presented to the regulatory authority either deliberately or by accident, between generation of data in the laboratory and presentation in the report. There is gradual but firm insistence by the regulatory and licensing authorities that any data submitted in support of product licensing application must be GLP-compliant. This, coupled with the international dimension of GLP given through the Organization for Economic Cooperation and Development (OECD), puts GLP in the dominating position.

ISO 9000 is general-purpose quality standard which essentially aims to guarantee customer satisfaction as far as possible. ISO 9000 places the onus upon the customer to define the specification which is to be met, and simply provides a management system to enable delivery to that specification to be under control. NAMAS is designed specifically to ensure the competence of testing laboratories. The common essence of these systems is the management of quality and a system which can provide documentary evidence for independent verification.

When companies contract out studies to academia or research institutions sometimes GLP and good clinical practice (GCP) auditing methods overlap. The production of bacterial vaccines and the method for testing them are quite different from that of the analytical laboratory. The requirements for using laboratory animals under defined controlled laboratory conditions can be translated from the existing GLP requirement for the pharmaceutical industries but it is the use of farm animals that causes major concerns.

The methods for testing in farm animals provide a number of problems. One of them is that it is difficult to test farm animals in a controlled environment. When conducting safety tests in cattle one of the measurements is recording body temperatures, but because cattle are housed in open loose boxes where there is no control of conditions, changes in environmental conditions may affect the results.

When farm animals are vaccinated the weather conditions may be different at each vaccination stage, for example it could be bright and sunny at the time of first vaccination and cold and damp during the second vaccination. In some antiparastic drug studies faeces samples have to be collected and this can sometimes prove to be quite difficult if the farm animals are at pasture, for example it could be raining, freezing or snowing, causing problems for the operator.

Unlike in toxicological studies where the animals are from accredited breeders and the history of the animals is known, this is not possible for large animals where in some cases they are bought at livestock auctions or directly from farmers. It is possible to buy some cattle from élite herds where the history of the animal is known but the cost of these animals is prohibitive and would be uneconomical.

The individual identification of farm animals can also cause problems in studies which can last up to 2 years or more. In a duration of immunity experiment where pigs were used, the main method of identification was ear tags: in one trial some pigs lost their tags and this affected the trial design. On top of that the farmer charged the company for repairing the pump which was used to remove sludge because the pump kept getting clogged up with ear tags. One way to overcome this is to use electronic tagging.

When a trial is conducted on a farm the records of calibration of the equipment in some cases are non-existent and the sponsor either has to address this or provide necessary equipment, for example a weighing balance. The type of balance, precision, and staff training to use this balance would be the responsibility of the sponsor.

For studies when animals are on farms, it is difficult to implement GLP requirements and quality assurance (QA) will have to follow the progress of the study all the way through. One of the main problems is the use of casual labour where the staff have no training in animal husbandry. The QA person has to be in constant contact with the study director and be present at all critical phases, checking the vaccines are stored properly and in accordance with the protocol. If the trial site does not have the right equipment, for example a fridge to store vaccines at the right temperature, then the sponsor may have to provide one. QA personnel would have to verify the recording of the raw data constantly.

The keeping of large animals on a farm is expensive and commands a large amount of space. The farmer's cooperation is vital, not only because the farm is tied up for the duration of the study but also because the farmer may have to delay sending the animals to market. Therefore he or she will have to be financially compensated, as well as for any medical treatment or death which occurs during the study. When large animals are kept in the field they are prone to parasitic infection while grazing, and will need to be treated; this will add additional costs. The study director will have to be convinced that this infection will not affect the integrity of the study.

The success of the vaccine depends on the efficacy of the results. This requires testing the vaccine on a percentage of the population, therefore the type of statistical test used is important. The study plan will be complex, involving quality control tests, analytical tests, immunogenicity tests, safety tests and efficacious studies.

Study director

For each study the management is required to appoint a study director. The study director has the primary responsibility in ensuring that the study is conducted to the highest possible standard. The study director will not be an expert in all of the scientific disciplines of the study but must have an overall awareness about the experiments. The study director will appoint scientists with relevant experience to conduct each part of the study. The report written by these scientists will form part of the final report and any inferences drawn from the study director's report should be with his or her consent and signature.

Conduct of the study (protocol)

The study plan should contain the following information but not be limited to it:

1 The title and objective of the study.
2 Identification of the test and any test or reference material to be used.
3 Name of the study director and the name and address of the testing facility or facilities, if applicable.
4 Proposed starting and completion dates for the experimental work.
5 Justification for selecting the test system, e.g. why a particular mixture of vaccine is used.
6 Procedure for disinfecting the animal housing before and after the study and the type of disinfectant used (Appendix 1).
7 Procedure for marking and labelling the test system, to establish identity.
8 A sealed envelope containing the identity of the vaccines used and the method of relaying this information to the study director in an emergency.
9 A description of experimental design, the units of measurement and transformation of the data.
10 Route and administration of the test substance/drug and the reason for choosing it.
11 The dose levels and/or concentrations to be used, together with frequency of dosing.
12 The type and frequency of the tests, number of times the animals are to be bled, how samples are to be labelled, and where they will be stored. Drug expiry date.
13 The species of animals, weight, age, sex, strain and reproductive status.
14 Diet.
15 Before the animals are used the veterinary surgeon must certify that the

animals are in sound health and fit to be used in the experiment. This certificate must be attached to the final report.

16 Allocation of the animals, i.e. how they are divided into groups.
17 Description of the statistical method to be used and the reason for using it.
18 Records to be maintained as raw data and to be signed and dated.
19 A description of the containment requirement for the biological studies, e.g. if the animals are to be isolated if infectious.
20 Names and qualifications of the personnel responsible for the experiment.
21 There should be a certificate stating that the protocol complies with the principles of GLP which should be checked by QA staff.

Manufacture of vaccine

Vaccines should be made to the good manufacturing practice (GMP) standard and the following information should be included in the records for the production of the vaccine and also in the protocol.

1 The bacterial vaccine strain and its history (Appendix 2).
2 The method of storage of the bacterial strains.
3 The passage number from the original strain used in production.
4 The number of seed passages before inoculation in the final fermenter.
5 The production method.
6 Type of medium used.
7 Method used for disinfecting fermenters, both before and after fermentation.

Some vaccines contain two or more strains of bacteria and therefore proof that these strains have been added is required. A standard operating procedure (SOP) for identity tests of these different strains is required.

8 It may be that these bacteria used in the vaccine are inactivated, therefore proof of inactivation is required.
9 If the bacteria are live then a different process would be needed, namely freeze-drying. Full details of this process should be included.
10 At each stage of the process quality control tests should be done (e.g. purity, identity, etc.) and records made available for inspection.
11 Full records of the blending process.
12 Once all the processes have been completed, then full quality control tests should be performed.
13 The method of storage of the vaccine.
14 The vaccine shelf-life.

15   Any contraindications and warnings about the vaccine.
16   Withholding time of the animals after vaccination.
17   The dosage of the vaccine.
18   The route of vaccination.
19   The age of the animal at vaccination and the type of animal.

Efficacy study

Vaccine has to be shown to be efficacious in target species, therefore there should be a facility for the purpose of containment of the challenge infection available. The disinfectant used must not be resistant to the challenge strain. A validation report must be available to confirm the effectiveness of the disinfectant. Wherever possible, animal history records should be available (Appendix 3).

Safety test

All vaccines used in a study have to be tested for safety. They are tested in the target species with twice the normal dose rate. The vaccine may need to be tested in pregnant and non-pregnant animals. The study has to be done to GLP standards and every aspect of the study will be audited by QA staff.

Study conduct

The study director:

1   will provide a protocol which will include all aspects of the conduct of the trial;
2   will select appropriately qualified and competent scientists;
3   will select a deputy study director if necessary.

The study director will be expected to cooperate fully with QA personnel and provide assurance that he or she has sufficient time to devote to the study. The study director should have adequate staff and facilities. Where the study director is not a veterinary surgeon, he or she will ensure that proper care is provided, the local veterinary surgeon is kept informed and access to suitable equipment is available in the event of an emergency.

The study director will:

1   obtain written consent from the animal owners if needed;
2   provide all relevant information to the staff and make sure that they are aware of their responsibilities and what is required regarding the recording of the data and the management of the study;

3 write the trial report and also check the validity of all data provided;
4 provide all raw data to QA – these should be signed and dated on the day when data were recorded;
5 ensure that any animal removed from the trial is documented, along with the reason for the withdrawal;
6 supervise when in certain cases sick animals are withdrawn from the trial for a limited period, treated and returned. This should be documented and confirmed that it does not affect the integrity of the study.

Quality assurance

Quality assurance staff should:

1 Check the qualifications of the study director and have a copy of his or her current curriculum vitae.
2 Visit the facility before and during the study to make sure that the trial is performed as stipulated in the protocol and ensure that all data are recorded properly and if needs be, verify them.
3 Make sure that the site for the study is adequate and the staff are properly trained.
4 Make sure that in an efficacy study, if animals are to be challenged then there are adequate facilities to isolate the animals for the challenge and the premises can be disinfected thoroughly both before and after the trial.
5 Check that storage, use of and recording of the test material is adhered to and all test material is accounted for.
6 Check that excess material is returned or properly disposed of.
7 Make sure that any adverse reactions of the animals are reported to the sponsor and other authorities if required.
8 Ensure that the method of recording data is adequate.
9 Check the quality of feed.
10 Check the quality of water.

Archiving

All protocols, reports and documents relating to communications with the study director, data on suspected adverse events and batch records need to be archived for 5 years from when the product was made. All data and documents will be made available if requested by relevant authorities.

In some cases when raw data are recorded in a farm situation they are really 'raw' and the paper on which these data are recorded has traces of mud and faeces and smell. The archivist will not be pleased with the raw data, therefore these documents can be photocopied and the QA person will stamp 'authentic copy', sign and date the copy.

In some cases the data will be in electronic form and all possible care must be taken to ensure that the data transformed are accurate. This can be checked with the hard copies. The hard copy must be signed and dated and can form part of the raw data. Steps should be taken to have back-up copies in case of accidents. All this information is to be kept in the archives with the final report.

Once the trial is completed the QA staff will ensure that the raw data and all reports, both from the study director and from the QA person are archived. The sponsor will ensure that the data are properly analysed, inferenced and a final report written and this should contain the signatures of all those involved in the study.

GLP audit

There are three main phases of GLP audit:

1 Protocol audit and checklist.
2 Audit of experimental phase.
3 Report audit.

The above reports will be circulated to the management in the following manner:

1 The QA department receives a photocopy of the report for auditing which is logged into the report audit book, and inspection number is issued from a consecutive number list.
2 A full and thorough inspection of the report is carried out. The raw data are verified by random checking and inspection of transcriptions from tables to figures and vice versa.
3 Following report inspection, the findings are discussed with the author and the agreed findings documented. This, together with copies of the highlighted areas for correction, is attached to the routing sheet and returned to the author who will implement the changes.
4 Once the changes have been implemented, QA will check that the requested changes have been made before completing the QA GLP compliance page.
5 On receipt of the issued report the master scheduling index is updated, the copy filed in the QA office and the original lodged in the archive.

Checklist and reporting to study management

It is the responsibility of QA to inspect each phase of the study periodically and to maintain written and properly signed records of each periodic inspection. These inspection reports should show the date of inspection, the study inspected, the phase or segment of the study inspected, the person performing the inspection and his or her findings and any problems, the recommended action taken to resolve existing problems; the dated report is then submitted to the management.

Any significant problems which are likely to affect the study integrity found during the course of an inspection should be brought to the attention of the study director and management immediately.

It is the responsibility of QA periodically to submit to management and the study director written GLP reports on each study. These reports should note any problems encountered and any corrective action taken. QA should determine that no deviations from approved protocols or SOPs were made without proper authorization and documentation. The final study report should be reviewed to ensure that each report accurately describes the methods and SOPs and that the reported results accurately reflect the raw data of the study. In each report, a signed statement should be included which should specify the date when inspections were made and findings reported to study management and the study director.

The responsibilities and procedures relating to these details and applicable to QA, the records maintained by QA and how such records are indexed should be in writing and maintained.

A designated representative of QA shall have access to the written procedures established for the inspection and may request testing facility management to certify that inspections are being implemented, performed, documented and followed up in accordance with the regulations.

Quality Assurance inspection programme

There are two main areas to be detailed here:

1 Experimental inspections and department inspections.
2 Report inspections.

Experimental inspection

1 The experiment checklist (Appendix 4) shows the items that should be checked at each inspection relating to each type of experimental procedure carried out. Each checklist details the items necessary to be inspected but not necessarily on each occasion. At the initial vaccination, and subsequent work-up procedure, certain areas may be completed and circulated to study management until the report is complete or the work is considered by the scientist to be terminated.
2 Department inspections carried out on a 6-monthly basis are detailed in a separate report and these show a facilities inspection only.

3 Follow-up inspections to both of the above points may be produced where circumstances dictate.

All reports on experimental and departmental inspections are sent to the study director, management and the head of the department (Appendix 5).

Report inspection
The QA inspection report contains a record of the review, the faults found, amendments made and corrective action to be taken. As with the experimental inspections, follow-up reports may be produced. These reports are sent initially to the author of the report to enable comments and signatures to be obtained, and then to the study director and head of department (Appendix 6).

Reporting to study management

As has been detailed, reports are produced and circulated to various persons in the management structure. A routing slip (Appendix 5) should be attached to each report produced by QA. This is divided into appropriate areas and also details the type of report, the inspection report number, and the date submitted to study management. The first area on this front sheet allows comments or action to be taken by the scientist or technician involved, his or her signature and a date to show agreement with QA. The second area allows for the same action to be taken by the study director and the subsequent areas for any comments, or action by the head of the department.

When these areas have been duly completed the inspection report is then signed off by QA (Appendix 7) and additional or follow-up inspection reports will be taken through the same procedure. The responsibility for carrying out these actions rests solely with the QA department.

Protocol approval and checklist

With regard to Department of Health Guidelines (Good Laboratory Practice and the role of the Study Director, Advisory leaflet no. 4, 1993) there are standard points which must be included in protocols. These, plus commonly occurring headings, are included in a checklist, shown below, for inspection and reference purposes.

1 Each study shall have an approved written protocol that clearly indicates the objectives of the work and all methods of study.
   1.1 This is, of course, essential where any part of the study claims GLP compliance.
   1.2 Most important of all is that no work should begin until a protocol

is approved and issued, duly signed by the responsible scientists, study director and QA manager.

2 The protocol shall contain, but not be limited to, the following information:

  2.1 Descriptive title and statement of purpose of the study.

  2.2 Identification of the test article by reference to name or code number.

  2.3 Name of the company and the address of the testing facility where the testing is conducted.

  2.4 Reference number of the document for archive retrieval purposes.

  2.5 The names of the author, study director and responsible scientist should be shown, plus their signatures.

3 Where applicable, the number, body weight range, sex, source of supply, strain, substrain and age of the animals utilized in the test system should be given.

  3.1 The method of identification of the animals used in the study.

4 A description of the experimental design, including the methods of randomization, control of bias, etc.

5 A description of the identification of the diets, housing and experimental route.

6 The type and frequency of tests, analyses and measurements to be made, with references to SOPs if applicable.

7 The records to be maintained, mentioning designated location if applicable.

8 The date of approval of the protocol by the study director and his or her signature.

9 Where applicable, a statement of the proposed statistical methods to be used.

10 Where applicable, the other department concerned with the study and the study directors in those departments should be noted, to allow complete inspection and liaison to be maintained.

11 All changes or revisions, and reasons for them, to an approval protocol shall be documented, signed by the study director, dated and maintained with the protocol. It is essential that this revision should be circulated to all those holding an original protocol.

12 Under normal circumstances relevant vaccine samples will be stored for a period of 1 year, or until the vaccine is regarded as of no scientific value.

Certain requirements for protocol content are detailed below and explanations for omission, if applicable, should be given in the policy statement.

13 The justification for selection of the test system.

14 Another area of importance is auditing of validation plans for software.

The plan should contain a number of points but not necessarily be limited to the following:

14.1   Purpose of the system.

14.2   A description of the test environment.

14.3   Any assumptions, exclusions and limitations of the system.

14.4   The start and finish dates with respect to the execution of the plan.

14.5   The validation data sets.

14.6   Validation plan execution, expected results and criteria for acceptance.

14.7   Error resolution.

14.8   Documentation to be produced as the plan is executed.

The total responsibility for the action detailed above lies with QA department. However, the compilation of the protocol and the ultimate responsibility of the study rest with the study director.

Checklist for report content and GLP compliance

With regard to the Food and Drug Administration and OECD regulations, there are standard points which must be included in reports. These, plus commonly occurring headings, are to be included in a checklist (Appendix 8), shown below, for audit and references purposes.

All reports produced are subject to GLP inspection and will be submitted in the final report format to the QA department for inspection.

The final format is the stage in report production when all items have been addressed and the author and scientists involved in the study have signed the report.

1   A final report shall be prepared for each study including but not necessarily limited to the following:

1.1   Name and address of the facility performing the study and the dates on which the study was initiated and completed.

   1.1.1   The correct front and GLP sheets must be utilized.

   1.1.2   Pagination must be correct throughout the report.

1.2   Objectives and procedures as stated in the approved protocol, including changes to the original protocol.

1.3   Characterization of the test material.

1.4   A description of the methods used. (Reference may be made to SOPs.)

1.5   A description of the test system used. Where applicable, the initial report shall include the number of animals used, sex, body weight range, source and supply, species, strain and substrain, age and procedure used for identification.

1.6 A description of the dosage, dosage regimen, route of administration and duration.

1.7 A description of any circumstances that may have affected the quality or integrity of the data.

1.8 The name of the study director, the name of other scientists, and the names of all supervisory personnel involved in the study.

1.9 A description of the transformations, calculations or operations performed on the data, a summary and analysis of the data, and a statement of the conclusions drawn from the analyses.

1.10 The signed and dated reports of each of the individual scientists or other professionals involved in the study.

    1.10.1 The *original* copy is retained by the departmental secretary and a photocopy provided for the QA inspection.

1.11 The location where all raw data and the final report are to be stored.

    1.11.1 Notebook and project file references must be included to indicate raw data locations and facilitate easy retrieval and auditing.

    1.11.2 Tabular display must be consistent.

    1.11.3 Date of injections must be shown on the reference page.

2 Corrections or additions to a final report shall clearly identify that part of the final report which is being added to or corrected, the reasons for the corrections or addition, and shall be signed and dated by the person amending the report. If amended after issue then this must be treated as a *report amendment* and should be in the same format as a protocol amendment with the same controls.

3 The report is checked as detailed in SOPs and the QA person signs to indicate that the document has been checked, both mathematically and for content, to verify that it complies with the protocol and that raw data had been checked.

4 Depending on the type of report, random data points will be checked in two ways:

(a) raw data to report.

(b) report to raw data.

4.1 Where there are a minimal number of calculations and they are able to be performed on a hand calculator, these will *all* be checked.

4.2 Where there are a large number of calculations, and they are able to be performed on a hand calculator, random numbers will be checked depending on the total calculations contained in the report. Random numbers can be generated by using the appropriate function key on a scientific calculator or using computer software.

4.3   Where calculations are unable to be checked on a hand calculator, review of the raw data and computer program with computer printout will be validated *in situ* with the responsible scientist.

5   Attached to the SOP are checking procedures for animal study reports (Appendix 9). The responsibility for checking the report for GLP compliance rests with QA, but the content, compilation and overall responsibility for the reports rest with the study director and scientists involved.

Conclusions

The quality of the data generated from research must be of concern to scientists, managers and regulatory authorities. The common goal must be that of reaching excellence – producing safe and efficacious products – and GLP is a good vehicle for achieving these goals. In time GLP will become the international norm for industries and other institutions for reporting data generated in laboratories. The influence of regulatory and licensing authorities will force it to be sooner rather than later.

Appendix 1: The following standard operating procedures should be available

- Requisitioning of animals
- Receipt of animals
- Certification of the animals for health status
- Cleaning animal accommodation
- Decontamination of animal accommodation
- Animal husbandry procedures (including daily cleaning, watering, feeding and monitoring)
- Procedure for informing about sick animals and treatment
- Procedure for dealing with the unexpected death of animals during study
- Method for removing carcasses
- Method for decontaminating infected carcasses (if infected)
- Procedure for entering challenged animal accommodation

Appendix 2:   Bacterial history

Type:
Name:
Strain:
Date isolated:
Animal isolated from:
Tissue isolated from:
History of the animal isolated from:
Passage no. from original strain:
Date freeze-dried:
No. freeze-dried:
Passage no. to be used for the production:
Date checked for identity:
Checked by:
Date checked for purity:
Checked by:
Growth temperature:
Solid media used:
Media for fermentation:
Person responsible for the custody of sample:

Appendix 3:   Animal history record form

Animal species:
Breed:
Source:
Age:
Sex:
Identity:
Protocol no. for the study:
Vaccine history if available:

Appendix 4:   Checklist for animal studies

Date of inspection:
Inspection no.:
Date:
Department:
Auditor:
Test material:
Study director:
Protocol no.:
Animal study no.:
Test material batch:
Animals:
Strain:
Species:
Date of birth:
Sex:
Weight range:
Vaccination route:
Dose:
Samples:
Records:
Comments:

Appendix 5:   Confidential – inspection report no.

Protocol inspection report   } For signature and return
Experimental inspection   } to quality assurance
Final report inspection   } *within 14 days*

Date submitted to study management:

Scientist/technician – Comment/action   Signed: Date:
Study director – Comment/action   Signed: Date:
Project leader – Comment/action   Section head   Signed: Date:
Head of department – Comment/action   Signed: Date:

Appendix 6:   Inspection record form

Date of quality assurance (QA) document issue: Document no.:
Date of inspection: Department:
Auditor: Vaccine:
Study director: Project no.:
Protocol no.:

Report

QA inspection report no.:
This report was reviewed by QA on the above date prior to distribution.

The document consisted of:

page(s)	Front sheet
pages(s)	Text
pages(s)	Tables
pages(s)	Figures
pages(s)	Signatures and Distribution

During the review the document was checked for mathematical and grammatical points and inconsistencies found are detailed below:

Appendix 7: Study report

Quality assurance (QA) unit

In compliance with the current good laboratory practice regulations and procedures, this study has been inspected and this report checked in conjunction with the appropriate QA standard operating procedures.

As this phase of the experiment was of a short duration, inspections have been limited to the raw data, the samples upon receipt and the final report.

Date of inspection   QA inspection no.   Date submitted to management

Signature: Date:

Appendix 8:   Report compliance checklist

1 Name and address of the facility performing the study.
2 Study start and completion dates.
3 Correct front and back sheet.
4 Correct pagination and document code.
5 Objectives and procedures, including changes to protocol.
6 Characterization of test article and control.
7 Description of methods used (standard operating procedures may be quoted).
8 Description of the test system – species, strain, numbers, etc.
9 Any circumstances affecting the quality/integrity of data.
10 Identification and signatures of study director, scientists and supervisors involved in the study.
11 Descriptions of statistical methods, transformations and calculations. Summary and analysis of data and conclusions.
12 Consistency of tabular display.
13 Notebook/study references for raw data.
14 Signed and dated reports of individual scientists.
15 Raw data and final report location.
16 Quality assurance good laboratory practice compliance and study director's statement.

Appendix 9:   Good laboratory practice inspection report

Date of document: Inspection no.:

Date of inspection: Department:

Auditor: Vaccine:

Study director: Protocol no.:

Vaccine batch no.:   Expiry date:

Materials and methods

Species: Sex:

Strain: No:

Vaccine dose: Vaccination route:

Samples:

Records:

Comments:

PART TWO

Preparation for good clinical practice – the investigator viewpoint

5   Good research practice – the way forward

R Brase

Preparation for good clinical practice – the principal investigator viewpoint – the involvement in a phase III multi-centre clinical study – problems and resolutions

This chapter describes the problems met during the preparations for and the participation in several large sepsis trials. It outlines some of the difficulties with which a clinical investigator has to cope when preparing and performing local clinical research in large multicentre trials. Investigators planning to participate for their first time in large trials will find assistance to steer them safely around the rocks and shoals on their course towards their first successful clinical trial.

The setting of multicentre trials

Clinical work, clinical research and lab work can be done in many different ways. As long as the research is performed by single individuals or a small group in a single institution, the investigators have the opportunity to set up their work according to their own style.

When clinical trials are done in a multicentre approach, local investigators have to work according to rigid protocols which often were developed without their participation. Protocol adherence and consistency in its execution are of major importance for the success of these trials. Individual approaches are only to be found in the integration of the trial into local clinical practice.

Clinical practice and documentation

In bedside medicine, the actual conduct of the work is of much higher value than its documentation – the paperwork. Pre-hospital emergency medicine is an extreme example. Emergency personnel rarely glance at their watches while receiving large amounts of information and working through many decisions. Protocols are filled out when the 'heat is off'. Descriptions given are brief and many data are imprecise when it comes to numbers and time-points, although the overall picture is correct. Hospital medicine has more resources allocated to documentation of data, but documentation still has a low priority when compared to direct patient care. Documentation again is imprecise and incomplete during phases of high workload in the unit: available information is often compressed to short written notes. Even good data documentation in clinical medicine has substantial information understood but unwritten or in a form which is not readily accessible by out-side personnel (routine orders, abbreviations, different source documents).

Each hospital has its own system of documentation. The system often represents more or less individual and sometimes contradicting solutions which differ from department to department and from unit to unit. The development of different documentation or protocols is timeconsuming. It is therefore often avoided or handled as a low priority.

Studies performed and lab work done in a single unit approach always represent a unique solution to the single unit's project. It can be regarded as the centre's best solution. Centres tend to be conservative when it comes to their procedures or documentation process. This approach must be changed when it comes to participation in multicentre trials performed under the recently introduced guidelines for good clinical practice (GCP).

Phase III multicentre clinical studies

Guidelines for GCP for trials on medicinal products impose standards on the pharamaceutical industry and participants in any of the four phases of clinical trials. The standards contain pre-established, systematic written procedures for the organization, conduct, data collection, documentation and verification of clinical trials.

Participation in externally created trials and especially in a large multi-centre clinical trial is a challenging project for every participating centre. These trials carry their own rules.

There is a group of participating centres with a large variety of settings. The variety is controlled through a rigid procedural approach (protocol). There is lot of paperwork to be done according to the rules of the protocol and GCP. We participated in three different phase III multicentre clinical trials for new agents in sepsis. The case report books for a single patient were voluminous in all trials. They contained between 41 and 83 pages, with approximately 18–40 data entry fields per page. Strict protocol adherence and a consistent approach towards the protocol had to be accomplished by each centre.

Although this is not known by most centres, each centre is checked on its performance and protocol adherence by the sponsor.

Some centres will be formally audited by the company's own quality assurance staff, by external auditoring firms hired by the sponsor and by regulating agencies. Protocol violations and failure to adhere to GCP guidelines endanger the results of the whole trial and carry the risk of consequences for the offender and the institution. Passing an audit without negative findings can be regarded as proof of good-quality work and can be used when applying for participation in future trials.

Planning your research effort

Research efforts should be planned after several questions have been answered:

1 Does the site have the right patients for the trial (according to the inclusion and exclusion criteria)?
2 How many eligible patients can be expected per year (minimum/ maximum)? There should be a deduction of at least 20% for consent denied, times of reduced staffing and other confounding factors resulting in non-enrolment of eligible patients. Calculate your patient enrolment on the basis of a minimal and maximal estimated enrolment rate.
3 Does the principal investigator have enough access to the patients to enrol them and enough influence on the care of the patients to avoid early or late protocol violations (e.g. entering the patients at the right time-point into the trial or avoiding confounding medical treatment during treatment or the follow-up phase)? According to GCP, the principal investigator is responsible for the provision of good medical care to each study subject during and after treatment.
4 Is there enough driving force and personnel available at the site throughout the entire study period to participate in this effort (which sometimes compares well with a long-distance run)? Will you have to hire extra personnel in order to do the work?
5 Do you have enough support from your department and management to conduct the trial?
6 Has the site the technical equipment and support necessary to carry out the work (infusion pumps, refrigerators, freezer, shelf storage space, etc.)?
7 What are the costs (workforce, lab work, equipment, communication/transportation, overheads) for the trial calculated on the basis of the estimated minimal and maximal enrolment performance? What are the costs per month and per patient? Expect a 20% increase in costs due to miscellaneous factors (see below).
8 What is the expected reimbursement per patient by the sponsor? What overall reimbursement can be expected calculated on the basis of estimated minimal and maximal enrolment?

9   Who is covering your expenses during the preparation for the trial (e.g. fee for Institutional Review Board (IRB) handling)?

10   What is the estimated schedule for the preparation and conduct of the trial at your site? How much time is necessary to get permission from the hospital management and the IRB (ethics committee)? Calculate the time taken for delayed IRB approval due to changes within the protocol or informed consent.

11   Are there other trials planned or underway which might interfere directly or indirectly with patient enrolment? In many sepsis trials, the use of another investigational drug or biomedical product in a patient within 30 days of the study period is regarded as an exclusion criterion. GCP requests you to make the statement that the trial may not be disturbed by any other trials performed at your centre.

Preparing your participation

Financial preparations and contracts

A financial calculation of the trial should be done according to the estimated minimum/maximum enrolment. A detailed work-up of the costs (personnel, material, overheads, communication, fees) assumed during the precalculation will evolve a better and more precise picture of the financial side of the trial. A safety margin of 20% (covering cost increases due to, for example, queries, audits, unevaluable and thus not reimbursable patients) should be integrated into the calculations. Do not underestimate the time and costs of unevaluable and thus not reimbursable patients, of resolving queries, preparing and conducting audits, study close-out and IRB-related issues. Reading this chapter and doing the proposed precalculations must be regarded as the overhead costs of the ongoing or forthcoming trials.

Your hospital administration may request some form of financial calculation before approval of the trial. When the above-mentioned safety margin of 20% of costs cannot be openly declared, it should be covered within defined parts of the calculations. The financial calculation of the trial will allow the investigator to decide on a rational basis about the participation, hiring of personnel and buying or leasing of equipment. A cost-benefit analysis for every trial should be done, although it is sometimes hard to define the immaterial benefit of a trial (e.g. scientific profile, follow-up trials).

Contracts with payments on a per-case basis carry risks in case of early study termination. A financial bail-out plan in case of premature study termination should be prepared.

After the planning phase has been successfully finished and the trial has been approved by the department on the basis of the study protocol and contract draft, the final study contract should be negotiated. The contract should contain the definite start and duration of the trial, estimated number of patients per site, payments and provisions in case of early termination of the trial. These should at least cover expenses for the equipment and salaries for personnel hired for the trial.

The outline of the contract conditions might already be a topic to be discussed during the first visit of a sponsor team at your site. For the sponsor, the major part of this visit is to verify that your centre is an appropriate investigative site for the conduct of the trial.

Laboratory and other diagnostic facilities

Some trials rely almost exclusively on the the work of an external central study lab. Other protocols require in-hospital laboratory data as a major part of the dataset gathered. In the latter cases, the cooperation of both the lab head as well as the lab technicians is important for the conduct of the trial.

Basic clinical lab work is regarded as important for patient care and therefore more or less available on a 24-hour basis. The lab data necessary for the case report of a trial have a much lower priority for the lab personnel. This can lead to problems during night times and weekends, especially when laboratory data outside the clinical routine are required. The cooperation of both the lab head as well as all the lab technicians involved has to be gained in advance in order to smoothen the conduct of the trial, avoid unnecessary extra work and perform well when it comes to an audit. The cooperation can be achieved by addressing their specific interests.

The lab head thinks in organization categories like distribution of workload, costs and budget limits. His or her cooperation can be gained by paying for the trial lab work and adding some extra funding for lab research purposes. If the sponsor is paying on the usual per-patient basis, your payments to the lab should also be done on a fee-for-service or per-patient basis to avoid unnecessary financial commitments. The lab technicians' interest in avoiding extra work can be overcome by information about the importance and the goals of the trial, e.g. during a brief presentation. Recognizing their sometimes high workload is mandatory; finding and negotiating a solution as to how the extra work can still be done is a challenge. This can lead to agreements which might have some lab work with the investigator group (e.g. centrifugation) and might contain extra financial support towards the lab.

The study protocol might request results of other diagnostic procedures and thereby the cooperation of other diagnosic facilities as well. Most problems arising when dealing with the clinical laboratory can be transferred to other diagnostic facilities. Solutions and agreements can only be achieved through negotiations which recognize the interests of both sides.

Not achieving the maximum goal in these negotiations might not satisfy the investigator, who routinely is used to having his or her requests fulfilled. But the negotiating efforts and some compromising can be expected to reap rewards during the long run of the trial, when the diagnostic work is done smoothly and the results come in reliably. The investigators will spend less energy on the retrieval of missing printouts and records, arguing with and convincing each single technician over and over again to do a test for the trial or browsing through their master files for single missing values or records requested by the their sponsors.

As part of the preparation of a site, the sponsor will request written statements from the heads of all diagnosic facilities involved about the methods they use and the local ranges of normal values. Asking the lab head in time will enable you to respond early.

Collaborators

In most trials the amount of work at a study site cannot be managed by a single person, when the individual has clinical responsibilities besides the trial. There are two general approaches to handling the workload:

1   Setting up a group of clinical collaborators (the local investigator team including a local study coordinator) which runs the trial beside their clinical work.
2   Employing study nurses or doctors for the conduct of the trial.

Each solution has its advantages and disadvantages.

The group of clinical collaborators offers the advantage of experience within the field and a limited financial burden for the trial. This holds true even when the collaborators are paid for some of their overtime. The disadvantage of this approach, even when having several collaborators results from the collaborators' occupancy with their clinical duties. This may sometimes result in a lack of workforce at critical points of high workload within the trial. A real team effort and high level of discipline are necessary to overcome these periods without weakness in the performance during the trial.

Employing study nurses, doctors or other dedicated personnel (one of whom should be nominated as local study coordinator) for the course of the trial has the advantage of having staff available for the conduct of the trial throughout the entire period. This theoretically enables the site to deliver its work at a more constant level of performance and eases many outside contacts due to the uniform availability of the site.

Employing only one person for the trial was not considered sufficient during the sepsis trials we participated in. Even with flexible working hours, complete weekend and holiday coverage cannot be achieved with a single-person approach. The problem of shifting workload and holidays might be solved by hiring two collaborators both working part-time.

A considerable disadvantage of hiring collaborators for the trial results from the relative uncertainty of the financial basis of their employment. At least in the German public health system, working contracts cannot be easily terminated. Some of the recent sepsis trials have been cancelled at very short notice during the course of the trial. The contracts provided payments on a per-patient basis. All of a sudden, some investigators faced the dilemma of having employed collaborators on a long-standing conduct of a trial which was suddenly stopped, leaving the investigator to pay monthly salaries for a study doctor who has no more work to do. Compared to this dilemma, the lack of work of a hired collaborator for weeks due to delays between the expected and actual start of a trial (late IRB approval, late study drug delivery, problems with printing the casebooks, last-minute protocol changes, etc.) is a minor problem and generated relatively little extra cost.

Your direct collaborators and the staff of the diagnostic facilities are only part of the group involved with the conduct of the trial. Your fellow staff doctors, nurses and other personnel have to contribute their share to your success. Adequate handling of blood samples and test articles is as necessary as correct drug application and avoidance of protocol violations by chance. Early information about the goal, inclusion and exclusion criteria and the practical conduct should be presented to the entire personnel. All colleagues who may encounter study candidates should be provided with abbreviated written enrolment and exclusion criteria. In case of continuous drug application, written guidelines for drug application should be prepared for use at every study subject's bedside. These guidelines should include clear instructions on whom to inform and how to proceed in case of errors or interruptions of drug administration, adverse events or major deviations from the protocol. You should encourage all personnel to contact the investigator team in case of any perceived problems during the trial. A dozen unnecessary questions and phone calls during the night are easier to handle than one severe protocol violation which is missed, because the intensive care unit staff didn't dare to disturb a member of the investigator team.

Communication

In order to ease contact with the sponsor, a dedicated phone number should be used throughout the trial. An answering machine is helpful. A dedicated fax number will further improve sponsor contact, especially when cooperating with sponsors from overseas.

The members of the investigating team, including their phone numbers, should be noted on the abbreviated enrolment criteria and the written guidelines mentioned above. During any phase of the trial, a member of the site team should be available on a 24-hour basis. A pager or cellular phone will be necessary. The phone number should be widely distributed within the research site, including the sponsor. Communication charges are part of the overhead costs. Communication will be necessary in four major circumstances:

1   Evaluation of new patients for the trial.
2   Problems with drug application during trials and continuous test article administration.
3   Mild or serious adverse events. Serious adverse events have to be reported within 24 h.
4   Questions about confounding factors arising from the standard clinical treatment of patients.

Encourage all staff to communicate with your investigating group to avoid protocol violations and to enhance overall performance.

Institutional Review Board

The IRB represents an independent group of experts and laypersons. The local investigator is responsible for the trial and has to apply for IRB approval. The letter should cover:

1   a brief description of a background of your trial;
2   a short outline of the protocol;
3   a description of your personal experience in the field.

A copy of the protocol, patient information and informed consent as well as the patient insurance certificate should be enclosed. The IRB office will copy your material and distribute it to the IRB members in preparation for their meeting.

The IRB will charge you for their service. Reimbursement from the sponsor should be part of the study contract. (The fee in 1996 for the local IRB in Bremen is 1400 $US per protocol.)

The IRB approval decides on the conduct of your trial. The IRB may offer you the opportunity to present your trial during their meeting. Prepare for this presentation and be ready to answer questions about the specifics of the field of research, the protocol and differences from other trials in the field as well as the protocol itself. Most IRB members, colleagues as well as laypersons, are unfamiliar with the specifics in the field of your trial. The

IRB therefore might ask consultants, usually local experts in your field, to look at the scientific integrity and value of your trial.

The potential hazards, possible risks and discomforts to study subjects are major topics of the evaluation of your trial.

Another focus of interest is the informed consent and patient information sheet. According to GCP, the principal local investigator is responsible for adequate information of all study subjects. In multinational, multicentre trials, the sponsor usually offers a standard informed consent and patient information to every site. An IRB request for changes in both forms is a common cause of delay in IRB approval and study start. The new version often needs approval at the next IRB meeting. You may avoid possible delay if you approach the IRB office as soon as you have a draft of the forms at hand. Get a good-quality translation using only expressions that non-medical persons can understand. Before or while you formally approach the IRB, its secretary may help you re-edit the drafts and get them into accept-able shape. The two papers have to be short as well as complete, easy to read and understandable for a layperson. Don't try to argue with the IRB about content or style – they have to OK it.

The informed consent has to contain a statement that the trial is a research project and participation is voluntary and free of any extra charge. It should be stated that the subject is free to deny or withdraw approval at any time during the trial without any negative effects on his or her treatment. It has to be noted that the patient information has been read, understood and any open questions have been resolved.

In case the patient cannot give informed consent due to underlying disease or medical treatment, a surrogate decision through his or her autho-rized representative (mostly next-of-kin) may be acceptable for the local IRB. The informed consent form should contain a part or separate page for this informed assent. Local regulations concerning the informed assent may be very restrictive if it comes to clinical trials. Assent through a guardian-ship court may be necessary. This question should be clarified with the IRB office before application for approval.

The patient information should contain statements about the type, goals and methods of the research project. Names and phone numbers of contact persons have to be noted. Description of the test article, randomization, use of placebo (if any) and all other treatment is necessary. The potential hazards, possible risks and discomforts to the patient should be described as well as any anticipated benefit. Alternative treatment, if any, should be explained. The voluntary character of the participation and all other terms of the informed consent/assent should be repeated. Measures taken to protect the patient's health and the confidential handling of all data should be clarified as well as the insurance and procedures for compensation in case of injury due to the participation.

The written approval of the IRB is a condition *sine qua non* for the start of the trial. Most sponsors require written IRB approval even before shipment of the test article. Unnecessary delay in the start-up of a site can be avoided by taking several measures:

1   Get a written statement from the IRB in advance about its working rules and a list of its members including their sex, profession and affiliated hospital (US GCPs require there to be women and non-scientific members in the IRB. Your sponsor will ask you for this letter).
2   Find out the working rules of the IRB, including deadlines for application.
3   Keep your sponsor contact informed about the deadlines for application.
4   Try to clarify as many as possible of the potential problems arising from your protocol before application for IRB approval (e.g. reshape the informed consent and patient information together with the IRB secretary into a version which will be accepted by your IRB).
5   Arrange for facsimile transmission of the IRB approval.

The IRB has to be informed about all protocol changes, changes of informed consent, adverse events occurring at the site, adverse event summaries provided by the sponsor and any significant event within the trial. Relevant new findings that become available during the conduct of the trial may lead to changes of the patient information.

The IRB file will be audited. Keep it updated and complete. In case of an audit, there is a 100% chance that the auditors want to look at the confirmed consent/assent forms of every patient. After termination, provide the IRB with a summary of the trial. This recognizes its important role and each member's contribution to the trial.

Your boss, your administration, other departments

You need their support. In order to assist you from the beginning, your boss has to be informed about your plans and the progress of the trial. Your administration, like the IRB, has its own working rules. Learn and respect its working rules and interests in the trial. Although this does not relate to GCP, good information and cooperation with your administration keep the trial progress on a smooth road.

Extensive information of other clinical departments enhances their cooperation. It may even increase patient enrolment through feedback about remote patients who might be considered appropriate candidates. It will definitely ease the retrieval of charts and access to patients' follow-up. Recurrent retrieval of charts will be necessary throughout the trial. Knowing the exact location of the charts of patients who are still in hospital will save you much time and energy. During audits, reviewers will ask for charts and other source data.

Prompt information of your administration and other departments involved about the study termination and its results will ease their co-operation in the next trial.

Drug supply and storage space

Drug shipment and subsequent storage is a bureaucratical issue. The sponsor will inform you about standard operating procedures concerning test article shipment and storage. Test article location and storage conditions will be explained within the protocol. If drug shipment comes from abroad, ensure that the shipment passes customs without delay We experienced a situation where the refrigerated drug supply was detained at customs on a mid-summer Friday afternoon. Only luck and good time avoided damage. Handle all paperwork related to drug shipment according to protocol and sponsor guidelines.

In contradiction to routine clinical work, where you discard empty vials and containers, GCP requires that every test article vial and container has to be returned to the sponsor for reconciliation with the delivery records.

The initial sponsor correspondence and the study protocol can be stored in only one single file. The enrolment of your site will be followed by a large demand for working space. Even the few patients enrolled into one of the sepsis trials required a working basis of at least 6–8 m². Ideally this should be an office or a storage room dedicated to the trial. Ensure that the test article is safely and properly stored and handled at your site. It should be located within or close to the intensive care unit and should be kept locked whenever not in use.

You will need a desk and several metres of shelf space for files, blood sample boxes, test article and space for the large shipment containers. Some drugs have to be stored in a refrigerator. Many blood samples need storage in a deep freezer (at –30°C or –70°C). If you don't use a pharmacy for test article storage and preparation and a lab freezer for specimen storage, provide space for it. If you use these facilities, gain their cooperation from the planning phase on. Regular (sometimes daily) checks of the storage conditions as well as safe and proper handling of test article and samples throughout the trial will be requested by the protocol. You will be held responsible for it. The freezer should have a safety system in case of malfunction. It should be hooked up to a central surveillance system or placed at a site where personnel will recognize and respond in case of dysfunction. Refrigerator temperatures should be monitored daily. If there is no surveillance system for the refrigerator, filling the shelf space with cool-packs will give additional cooling in case of dysfunction. Your adequate test article, files, blood and other sample storage as well as the limitation of access to the test article will be reviewed by monitors and auditors.

Case record forms (CRFs) and other source data have to be stored for at least 15 years after the end of the trial. Provide adequate archiving space.

The start-up phase

Training and local working rules

The time between signing the contracts and the first enrolment should be used for the training of the collaborators and establishing of local working rules. The training and local working rules have to focus on the critical path of the trial. As a rule of thumb you may expect that 10% of the protocol and your part in it decides about 80–90% of the overall result of the trial. Another 80% decides about 10% of the results and 10% has no impact on the result at all. The task is to identify the critical path.

CRF drafts should be requested from the sponsor. Sham enrolment performed on the basis of real patients is advisable. While enrolling these patients with zero-numbers, the local group of investigators should go through every step of enrolment, treatment and follow-up. Each step should be discussed with the practical problems evolving and solutions or agreements on how to handle it should be made. Major goals in this training should be protocol adherence and consistency within the group. The agreements should focus on the critical path, practicability and easy retrieval of the complete information during monitoring and auditing. A system allowing easy and complete retrieval of information will save the group a lot of time during the completion of the CRFs, the monitoring visits and give a good first-glance presentation during audits. Topics agreed upon should be:

1 How to obtain informed consent.
2 How to record in the patient charts that the subject is participating in a clinical trial. Drug administration date and time, protocol number and test article module should be noted. Although not requested by GCP, we always stated in these notes that informed consent/assent was obtained prior to enrolment.
3 How to highlight the data in the source document which are transcribed into the CRF (e.g. text marker, underline, colour).
4 How to mark pending data within source documents and CRF.
5 How to label complete pages in the CRF. This proved to be a very time-saving approach during our recent trials.
6 How to make corrections in the CRF or other hard copy. How to insert, initialize and date these corrections.

7   How to refer to different and sometimes slightly contradicting sources (e.g. chest X-ray result on typed radiology report or the hand-written notes on the intensive care unit flowsheet).

8   How to evaluate, mark and comment upon values outside the clinical accepted range.

9   How and where to comment in the source documents about specific events (adverse events, enrolment, study termination, physical exams, protocol violations).

10 How to handle and whom to inform during special events (e.g. adverse events, protocol violations, drug application errors). The appropriate measures to protect subjects in case of adverse events should be known to every collaborator.

11 How to handle and process blood samples. Standarization of specimen sampling increases the value of laboratory data. This becomes a crucial point if the protocol looks for fragile substances like fibrinogen split products, endotoxin, mediators. Keep everybody informed about changes in the arrangements made with the lab and other facilities.

12 How to cooperate with the monitors and how to prepare for their visits.

13 The importance of the management of code procedures, adherence to the randomization procedures and the documentation of test article administration cannot be overestimated. The investigator team has to ensure that the treatment code is only broken according to the protocol. A real necessity to break the code is extremely rare.

14 How to guarantee the confidentiality of all information relating to the study subjects and the information provided by the sponsor. Parts of the study protocol, the investigator brochure and sponsor communication are regarded as confidential. Clinical research is a competitive business.

15 How to notify your collaborators within the group about blood samples to be drawn and other pending work to be done.

16 How to arrange the work during nights, weekends, holidays and illness.

The training and the setting of local working rules should be not be underestimated. It ensures good performance of the site from the start on. Pre-established working rules, thoroughly focused on critical path, practicability, importance and easy retrieval of information, will reduce the workload of the group in the long run. The joint training and creation of local working rules offers every team member a platform for his or her personal contribution towards the local shape of the trial. This might be the crucial point where the trial changes from a project more or less dominated by the principal investigator to a team effort involving all participants.

Investigator meeting

The sponsor will visit your centre before accepting it as the investigative site. Many topics described above will be discussed during this visit. Parts of the contracts might be negotiated as well. Besides this visit, the sponsor will distribute information about the trial and the protocol through mail; the sponsor is also obliged to hold an investigator meeting prior to the start of the trial. This meeting should be attended by all collaborators and offers several opportunities:

1 Learning about the specific background of the trial, the protocol and its purpose. The medical background of the trial and some of the latest, sometimes as yet unpublished data and reasoning will be presented.
2 The concept of the trial, the protocol and the inclusion and exclusion criteria as well as the sampling and documentation will be discussed stepwise. The randomization procedure and the statistical analysis will be explained.
3 The estimated timetable of the trial will be presented. The expected enrolment rate will be given. Test article supply and other shipment modalities will be communicated.
4 All collaborators will have the opportunity to meet the sponsor's representatives and other investigators. Sponsor contacts in case of emergency will be presented. The investigators and their collaborators may get a better impression of the person at the other end of the line. Contacts with investigators from other sites may generate first new working links for the following trial. Plans about mutual subprojects or support (e.g. IRB approval, sample handling) may be established.
5 Investigators have the opportunity to discuss forthcoming problems with the collaborators from their site as well as to meet them on an informal basis (the talk on the plane, after dinner or at the bar), thereby enhancing the team spirit.

The first enrolments

The enrolment of the first patients, the first rounds of the race, offers several opportunities:
1 To familiarize your collaborators and yourself with the enrolment process, test article preparation and administration, specimen sampling and stepwise data collection. Discuss the forthcoming problems in the protocol and your local working rules as well as flaws in the local handling of the trial with your collaborators in order to ensure a further coherent approach of your team.
2 Enrol the first patients with the complete group, at least with your inexperienced collaborators. This will enhance their performance.

3 Obtain the first informed consent/assent together with your collaborators. Discussing the informed consent/assent with critically ill patients or their relatives has been a challenging experience in past sepsis trials. Inexperienced co-workers should be trained, as well as guided and supervised during their encounters with patients and relatives.

4 Discuss systematic problems within the protocol with your sponsor contact.

5 A part of your local working rules might be too complicated, overorganized or just unnecessary. Eliminate unnecessary parts and reshape the working rules in a group approach.

6 Most trials start slowly. Use the time available to update your files from the preparation period. There won't be much time left to do this after enrolment speeds up.

7 Use the first patients to distribute information about the protocol and the practical conduct of the trial to your colleagues, nurses and technicians. Ensure their collaboration. There are always many people out there (returning from holidays, leave, etc.), who are not familiar with the trial and whose cooperation is needed for the smooth conduct of your project.

8 Keep yourself organized from the start on: keeping every CRF updated. Keep track of the patient charts. You might need them suddenly.

9 If you are one of the major enrolling sites, realize that this will increase the interest in the quality of your work even more. The impact of major flaws in the performance of sites on the overall quality of the trial is correlated to the number of patients involved. A fast enrolling centre is therefore more important than a site with very few patients. Prepare for an early audit.

The long stretch

When the trial is well under way, your group will develop a more routine approach. Enrolment rate tends to vary over time, giving you periods of more or less work to do. Your focus of interest has to change:

1 Don't lose your pace (working rules). Stay within your schedule. This is sometimes hard to achieve during periods of fast enrolment. Consequently, use periods of slow enrolment to work-up your files and close gaps in your documentation. If you realize there is a large, steady or even increasing gap between enrolment and completion of files, you should discuss this openly with your sponsor. The sponsor is interested in fast enrolment, fast progress of the trial and fast and complete documentation. Only complete patient data are evaluable datasets. You might get some extra support.

2 Listen to the advice and comments of the monitors. They are profes-

sionals in their business and oversee a large number of sites. Critique from their side, even though the monitors might be employed by a contract research company, should be regarded as coming from the sponsor. They will report their visits and comment about your performance.

3   Don't burn out by going to fast. The fastest long-distance runner cannot perform at maximum speed during the entire race. Your collaborators and you need some rest periodically. Research should be fun. In some circumstances, it might be necessary to reduce enrolment to handle the workload.

4   Stay in contact with other investigative groups. Talking to them will give you new insight into the mutual project and things going on. Information about their problems and solutions will relieve you and your team from regarding yourself as being on a lonely stand. You may be able to support each other within subprojects. Sometimes you will learn about new aspects of the project outside the perspective of your regular sponsor information.

5   Be prepared for an intermediate audit. Although auditors will not come without prior notice, due to your changing clinical workload, the effective time left to prepare your site for the audit might not be long.

6   Successful participation in an ongoing trial will inevitably give you expertise and experience in the practice of clinical research in the field. If you regard your site as appropriate for future trials, you should plan your future research efforts while the ongoing trial is still under way. Talk to your sponsor about future projects and get into contact with other groups or companies performing research in your field of interest.

The end

After the last patient has been enrolled, the IRB, your boss and your administration should be informed about the upcoming end of the trial. Your collaborators in your hospital, the lab personnel, your fellow doctors and the intensive care unit nurses should be informed when enrolment stops and the upcoming close-out process. Take the opportunity to thank everybody for their contribution and celebrate the end of the trial within your group.

Don't wait too long before you proceed to clean up your files. Nothing is as boring and time-consuming as retrieving data from patients who were treated months ago. Prepare for queries. As long as the database is not closed, you might encounter minor or major amounts of queries coming in by fax or mail. Keep the archive of queries up-to-date. They are part of the trial documents and will be checked in case of an audit. The sponsor and regulatory agencies might audit sites with delay.

The close-out visit by the sponsor has to be prepared by updating all documents, including IRB documents. If you don't need the study data for subprojects, they should be prepared for definite further storage. Retrieval and later access might be requested. The files should be in a form which allows fast access. Returning the files to the sponsor when storage space is lacking limits your access to the data and cannot be recommended.

Summary

The introduction of the *Guidelines for Good Clinical Practice* resulted in a substantial change in medical research through clinical trials.

Although this cannot be quantified, it is the opinion of the author that the introduction of GCP guidelines inflicted a large increase in the workload of clinical trials. The guidelines standardize the approach towards clinical trials throughout the EC and enable data gathered in trials to be compared. The enormous increase in documentation combined with the extensive monitoring and auditing process imposes a heavy burden upon every clinical investigator. Some clinical investigators will refrain from participating in trials after recognizing the enormous amount of work which is hidden in the protocol and case report form. Every investigator should precalculate every trial according to the descriptions given above. Compared to the legal requirements before the introduction of the GCP guidelines, the investigator nowadays has to expect to do much more work for the average clinical trial. Acceptable compensations for each study site have to be negotiated. This inevitably leads to a cost increase in clinical research.

Another potential problem arises from differences in funding of clinical trials. Drugs with high anticipated earnings after market introduction might be studied more deliberately than generic products. The introduction of fees for local IRB approval already reduces the ability of some low-funded departments to perform clinical trial for low-cost drugs.

Despite these drawbacks, the author regards the recently introduced GCP guidelines as the key to a substantial increase in the quality of clinical research. The inherent cost increases will be recouped through a better basis for the licensing of drugs as well as an increased overall standard of medical research.

Reference

EEC Note for Guidance: Good Clinical Practice for Trials on Medical Products in the European Community. (1990) Luxembourg: Office for Official Publications of the European Community.

6 Conducting clinical trials in Slovenia

B Rozman

Introduction

Slovenia has a relatively strong pharmaceutical industry, 35% of which is based on licensed products. This kind of industry demands studies of bioequivalence and bioavailability. Usually, 12–24 volunteers from 20 to 40 years of age are included in blind, randomized, crossover trials. In the years preceding the Slovenian attainment of independence (in 1991), many compulsory clinical trials were carried out only in order to satisfy regulations and in order to license products before placing them on the market. The majority of these clinical trials were not performed following the introduction of good laboratory practice (GLP) and good clinical practice (GCP). Such local trials became less frequent as our authorities recognized the quality of pre-registration trials performed in the west and accepted them as adequate from the point of view of safety and efficacy with regard to the new drug.

So far, the research phases I, II or III conducted in Slovenia were very rare. After the attainment of independence, the Committee of Drugs at the Ministry of Health received fewer than 20 requests to approve such clinical trials (five of them were from the Department of Rheumatology), and they concerned mainly phase III studies, i.e. testing an already registered drug. Some of the reasons for the infrequency of such trials are quite obvious. Our pharmaceutical industry is hardly in a position to investigate a promising new chemical entity and to finance the whole procedure, beginning with isolation and continuing to the stage of being offered to human beings. Foreign pharmaceutical industries are still sceptical about performing the phase II or early phase III studies in Central and Eastern Europe, including Slovenia, believing that in these countries clinical trials cannot be performed according to international standards or rules. Some objections relate to poor infrastructure communications with investigators. Some obstacles are caused by drug laws and other regulations in the West, not allowing Central and Eastern European countries to be included in multicentre studies. These facts have become less important as the leading European auditors and consultants confirmed that some of the best clinical trials, performed over the past few years, were carried out in the countries of Eastern Europe, Slovenia included. Together with many project managers, they could perceive advantages, such as drug-naïve population, quality and motivation of investigators, and patients' excellent compliance.

Current regulations in Slovenia covering clinical trials

Currently used regulatory proceedings about clinical trials including GCP and GLP recommendations date back to 1986. Before starting phase I, II or III studies, the principal investigator should get approval from the Ethics Committee and the Committee of Drugs at the Ministry of Health of the Republic of Slovenia. Usually, the approval is first granted by the Ethics Committee and the final decision depends on the Committee of Drugs at the Ministry of Health. The phase IV studies can be conducted on the basis of the Ethics Committee approval, with the Committee of Drugs only being informed about it.

The Ethics Committee consists of 13 members, one of them appointed president. Currently, there are nine medical doctors, six of them affiliated to the Medical School of Ljubljana, while three members are of non-medical profession. The committee includes four women members. For a long time, the Ethics Committee's approval was indispensable for performing clinical trials in Slovenia. However, our Ethics Committee had no experience in giving approval to phase I and phase II studies. As a rule, the committee meets every 2 months.

The Committee of Drugs is a highly professional body appointed by the Ministry of Health, currently consisting of 11 members, who are experts on clinical medicine and pharmacy. The approval for conducting trials is given on a basis of consensus and after a thorough examination of the following documents:

1 Results of the preclinical investigation of the drug.
2 Pharmacological report with the name and chemical structure of the active substance, name of producer, critical referee of preclinical investigations, description of pharmacodynamic action mechanism, pharmacokinetic data and detailed report of all the tests that will be carried out on patients.
3 Protocol of the clinical trial.
4 Names of the countries (centres) where the clinical trial will take place.
5 Approval of the Ethics Committee of Slovenia.
6 Experts' report on chemical, pharmaceutical and biological documentation.

There are some local committees of drugs in the hospitals. Usually, the principal investigators inform them about clinical trials, but otherwise they have no role in assigning the approval. According to the draft law, the hospital committees of drugs are held responsible for supervision of the trial plan and evaluation of the results.

In Slovenia there are no formal criteria or verification systems for monitoring principal investigators and medical institutions while conducting clinical trials. In what concerns international studies, the sponsors' requirements about experience required in a research topic, an adequate number of highly qualified investigators, appropriate facilities and equipment are very strict.

The new Slovenian drug law is now in its final stage of parliamentary procedure. A special chapter deals with clinical trials and, together with other corresponding instructions, the inadequate or missing parts of current requirements and regulatory procedures governing clinical trials.

Conducting clinical trials to GCP

Experience of the Department of Rheumatology

The Department of Rheumatology represents a section of the Medical Centre of Ljubljana and is the only University Rheumatology Department in Slovenia. After having performed many phase IV clinical trials before marketing non-steroidal anti-inflammatory drugs and disease-modifying antirheumatic drugs (DMARDs) and having collaborated in some trials of clinical bioequivalence and pharmacokinetics of antirheumatic drugs, in 1990 we started international multicentre clinical trials of non-registered compounds which are potentially effective in rheumatoid arthritis. From that time on, we have been perfectly aware of GCP rules and we act accordingly.

So far phase II and III studies have been performed with products for rheumatoid arthritis, sponsored by German and American pharmaceutical companies, as part of international, double-blind, randomized, placebo-controlled trials. The initial 6-month studies were usually followed by 12–18-month extension trials. From 30 to 70 rheumatoid arthritis patients were included in a special trial. Substudies on magnetic resonance imaging as a new 'gold standard' for monitoring inflammatory changes in sinovial tissue of small hand joints represented a very important part of several clinical trials. The efficacy and safety laboratory tests were carried out either in local laboratories or in a laboratory outside Slovenia (a central laboratory for all participants).

Our local laboratories are permanently under control. Four times a year they are controlled by the state institute, twice a year by the Institut für Standardisierung und Documentation im Medizinischer Laboratorium (INSTAND) from Germany, and throughout the year by the World Health Organization. The methods are standardized by the International Federation of Clinical Chemistry (IFCC). However, we meet some problems while performing tests in local laboratories. The tests for rheumatology studies are not performed in one laboratory, therefore the material has to be sent to different places. All the results have to be copied to case record forms (CRFs). We believe that the sponsor's most important problem with this kind of work is the fact that different kits and even different units were used in investigators' centres. We could see that there was no uniform agreement on using SI units. The method of using a central laboratory seems to be a much better solution, in spite of minor technical problems that may occasionally appear during this collaboration.

Ethics Committee

There were two major essential problems which the Ethics Committee raised so far, the most important being the question of participation of women in their fertile period in early-phase clinical trials, in spite of having adequate birth control. Our Ethics Committee's firm suggestion was to exclude women in this condition from trials. The investigators of many rheumatic diseases, except osteoarthritis, would not accept this suggestion, as the main incidence of the diseases is somewhere between 20 and 50 years of age.

The second concern involves X-ray examinations, which the Ethics Committee suggested should not be carried out as frequently as at usual trial plans. For rheumatologists the X-ray of hands and feet is evidently a method that should be performed at the beginning and at the end of the trial, in spite of only 6-month follow-up. This is the only method to evaluate the destructive changes of joints, and as the exposure is very small, a 6-month interval seems reasonable even for routine work.

The committee required other additional information as summarized below; this meant that the whole procedure of final approval took approximately 3 months:

1 How are patients treated in the so-called placebo group? Is this acceptable from a medical point of view?
2 How do you avoid overdosage in the case of subcutaneous injections?
3 How do you control the taking of tablets?
4 How do you use the experimental drug after the conclusion of the clinical trial?

5   Details of extended studies.
6   Details on indemnity.
7   Details of centres involved.

Subject selection

The patient recruitment in our centre was reasonably successful. The rheumatologist investigators invited selected patients to participate in the studies. No advertisement was used to attract patients; nevertheless, there was some information in daily newspapers about the role entrusted to the Department of Rheumatology in testing new antirheumatic drugs. We were never short of the drugs usually prescribed against rheumatoid arthritis, but we were, as everywhere else, faced with lack of efficacy and with the side-effects of these drugs.

Therefore, many a patient needs an alternative treatment, and testing a new drug offers him or her a new chance. A small proportion of patients, who were given a chance to participate in clinical trials, refused to take part in the study. The patients who refused were usually those without much experience in drug therapy and they usually expressed their fear of the 'unknown' drug. Placebo-controlled studies didn't represent a major problem for our patients, especially when extension trials, excluding the placebo, were offered. Different ways of taking drugs, like subcutaneous injections, did not have a negative influence on our patients. The remoteness of the patients' home from our department was an objective reason for not joining the early-phase studies, requiring numerous visits during the trial. When less mobile patients were concerned, this obstacle was even more evident. Sometimes there were also some technical problems about directing patients to our department from another administrative region. So far, we have been very careful not to accept studies where subjects and facilities were in substantial contrast.

Clinical studies become more and more complicated. The groups of patients have to be more homogeneous, and besides, patients with extremely serious diseases are put under study. Therefore, it is expected that in the future, fewer and fewer patients will be available for studies in particular centres.

Informed consent

The principal investigator translated word for word into our national language all the information for patients involved in trials, including informed consent, from the original sponsor's proposal. The information pointed out the possibility of placebo treatment and the patient's right to withdraw from the study at any time, without consequences for future treatment. The confidentiality of the patient's personal and medical data is placed very high on the list of patient information. Sometimes, one could feel that the informed consent as proposed by the sponsor included some repulsive and pessimistic words or sentences. Every patient was given written and oral information at least 1 week before joining the study in order to think over the relevant information and to consult his or her relatives. We also encouraged discussion among the enrolled patients. The cooperation among those patients was extraordinary.

Responsibilities

The responsibilities of sponsors and investigators overlap during a large part of a clinical trial. A fair and good collaboration between two partners is a condition *sine qua non* for performing successful clinical trials, with special emphasis on the contact with monitors. We had the opportunity to collaborate with the sponsor's monitors and we had no objection to such a collaboration. There are no contract research organizations in Slovenia and local monitors never participate in our studies. It is evident that both partners – sponsors and investigators – can easily make mistakes before and during the study. Even during carefully planned clinical research, one can meet with vague questions and indeterminate statements, presented at the beginning of practical work. The early monitoring is of crucial importance for defining such problems. Some other data appearing during the trial demand reconsiderations, some of them even amendments to the study.

In the area of rheumatology, the investigators are faced with different protocols and CRFs even in clinical trials with similar study drugs, because there is no consensus in a number of clinical and laboratory efficacy and safety tests.

Our investigators were fully aware of their personal responsibilities for the patients in the trial and the trial's vital meaning for the safe and effective drugs to become clinically used. Withdrawal of the patient, with or without breaking the code, is a crucial and most delicate decision to be made by the investigators which cannot be prescribed only by the regulations; it is also a result of medical experience and moral qualities. Such decisions were fortunately rare and they were always discussed with the whole team of investigators. Sometimes, however, it is not enough to follow strictly all the GCP guidelines, the ethical and moral recommendations. A high level of discipline, especially when more than one clinical trial is performed, is more than necessary. In our centre, certain days of the week were fixed for patients to be accepted, i.e. different days for each trial. Fixed days were used for substudy tests and accompanying investigations as well.

The international multicentre trials have been established and are only performed by highly qualified clinicians (specialists of internal medicine), trained in rheumatology and having access to Western European technology and expertise. No assistance staff were engaged at any stage of the clinical trial and no subcontracts were made. In spite of standard operating procedures, established by the sponsor in evaluating clinical data, a flexible approach by different investigators is possible. Therefore we permanently compare the evaluation of clinical data among the investigators that are in no relation with clinical trial, in order to ensure valid and reproducible results. A thorough coordination between the investigators and other collaborators (laboratory and X-ray technicians) was established. The supervision of collaborators is very strict from the beginning to the end of the study. In case of a central laboratory system with rather complicated sampling, all the procedures were done by the investigators.

Investigational medicinal products and accessory material were sent by sponsors directly to investigators. Currently regulations are not optimal for a quick customs clearing. The study drugs were received and stored by investigators in the hospital pharmacy and dispensed in 1–4 weeks to trial patients in specially prepared vials, boxes and blisters. All unused medicinal products have been controlled by sponsors and officially destroyed in Slovenia.

Data handling

So far our investigators have had experience with CRFs only. Notes were made directly to CRFs as the trial patient was examined. Some minor mistakes were inevitable; therefore the monitoring procedure every 4–8 weeks was an important corrective. All parts of the study books which have to be filled in by the patients were translated into our national language. We had experience with health assessment questionnaires only, but it has not been put into force yet. Requirements for source documentation differ from sponsor to sponsor. There is an impression that too much study entry note and ongoing evaluations should be repeated in patients' documentation and CRFs. The master files also differ from sponsor to sponsor and represent a minor problem for principal investigators to keep it up to date.

Statistics

The design of the trials, randomization and blinding procedures were prepared by sponsors and seem reasonable in all international multicentre studies. Besides, no special biostatisticians are available in our medical centre. All statistical analyses were performed by the sponsors.

Quality assurance

Our centre has been chosen three times for independent auditing. With regard to the documents available, a high degree of adherence to GCP was confirmed.

Conclusions

Clinical research in the Department of Rheumatology, Ljubljana, Slovenia is well-organized. The quality of data obtained is high, and trials can be conducted efficiently thanks to satisfactory patient availability and compliance and good investigator motivation. The facilities for performing the research are generally adequate. The performing of phase II and early phase III studies was an important stimulus for rheumatology research in Slovenia. We believe that at least early-phase studies are to be conducted by doctors. We strongly support the idea of multicentre international studies to use central laboratory and to examine other investigations centrally.

As a new country, expecting new drug laws and other instructions concerning clinical trials, some uncertainty is still present in the relation between responsible bodies for the approval of clinical trials and investigators. In future the suitability and competence of investigators and the appropriateness of the location for the trial should also play an important role.

In spite of the fact that the status and work of the Ethics Committee are governed by national regulations, we have the impression that some questions raised by experts are not (but should be) solved uniformly in Europe. We urgently need a Council of Medicine in Europe in order to follow the goals of national ethics committees and coordinate their activities. The council should also take into consideration the investigators' remarks in trying to find an acceptable solution for a particular country. It is evident that the bodies responsible for the approval of clinical trials should shorten the intervals between their meetings or include pre-session consulting interviews to make quick decisions possible. Some parts of the study, especially the extension trials, are performed under heavy pressure of time.

Finally, we would like to point out that the import procedure for test drugs and accessories for conducting trials should be simplified.

Acknowledgement

I thank Prof. Franc Kozjek, PhD, president of the Committee of Drugs at the Ministry of Health of the Republic of Slovenia for his suggestions after reviewing the article.

7 Dealing with, and setting up, clinical trials through a contract research organization – a guidance document

S Ollier

Contract research is a growth industry, with numbers of contract research organizations (CROs) continuing to increase significantly. Worldwide there are now thought to be over 1000 CROs, with 40–50 operating as multinationals. At present the largest density of CROs exists in the UK, whereas the largest organizations in terms of size tend to be based in continental Europe and the USA.

The reasons for the growth of contract research are many and varied. Obviously, whenever pharmaceutical companies face pressure on staff resources, for example, as a result of head count freezes, or of time, managers may turn to outside contractors. However, this is by no means the only reason for the increasing use of CROs as partners in product development. Some of the market force must be attributed to the increasingly stringent requirements of good clinical (research) practice (GC(R)P), including recent increased requirements for independent audit of studies. The result has been an increase in the number of quality control/quality assurance (QC/QA) personnel required to coordinate a study and, often, an overloading of in-house resources.

As Japanese companies turn increasingly toward Europe for product development, biotech companies, the medical device and diagnostics industry move toward more regulated clinical trials, and companies in the cosmetics and toiletries sector, as well as companies producing allergen avoidance products, also opt for trial evidence to support claims, the pressures on the industry seem set only to increase. As pressures on resources increase so, almost inevitably, will the contract sector play an increasing role in product development.

As long ago as 1990, a meeting of the British Association of Pharmaceutical Physicians (BRAPP) agreed that in the long term, it is not cost-effective for even the largest company totally to exclude the services of contract clinical research (Anonymous, 1990). However, CROs have always attracted adverse comment from a proportion of sponsoring companies. Although, as in any industry, a small percentage of CROs perform inadequately, by far the most common reason for the perception of a below-standard performance by the CRO is the failure of one, or both, partners to state clearly at the outset the terms and conditions of the contract. Without mutual awareness of the other party's expectations, in terms of the nature and size of the delegated task, well-defined end-points and time frames (and their relation to payment schedules), there will be trouble ahead.

In any collaboration between pharmaceutical company and CRO, the aim is to conduct clinical trials conforming to GCP standards as efficiently as possible. It is surprising, therefore, that a survey undertaken by the Association of the British Pharmaceutical Industry (ABPI) only a few years ago, found that as many as 16% of study sponsors had little or no information on the structure and operating practices of the CROs with whom they were collaborating (Anonymous, 1990). This chapter seeks to provide guidelines for both study sponsors and CROs which may help to ensure that projects are completed to the mutual satisfaction of both parties.

Most CROs offer a wide range of services including study design, protocol writing, case record form (CRF) design, monitoring, statistical analysis, QA and report writing. Sponsors should be clear at the outset which services they wish to use before selecting a CRO.

At a very early stage the study sponsor should take time to consider the following questions:

1 *Are we asking the impossible?* If the project to be contracted out has already caused major difficulties in-house, is it realistic to expect the CRO to perform better? This situation may be further complicated if the sponsor's initial attempts at the project have already eaten into some of the time allowed in the overall development programme, leaving the CRO expected to outperform the study sponsor – and within a reduced time frame!

2 *Are we being realistic about costs?* Finance is always a contentious area. Although some CROs are undoubtedly expensive, it was, until recently, rare for staff of a sponsoring company to appreciate the true costs of projects which they themselves run in-house. Internal product development budgets may exclude such items as rent, rates, heating and lighting, professional liability insurance and purchase/maintenance of basic office equipment such as photocopiers, word processors, etc. A CRO will propose a cost estimate which must, of necessity, include allowances for a proportion of all these outgoings. This makes it difficult to make a fair comparison of costings prepared by contract houses and estimates for the same work prepared in-house.

However, it is clear that, even taking all the above into account, some CROs are overpriced. Study sponsors are able to describe situations where quotes varying by as much as 500% have been received for the same work. This belies an unjustified costing policy on behalf of a few

CROs, which does nothing to engender sponsor trust or to enhance the reputation of the contract sector as a whole.

3   *Has the degree of direct involvement we wish to have been considered and agreed?* Is there agreement on the time lines to be asked of the CRO in respect of study conduct, data processing, draft and final report and any other study-related activities?

CRO selection

The first step from the sponsor's point of view, and almost certainly the most important, is that of CRO selection. Ideally, previous experience or the recommendations of colleagues will make this process a rapid one. However, often it is necessary to begin the process 'from scratch'. Dr Laura Brown writing in *Good Clinical Practice* (1994) suggests that, although cost is obviously important in CRO selection, other factors are equally important. Some factors, such as ensuring that standard operating procedures (SOPs) are in place and compatible with the study sponsor's GCP requirements, are unlikely to be overlooked but other points highlighted by Dr Brown may be less obvious. For example:

1   The sponsor should ensure that it is confident of the CRO's organizational and financial stability (perhaps via a search, e.g. Dunn and Bradstreet or equivalent).
2   Details of the CRO's size and history should be considered.
3   The sponsor should take steps to ensure its confidence in both staff stability within the CRO and the scientific and clinical expertise of the key personnel. Meeting the responsible staff is mandatory. Relevant curricula vitae should be requested and assurances sought regarding ongoing training. The sponsor's in-house audit term can be invaluable in checking the experience and capabilities of CRO personnel.
4   References should be requested (and followed up!).

Cost-effectiveness, rather than cost *per se* should be the goal. It is certainly false economy to commission work from a CRO whose quote is cheapest but whose facilities and staff are inadequate for the requirements of the project delegated to them. Such an action may be expensive in the long term if the sponsor is forced to re-run a failed project.

Clearly, obtaining several quotations is essential and, in order to compare costs effectively, CROs selected to offer cost estimates should all receive identical and detailed information. Asking for a quotation for a study of 100 arthritis patients is pointless and invites a wide range of uninterpretable costings. CROs need to know: what type of arthritis? is the study hospital or general practice-based? how many centres? in the UK or Europe-wide? for which aspects of the study will the sponsor retain responsibility? what is the duration of treatment? what is the projected time scale? etc. The value of time spent preparing the project specification cannot be overemphasized. The future management of the whole project, in both scientific and financial terms, will depend upon both the CRO and sponsor understanding each other's needs as fully as possible before even a provisional agreement to place the study is reached.

There should always be a site visit to the CRO by the project management team before provisional agreement is reached to place the study. In addition, before the placement is confirmed and contracts exchanged, a QA audit of facilities, competence and experience of personnel, and SOPs should be undertaken. If there is reluctance to allow QA personnel to conduct a systems audit or to sign a secrecy agreement, this may be indicative of future problems in conducting collaborative research to GCP standards.

It is important that the CRO/sponsor collaboration is one with which both parties feel comfortable. One sponsor may find a small organization ideal, whilst another may need the greater resources of a larger, or even multinational, organization. Often, the larger the CRO, the more bureaucratic and inflexible may be its operations. If a sponsor's need is for maximum flexibility, a smaller CRO may be a better option. Any sponsor should take great care to select a CRO which will fulfil its own specific needs in relation to each contracted-out project.

Defining responsibilities

During initial meetings the following are some of the major issues which should be discussed:

1 For what purpose is the trial being undertaken? If data are to be used for registration worldwide, trial procedures will need to take into account the requirements of regulatory authorities in the USA and Japan which differ from European requirements.
2 Will the CRO or sponsor:
    (a)   design the protocol?
    (b)   design the case record form (CRF)?
    (c)   identify investigators?
    (d)   arrange a pre-study investigator meeting (if required)?
3 Financial arrangements:
    (a)   staging of payments
    (b)   the proportion of costs payable on early termination or cancellation of the project by the sponsor

(c) any financial penalties for inadequate performance by the CRO, etc.

Sponsors should ensure that funds payable to the CRO, as per their contractual arrangements, are transferred promptly. A CRO will have financial commitments to ethics committees, pathology services, etc. and delayed payments from the sponsor can eventually cause problems for the efficient execution of the study.

It is essential at this initial stage to identify *one* primary contact from both sponsor and CRO who will liaise on a day-to-day basis about project progress and coordination. Most delays in collaborative projects result from misunderstandings of the expectations or capabilities of the project partner. Good communication is vital. The primary contacts need not be the respective medical directors, who may sometimes be difficult to contact. A suitably experienced study coordinator who is always available may be invaluable in undertaking this role.

It is essential to clarify whether the SOPs of the sponsor differ significantly from those of the CRO and, if so, to document whose SOPs are to be used for each task delegated. If a sponsor requests that a CRO work to the sponsor's internal SOPs, those procedures relevant to the delegated tasks must be made available to the CRO's staff at an early stage. It has been known for major multinationals to request such compliance to their own SOPs whilst simultaneously refusing the CRO sight of these documents on the basis of confidentiality!

Regardless of whether the sponsor or CRO will be conducting pre-study investigator meetings, it is wise for the sponsor always to arrange a training session for the chosen CRO. This will ensure that all the CRO staff are familiar with product and the purpose for which the trial is being undertaken. In particular cases, where the sponsor wishes to build a good customer relationship, it may be important for the CRO to work as an extension of the sponsor and for the CRO staff to be able to pass on any queries or comments from the investigators to the relevant personnel at the sponsor's site.

The following sections consider in detail various aspects of clinical trial designs and procedures where the role of the CRO/sponsor should be clarified.

The study protocol

If protocol design is to be delegated to the CRO the following points should be clarified:

1 The number of centres, number of patients and number of patients per centre.

2   Procedures for follow-up of patients withdrawn from the trial prematurely – the sponsoring company's SOP may define specific actions to be taken.
3   Type of investigators to be involved (e.g. hospital or general practice, or both).
4   Whose protocol guidelines are to be followed (those of the sponsor or those of the CRO)?
5   Who is to provide statistical input into the protocol design, establish the statistically necessary number of patients/subjects, and perform power calculations?

Even if the protocol is designed and written by the CRO, the sponsor should always authorize the protocol by signing off the final version. As Richard Gill (1994) has pointed out, this is to the advantage of both parties; the sponsor is reassured that the protocol to be implemented fully meets with its specifications and the CRO may find reduced premiums for errors and omissions insurance if it is able to confirm that every protocol will be authorized by the company ultimately sponsoring the study.

Design and production of case record forms

If the CRO is to design the CRF:

1   Are there particular sponsor requirements, particularly relating to the layout of questions pertaining to adverse experiences?
2   Does there need to be provision for the investigator to sign *every* page of the CRF (this may be mandatory for data use in certain territories)?
3   Is the format of CRF NCR paper or plain paper? (This question and the methods of collection of completed CRFs/individual 'clean' pages may have implications for monitoring time and associated costs for the CRO).

Trial supplies

The following points should be agreed:

1   Who will arrange the packaging of the trial supplies?
2   How are the supplies to be labelled?
3   How are the supplies to be packaged?
4   Is the study medication ready to be shipped? Is a release date already known or will its preparation possibly delay the start of the trial?
5   Are the expiry dates of the medication sufficient to cover the anticipated trial period? If not, is testing underway relating to extension of the dates?

6 Are there any specific storage requirements relating to light, temperature, etc. of which the CRO will need to make each study site aware?

7 If the supplies are likely to need dispensing 'out of hours', the practicalities need to be considered. It may be necessary for the sponsor to finance an on-call pharmacist especially for this purpose.

8 Frequently, especially in multinational studies, pharmacies may wish to relabel supplies to comply with local regulations. Occasionally, repacking may also be suggested, for example into childproof containers. Procedures covering this eventuality should be discussed between the CRO and the study sponsor. Problems can, of course, be avoided if the study sponsor is aware of local regulations at all study sites and arranges packaging and labelling of supplies accordingly.

9 Does the sponsor have specific drug accountability requirements over and above those already in place according to the SOPs of the CRO?

10 Will the CRO or sponsor be responsible for the destruction of unused drugs on completion of the study?

Potential investigators

1 Do the sponsors have any investigators whom they particularly wish to include (or exclude!)?

2 What, if any, geographical constraints are there?

3 Does the sponsor wish to approve the names of all potential investigators before they are approached by the CRO?

4 Are centres which change institutional overheads at percentage rate, over and above the basic study costs, acceptable?

It is common knowledge that even the best-designed study can fail unless suitably qualified, experienced and reliable investigators are selected. CROs will often have worked for several sponsors in a single therapeutic area and may have invaluable knowledge regarding the most appropriate investigators to approach. Sponsors should listen carefully to the advice of the CRO in this respect (and should acknowledge that this expertise is something which CROs do not have an opportunity to include in their cost proposals but which may be invaluable in saving time and money which can so easily be wasted if inappropriate investigators are used).

Ethics review committee, informed consent and regulatory approval

1 What is the regulatory status of the compound under study?

2 What form of indemnity is the company prepared to give to CRO/potential investigators? Will this be 'no-fault' and what are the sums indemnified?

3   Many health authorities in the UK expect study sponsors to sign their own standard statement of indemnity, which may differ significantly from that of the sponsors. A great deal of CRO time may be wasted setting up a study site where such a request is made and the sponsor then found to have a policy of not signing these statements.

4   Cases are known where ethics committees have found the wording of the sponsor's indemnity statement acceptable but failed to approve the study on the basis that the sponsor's insurance policy was effected with a foreign insurer. The legality of this course of action, particularly within the European Union, is unclear. However, CROs should be aware of this rare eventuality so that sponsors can consider their position *vis-à-vis* their insurers.

5   Is the trial to be conducted under an Investigational New Drug (IND) application? If so, there may be constraints upon the number of ethics committees whose constitution qualifies them to review the protocol (and details of their constitution and the affiliation of their members *must* be publicly available).

Monitoring activities

1   Does the sponsor have specific requirements for monitoring frequency which might require more site visits than would normally be expected under GCP guidelines? (If so, these must be advised to the CRO.)

2   Does the sponsor company have different requirements for source data verification than would normally be expected under GCP guidelines?

3   Will the clinical research personnel from the study sponsor wish to visit the investigators with the CRO's monitors during the course of the study?

4   How are data to be transmitted to the sponsor (e.g. is each visit to be collected separately or only completed CRFs to be transmitted)?

5   The method of notification of data errors from clients to CRO should be defined, as should procedures for subsequently correcting these either on returned original CRFs or on data clarification sheets.

6   The CRO should expect to be informed when the sponsor is happy to accept the data as clean and to 'lock' the database. If the sponsor normally issues a 'Data clean' certificate, this should be stated.

Adverse events

1   Where two parties are coordinating a study, there is potential for misunderstanding by the investigators regarding the primary reporting point for serious adverse events. It is of paramount importance that there is no confusion.

2   Relevant contact names and telephone numbers of the responsible CRO staff and medical staff within the sponsoring company should be clearly defined, preferably within the study protocol.
3   There should be clearly defined time scales for reporting of serious adverse events – any reporting procedures required by the sponsor additional to those outlined in the SOPs of the CRO must be clearly defined.
4   There should be agreement concerning which party is compiling the adverse event database relating to the compound (this would normally be the study sponsor, but a duplication of this at the CRO may occasionally be requested).
5   The frequency of transmission of updates on the occurrence of non-serious adverse events to the study sponsor should be decided.

Trial administration

1   It should be established how frequently the sponsor will expect to receive status reports regarding recruitment levels, etc. The exact topics to be covered in each report should be defined.
2   Procedures for introducing protocol amendments should also be clearly agreed.

Quality assurance

1   The sponsor's auditing requirements should be established at the time of contract agreement.
2   The CRO should confirm the extent and scope of proposed audits (the CRO, investigator sites, data management facility, etc).
3   If the sponsor wishes the CRO to arrange for independent auditing of study sites, it should be established whether audits are expected in-process or post-process. CROs will need to budget carefully for subcontracted auditing and should keep abreast of the likely rates charged by independent auditors.
4   Many CROs now have their own QA facility in-house. Prior to contracting a study, the sponsor should, as part of the CRO systems audit, assess the experience and function of the CRO's QA team. The respective roles and interaction of sponsor and CRO QA personnel should be established at an early stage.

Data management/statistical analysis/trial reporting

1   Who will assemble the database for the study (sponsor or CRO)?

2   Does the sponsor have any specific requirements for how data are handled or the hardware/software to be used?
3   Who is to be responsible for statistical analysis?
4   Statistical methods to be used should be agreed and included in the relevant section of the protocol.
5   The target variable should be agreed at an early stage.
6   Who is to write the final report?
7   Does the sponsor have any internal SOPs relating to the format of final study reports or should the CRO produce these according to its own standard format? This point is important to discuss at an early stage since the CRO's costings may partly depend on the complexity of the final report formatting imposed by the sponsor.

If all the above points are adequately addressed and a contract devised on this basis, it should be possible for the sponsor/CRO relationship to proceed smoothly to the benefit of both parties in the collaboration. However, some contractual problems may still arise. Many CROs, particularly those of medium-to-large size, now have a standard contract or statement of standard conditions, which sponsors are requested to sign. All sponsors will be constrained to present these for review by their own legal advisors prior to signature. Thereafter a lengthy process of amendment and approval may be engendered. In this situation some CROs cope better than others. Perhaps a better way of coping with this increasing problem would be for CROs to include, in their SOPs, guidelines as to the points they expect to see addressed in each contract and to leave the actual contract generation to each study sponsor.

The future

Alongside the vast majority of sponsors who now routinely collaborate with CROs are some who still regard CROs as a non-cost-effective option and prefer to contract in staff to work within their own system. Another option is for a company to delegate work to one of the increasing number of experienced clinical research personnel working independently as consultants, without the infrastructure (and overheads) of a fully fledged CRO. Some sponsors see a number of advantages in this type of collaboration. For example:

1   The consultant may be asked to work independently, with minimal supervision, or to work in-house alongside the sponsor's own staff depending upon need.
2   Sponsor/investigator contact may be more closely maintained.

Disadvantages are few but may include uncertainties about the responsibilities imposed by GCP upon individual consultants, particularly with regard to study documentation. The EC *Note for Guidance, Good Clinical Practice for Trials of Medicinal Products in the European Community* (111/3976/88-EN) which was issued by the Commission of the European Communities (Brussels) 1990, defines a CRO as 'a scientific body (commercial, academic or others) to which a sponsor may transfer some of his tasks and obligations'. Whilst an independent consultant undoubtedly falls within this definition, there are obviously differences in sponsor expectations of the role which a consultant will play, in comparison to a larger CRO, and this is an area of potential confusion. For example, although the EC *Note for Guidance* gives responsibility to the study 'sponsor or subsequent owner' for archiving of all original documentation pertaining to trials for the lifetime of the product, it is undoubtedly true that many sponsors routinely expect CROs also to keep copies of all study documents (including CRFs) for at least 15 years following completion or discontinuation of the trial. Sponsor QA departments often wish to check the documentation housed at the CRO and expect this to reflect much of the data archived by the sponsor. How far maintenance of such comprehensive documentation is required of independent consultants is an area which requires clarification. Clearly, auditors will keep copies of audit reports, correspondence, etc. according to normal office practice. If, however, individuals to whom monitoring is subcontracted are constrained to keep copies of all CRFs and associated documentation, an immense problem of secure storage arises which may limit future activities

An approach which has recently been proposed in order to allow smaller CROs to offer a more comprehensive service whilst retaining the flexibility which makes them attractive to sponsors is the concept of the virtual corporation, (1993; Gill, 1994). This concept hinges on a temporary association of companies, linked via information networks, designed to work together on an individual project. As each company could contribute its particular competence and expertise, an organization could be created which would offer the best of both worlds to each project. Dr Richard Gill proposes this concept as worthy of consideration as a cost-effective approach to the future conduct of clinical studies as well as a means of ensuring compliance with GCP. The questions of documentation and archiving, raised above in relation to independent contractors, would obviously also need to be addressed before virtual corporations become a reality in pharmaceutical research.

This chapter has focused specifically on collaborations in phases II and III of product development but may be extrapolated to collaborations involving phase I contract houses which now regularly provide the specialist facilities required for the labour-intensive early volunteer studies which have a key role in the development process.

References

Anonymous (1990) CROs: 'A quality product?' *SCRIP* **147**: 4–5.
Brown L. (1994) Checklist: selecting CROs. *Good Clinical Practice* **1**: 46–47.
Gill, R. C. (1994) Can CROs work to GCP? *Good Clinical Practice* **1**: 12–16.
Byrne, J. A. *et al.* (1993) The virtual corporation. *Business Week* **8**: 98–102.

PART THREE

Clinical trials and good clinical practice

8 Preparation for an FDA inspection for clinical studies conducted under a US IND

T Ott

Introduction

This chapter will review how to prepare for a successful Food and Drug Administration (FDA) inspection for studies conducted under a US Investigational New Drug (IND) application.

The most critical time to prepare for an FDA audit is before starting the study. By putting the appropriate controls in place you will be able to generate quality data that will be substantiated by source information. Also the subjects entered will be treated ethically and will have been given the opportunity for proper informed consent.

As defined by the FDA, the following information was provided to industry to show what constitutes a good study:

1   Adequate safeguards for the welfare of study participants.
2   Adherence to institutional review and informed consent guidelines.
3   Clearly stated objectives.
4   Well-defined selection criteria.
5   Strict adherence to protocol with modifications documented.
6   Rigorously defined response variables to measure the responses of subjects to the effects of the drug.
7   Objective methods of observation.
8   Description and documentation of statistical methods used.
9   Identification and analysis of unanticipated results or conclusions.
10 Provision for follow-up and analysis of problems and drop-outs.

I will review the FDA *Statement of Investigator Form (FDA-1572)* and the *FDA Compliance Program for Clinical Investigator* to give a sense of the obligations of working under an IND and what the FDA investigator is reviewing when he or she performs an audit. If you are aware of the criteria that will be used to evaluate the conduct of a clinical study then you can modify your programme appropriately.

Statement of Investigator Form (FDA-1572)

The signing of this form by an investigator allows the shipment of an unapproved drug to cross state lines (interstate shipment) and not be in violation of the law (Food, Drug, and Cosmetic Act Part 505i). There is a statement to this effect in the upper right-hand corner of the *FDA-1572* that states, 'No investigator may participate in an investigation until he/she provides the sponsor with a completed, signed Statement of Investigator Form'.

Who can sign the FDA-1572?

The individual (investigator) listed in block number 1 and whose signature appears on the back is responsible for all aspects of the study. This individual can delegate authority to the subinvestigator(s) listed in block 6.

If there is more than one investigator per site who has signed off on his or her own *FDA-1572* and shares responsibility equally, he or she is referred to as a co-investigator for a site. However in the Code of Federal regulations (CFR) the term co-investigator is not defined. Situations that may warrant using a co-investigator are when a clinical practice is being shared by physicians, there are satellite sites removed from the primary sites or you are using a well-known decision maker who may not be willing to devote sufficient time to your research programme. Also if you use a Doctor of Pharmacy (Pharm. D.) as an investigator you will need a physician either as an investigator or subinvestigator to make medical interpretations.

The *Statement of Investigator Form* is provided by the sponsor, signed by the investigator and information from this form is extrapolated and added to a cover letter filing this investigator and site with the FDA.

It is not uncommon for the sponsor's representative (clinical research associate (CRA) or clinical scientist) hastily to have the investigator complete and sign this form without a proper explanation of the commitments listed on the back of the form. What is listed are the conditions that the investigator is agreeing to in order to receive and work with an investigational drug.

The general responsibilities that the investigator is committing to are:

1 Sign the investigational statement (the *FDA-1572*).
2 Follow the investigational plan, which is the protocol.
3 Adhere to all applicable regulations and guidelines, 21 CFR 50, 56, 312.
4 Protect the rights, safety and welfare of the subjects.
5 Administer drug only to subjects under the investigator's control.
6 Maintain control and disposition of the drug.
7 Return all unused drug to the sponsor at the end of the study.

8 Obtain written informed consent prior to performing any study-related procedures on the subjects.
9 Prepare and maintain adequate case histories.
10 Furnish reports to the sponsors.
11 Promptly report adverse events to the sponsor and the Institutional Review Board (IRB).
12 Obtain initial and continuing IRB review.
13 Allow inspection by the FDA.
14 Maintain proper drug storage and for controlled substances maintain under locked storage conditions.

FDA compliance inspection programme

The FDA inspects clinical investigators under the FDA's *Compliance Programme Guidance Manual*, Chapter 48: Bio-Research Monitoring: Drugs and Biologics, 7348.811, Clinical Investigators. Also found in this chapter are: 7348.809, Institutional Review Boards and 7348.810, Sponsors, Contract Research Organizations and Monitors. As defined in the programme, the objectives are twofold.

First, obtain compliance of the clinical investigator with the regulations and second, assess through audit procedures whether data submitted to FDA are substantiated by records. The FDA investigator will compare the source documents at the investigational site with information that had been submitted to the FDA. This could be in the form of case report forms completed by the investigator or his/her staff or data listings that have been extrapolated from the submission (new drug application (NDA) or supplemental new drug application (SNDA)) that pertains to this particular site.

There are seven parts to each compliance programme.

1 Background – giving an explanation why the programme was written.
2 Implementation – how the programme is to be carried out.
3 Inspectional – instructions on what to check and areas to be reviewed.
4 Analytical – for sample collection and laboratory analysis.
5 Regulatory/administrative strategy – sanctions that can be applied for non-adherence to the regulations.
6 References/attachment – background information that supports the compliance programme.
7 Headquarters responsibilities – responsibilities of headquarters personnel in evaluating the inspectional operations performed by FDA field personnel.

The focus for this chapter will be on the FDA inspectional process (part III).

Operations

As stated in the programme, the nature of these inspections makes unannounced visits to the clinical investigator impractical. An FDA investigator will usually call the investigator to schedule an appointment to perform the audit. Please note that this is done for the convenience of the FDA and not for the investigator, therefore the investigator should cooperate with the FDA representative. This is the only type of inspection of which the FDA will give advanced notice. A reasonable timeframe from the time of the call to the actual visit is 1–2 weeks. This will allow the investigator time to collect the administrative/regulatory files and the patients' source documents. At many institutions hospital record rooms need from several days to a week to pull charts from their files.

During the inspection the FDA can have access to and copy all records affiliated with the study. The FDA is obliged to protect the confidentiality of the subject and therefore will not routinely take patient-identifying information. The only exception is when the FDA suspects fraud and may need this information to interview the subject to determine if he or she took part in a clinical research study.

If the IRB has not been inspected within the last 5 years, the FDA may perform a concurrent inspection of the IRB under *compliance program* 7348.809.

Also requested would be a listing of all studies performed by the clinical investigator, including those for government agencies and commercial sponsors. It is good policy for the site to maintain a current list.

At the conclusion of the inspection, the FDA investigator will issue a list of observations on an FDA-483 form. Items that would be listed would be deviations from the regulations (21 CFR 50, 56, 312) and from the protocol.

Authority and administration

How did the monitor explain to the clinical investigator his or her obligations in conducting studies under an IND, the status of the drug and the protocol?

Was it documented through attendance at an investigator's meeting, through a pre-study visit, a teleconference or correspondence? Whatever means was used should be documented and available for review.

The FDA investigator will determine if authority was delegated properly and whether the clinical investigator retained control of the study. This is especially critical when satellites are used. If there is more than one site, then you need to know how involved the clinical investigator is with these secondary sites. What is the frequency of visits to these other sites? Is the clinical investigator actively involved in seeing subjects and is it documented in the clinic chart? Did the clinical investigator explain the consent to the subject? If the clinical investigator was not involved in these secondary sites, than a physician from this site must be listed on the statement of investigator form.

If a laboratory facility is analysing samples as part of the protocol requirements, than a review of the laboratory is warranted, especially if the laboratory is analysing samples not only for safety but also for efficacy. The laboratory that was used should be the same as the one listed in block 4 of the investigator's *FDA-1572*. As a minimum the laboratory should be checked to ensure that it has been certified to perform the testing required, that there are written standard operating procedures (SOPs), organizational charts and training records. Also, that the facility has sufficient space, that equipment is clean and functional and that samples are properly identified and traceable throughout the analysing process.

If the investigator analyses samples in his or her office, than he or she must show how the equipment was calibrated and that the results generated are reliable.

Protocol

For the initial protocol and any subsequent modifications or amendments there must be IRB approval, including dates. All changes, except in the case of a medical emergency, must first receive IRB approval prior to implementation.

Did the protocol remain unchanged regarding:

1 Subject selection and number? If the IRB approved a specific number of subjects, you must receive approval before exceeding the specified number.
2 Frequency of observations and dosage? What is listed in the protocol must be followed and the investigator must adhere to the dosage specified.
3 Route of administration?
4 Blinding procedures? If there is a randomization plan then it must be followed. The investigator cannot modify the randomization schedule from what was received from the sponsor.

Violations of protocol are not changes in protocol

Any changes to a protocol must be documented. If it is necessary for an investigator to modify a protocol then it may indicate that the protocol as written may be too stringent. Many times a sponsor will institute a protocol that has strict controls built into it, so that subjects that are enrolled will fit into defined areas. The problem with this concept is that it may be difficult for a clinical investigator to find subjects for the trial who meet the protocol requirements. The investigator then enrols subjects who may only partially meet the criteria listed. The end-result is un-evaluable subjects who will not support the indication being sought by the sponsor.

Subjects' records

For a clinical trial the source documents are the first place where information is recorded on a subject on a clinical trial and are the raw data files. Information from these source documents is transferred on to case report forms (CRFs), entered into the sponsor's database and incorporated into the NDA or SNDA for submission for regulatory approval. If information is not accurately transferred or is not complete, then the data trail will be incomplete and the study results could be jeopardized. To see the importance of this one only needs to review the number of drugs that were removed from the market in the 1980s due to serious adverse events that were not properly captured during the clinical trial phase.

Examples of source documents are office charts, clinic charts, hospital records, laboratory slips, electrocardiogram tracings, exercise printouts, dietary records, anxiety and depression scale ratings, quality of life interviews and pharmacy records.

During an FDA audit they will describe in their report the raw data files. Since audits may take place years after the trial has ended, it is important that the information should be captured appropriately. The use of sticky yellow notes, scraps of paper and other non-conventional source should be discouraged. The investigator with his or her staff should record information on records that are part of their routine office procedures. Information should not be recorded directly on to the CRFs except when collecting detailed information that could result in transcription errors, such as a series of blood pressure readings. When information is recorded directly on to the CRF, there should be a reference to it in a progress note in the subject's chart. This same concept will also be valid in central nervous system studies when you are having the subjects complete questionnaires or anxiety or depression scale ratings.

Records should support the fact the subject exists and that there is a history for a given subject for the disease state being studied. Examples would be a subject with a 10-year history of hypertension or one with a 20-year history of psoriasis. If these subjects are not under the routine care of the clinical investigator, then there should be a referral letter along with progress reports to the subject's primary-care physicians for the purpose of providing updates. Records that support the fact the subject exists would be documents such as appointment books and individual subject files with back-up documentation. For research centres where there would be 'walk-ins' who respond to recruitment advertising, a medical history needs to be recorded. Again, it is encouraged procedure to determine their primary-care physician to inform them that their subject is on a clinical trial and to verify the subject's history.

A comparison of the raw data files will be performed against the CRFs. In doing a review you should always go from the source to the CRF. The reason is, that if you go from the CRF to the source, you will verify only information on the CRF. You will not pick up information such as concomitant medication and adverse events that were in the source but not transferred on to the CRF. You need to review all available source documents, then compare them against the CRF.

Close attention should be given to the occurrence of adverse events. Were they anticipated in the investigator's brochure? It must be noted that all adverse events, regardless of causality, have to be reported to the sponsor. The investigator cannot decide what needs to be reported. Adverse events need to be reported from the time the subject enters the trial to a set time following study completion. This period is usually several weeks to ensure that the drug has been washed out.

In addition to adverse events, concomitant medications and intercurrent illness need to be listed. Both situations may have some types of study effect, such as drug-drug interactions or, as an example, a renal clearance problem that could affect the excretion of the drug.

Inclusion/exclusion criteria listed in the protocol should be checked against actual patients enrolled. If the proper subjects are not entered, then at the time of data analysis you may lose these subjects for efficacy, which could weaken your submission by losing a potential indication or a delay in drug approval. If protocol criteria are restrictive then enrolment will be slow and those enrolled may not fully meet the inclusion requirements. If this happens, the investigator may want to communicate back to the sponsor and see if the protocol can be modified.

Other study records that the FDA would be interested in reviewing are a comparison of the number of subjects reported by the sponsor and by the investigator. The current trend is for the FDA to download data listing information for a particular investigator and compare it to what is on file at the investigational site. The FDA will usually concentrate on pivotal protocols. Comparison will be made for the following:

1 Number of subjects entered.
2 Number of dropouts.
3 Number of subjects who are evaluable/unevaluable.
4 Number of adverse reactions and deaths.

The purpose of this comparison is to ensure that all subjects who entered the trial were reported to the sponsor and were listed in the regulatory submission. If subjects dropped out, what are the reasons for their discontinuation? Could it have been caused by the study drug? Also the number of adverse reactions and deaths must match what the sponsor has reported.

Equipment

Today, as technology continues to increase and become more complex, we rely to a greater detail on machines to support our decisions in making evaluations. This fact is especially true in the clinical research area. Any equipment that provides the clinical research personnel with information concerning a subject needs to be evaluated. The purpose is to ensure that the equipment can provide you with the required information and is working properly. Simple equipment such as treadmills and other exercise machines, X-ray equipment, refrigerators and freezers need to be checked to ensure that they are working within the specifications for which they were designed. This is especially true if polling data from multiple sites and the calibration at a given site is off slightly. When the data are merged this could have an effect on the overall study results.

Consent

FDA regulations require written consent to be obtained for all subjects prior to their entry into a study (21 CFR part 50). Prior to entry into a study has been defined as before protocol-required procedures are performed on the subject. The consent must have all the elements required by the regulations. This includes the following:

1 Statement of the purpose, that it involves research; duration of subject's participation, identification of experimental procedures and description of procedures to be followed.
2 Complete description of the risks and discomforts likely to occur.
3 Description of any benefits to the subject.
4 Disclosure of alternative procedures available for treating the illness.
5 Statement regarding confidentiality of records, indicating that the sponsor and/or sponsor's representative will review the records and the FDA may review the records at the time of an inspection.
6 Statement of compensation and/or medical treatment available if the subject is injured during the study.
7 Name and telephone numbers for the subject to contact regarding:
    (a) his/her rights as research subject;
    (b) questions about the research project;
    (c) whom to contact in the event of research-related injury.

8   Statement that participation is voluntary; that there will be no penalty or loss of benefits if they refuse to participate and that they may withdraw at any time.

There are six additional elements that may need to be included in the consent form in certain circumstances. These elements are:

1   Statement that there may be unforeseeable risks including risks to the fetus should the subject become pregnant during the study.
2   Statement that the subject's participation may be terminated by the investigator and circumstances under which this could be done.
3   Statement concerning any additional costs to the subject.
4   Description of the consequences if the subject withdraws from the study.
5   Statement that significant new findings which may have an impact on the subject's willingness to participate will be provided to the subject.
6   Statement concerning the approximate number of subjects in the study.

The subject must be given an opportunity to review the consent form, ask questions and decide if he or she wants to sign it. The investigator or study staff must be available to explain the consent and to answer any questions the subject may have. The consent must be in the subject's primary language.

The subject must sign and date the consent form and be given a copy. The investigator must keep as part of the study records the original signed consent form.

If the sponsor and/or IRB (or ethics committee) requires the signature of the investigator and/or a witness then these must be completed on the form. The witness should sign and date the form at the same time as the subject.

The FDA has provided the following pointers regarding informed consent:

1   There should be no reference to the drug being approved elsewhere.
2   Use the words 'may' and 'can' rather than 'will'.
3   Avoid technical language and complex words. The consent should be written in language that a person can easily understand.
4   Avoid using standard wording for alternatives.
5   Address the subject as 'you'.
6   Use normal conversation in presenting the consent to the subject.
7   State in the consent: 'I have been given a copy of this consent'.
8   Spell out clearly whom to contact with questions regarding the research, the subject's rights as a research subject and whom to contact if injured during the study.

9   State that funds are not available for compensation if this is the case.
10   State that 'by signing this consent I have not given up my rights'.

The consent form must be reviewed and approved by the IRB before being implemented. If the protocol changes during the course of the study or new information becomes available that would have an impact on subjects, the consent form must be revised to reflect these changes. In addition, the revised consent form must be reviewed and approved by the IRB.

If the consent form needs to be revised during the course of the study the subject may need to sign the revised consent, if the revisions have an impact on the subject's continued participation in the study.

Institutional review boards

FDA regulations require that IRBs review and approve all studies before they are implemented (21 CFR part 56). FDA regulations define an IRB as 'any board, committee, or other group formally designated by an institution to review, to approve the initiation of, and to conduct periodic review of, biomedical research involving human subjects'. The primary purpose of the IRB review is to ensure that subjects' welfare and rights are protected.

FDA regulations require that an IRB consist of at least five members who possess varying backgrounds and diversity in race, gender, culture and sensitivity to such issues as community attitudes (21 CFR part 56.107). Each IRB must have at least one member whose primary interest is non-scientific as well as one member whose primary interest is scientific. An IRB member may be conducting research in the institution and have protocols reviewed and approved by that IRB but the member cannot vote on any protocols with which he or she is involved.

The IRB approval must be obtained for the final version of the protocol before being implemented. The IRB should be provided with all reports of prior investigations for their review of the protocol. This is generally in the form of the investigator's brochure and subsequent updates to it. The IRB must approve any modifications or changes to the protocol and must approve all materials used to obtain the subject's consent to participate. This is generally the informed consent form but may include other information that the investigator will provide to the subject.

The IRB must review and approve all the advertisements used to recruit subjects into the protocol. This includes posters, radio and newspaper advertisements, and 'infomercials' on television. Press releases from universities, if these releases provide contacts for potential subjects to call if interested in the study, must be viewed by the IRB.

The IRB approvals must be in writing and signed by the chairperson of the IRB or his or her designate. The approval should state clearly the protocol being approved and the date of approval. Amendments should be identified by number or letter or other method providing clear identity of the specific amendment.

The IRB must be notified of all deaths and all serious, unexpected adverse experiences occurring during the study. This information is provided to the IRB to give them an opportunity to review the information and decide if the study should continue.

The investigator must provide the IRB with a report on the progress of the study at least annually. Some IRBs require reports quarterly or half-yearly. The investigator must comply with the specific IRB requirements if they request more frequent reporting. The IRB must be notified by the investigator of the closing of the study. The investigator should provide the IRB with information summarizing the study, including number of subjects and adverse experiences. The investigator should maintain a copy of this notification for his or her files.

IRBs must maintain records showing what protocols, consents and advertisements were reviewed, which members were present and how each member voted on the material reviewed. All of these records should be available for FDA inspection.

Sponsor interactions

The sponsor is required by the regulations to see that the study is moni-tored at established intervals by individuals with the appropriate back-ground and training. The sponsor should review the monitor reports for adequacy, problems and frequency of monitoring.

The sponsor or the sponsor's representative should review the consent form for each investigational site to determine that it contains all the required elements, does not contain exculpatory language and is in agree-ment with the protocol.

The sponsor and/or the sponsor's representative should review com-pleted CRFs in a reasonable timeframe after receiving them from the site. Industry practice is generally to review them within 3 months of receipt. This review is to determine that the CRFs are being completed correctly and completely, that there are no unanticipated problems or adverse experiences that have not been previously reported, and to look for trends or patterns in adverse experiences or problems with use of concomitant mediations or therapies.

The sponsor should review all deaths and serious, unexpected adverse reactions in a timely manner. The sponsor's review is to determine that all information has been submitted and to look for new trends or unantici-pated problems. Reviewing the information in a timely manner may avoid unnecessary additional problems or reactions and placing the subjects at additional risk.

Sponsors should review information on study dropouts to determine the cause for the subjects ending their participation early and this may provide additional information on the conduct of the study and/or the investigational drug.

Drug accountability

The FDA will determine who is responsible for administration of the drug. Is it the same individual listed on the statement of investigator form or has the investigator delegated this responsibility to a subinvestigator?

An agreement will sometimes be made between an investigator and the on-site pharmacist to assume control over the drug both for proper storage and for accountability purposes.

Since the drug is under investigation there must be a system in place to show how much drug was received, how much was dispensed and at the end of the study how much was destroyed or returned to the sponsor.

If someone other than the investigator's staff has assumed responsibility for the study drug then it is important for this individual to understand that the accounting procedures must be documented and that the investigational records must be stored for the required time period. The records also must be able to be retrieved if requested during an inspection. One good system is for the pharmacist to dispense only upon receipt of a prescription from the clinical investigator. At the end of the study the pharmacist will transfer all records to the clinical investigator for storage with the study files.

The storage area for the investigational drug should be of sufficient space so that there is no possibility of mix-up with other investigational products. The storage area should have limited access and be available to only the investigator and his or her staff. The only requirement for drugs to be stored under locked conditions is for controlled substances. However, it is good practice that all investigational drugs should be stored securely. This will help prevent drugs that are in demand from being diverted.

If during or at the end of the study drugs are to be destroyed on site, records documenting this destruction must be maintained. The records of destruction should contain a complete inventory of what was destroyed, the method and date of destruction and a witness signature. By building in these safeguards you may discourage drug diversion by accounting fully for the drug.

Investigational drugs may have a reassay or expiry date. It is important for the investigator to be aware of any time limitations on dispensing the drug. Before the drug becomes outdated, contact the sponsor to determine if use of the drug can be extended. You do not want to cause any interruption in patient care while you are waiting for a new supply of drug.

During an audit, the FDA may perform an individual count to see if the number ingested matches what is left in the subject's supply and what is recorded on the CRF. They would also verify the blinding procedures, labelling of the drug, lot number and whether this information agrees with the shipping records to the site.

Record retention
FDA regulations require that all records pertaining to studies conducted under an IND be retained for 2 years following approval of the marketing application for the product; or 2 years from the date the FDA is notified that there will be no application submitted; or 2 years from the date the sponsor is notified that the application is not approved. This requires all records pertaining to the study be maintained, at the sponsor, at the investigational site and at a contract facility if one was used.

When closing out an investigational site, the monitor should remind the investigator of his or her responsibility to retain the required records. The investigator should notify the sponsor if he or she moves or retires or relinquishes control of the records. Appropriate procedures must be implemented to ensure that the records will be adequately maintained and available for a regulatory audit. Records would include CRFs, source documents and all adminstrative or regulatory documents.

Computer/electronic data system

As part of an ongoing information-gathering programme, the FDA realizes that newer techniques for capturing data have emerged in the industry, such as remote data entry. In order to develop meaningful regulations the FDA wants to determine what the current industry standard is for the types of computer systems and software in use. Are they used for gathering, storing or transmission of data and how are the data transmitted to the sponsor?

For information entered into the computer, what is the source of the data? Is it directly entered, taken from the CRF, office or clinical records or extrapolated from a form designed for the specific study?

Is the information entered by the specific individual or by anyone on the investigator's staff? What type of audit trail is maintained and who can make corrections? Are there security procedures built into the system?

Does the investigator retain a copy of the electronic data and can it be viewed or printed well after study completion? The FDA stated that at the time of an audit they need to be able to access all available sources of information.

Project notebook/study files

As is the case in any clinical trial, documentation of the study events is key to supporting the facts that have been developed. A famous FDA quote is, 'If it isn't documented, then it did not happen'.

One of the important parts of documentation is the administrative/regulatory files associated with a clinical trial.

Over the years a system has evolved whereby these files were centralized into a ring binder or into folders placed in a banker's box.

Centralizing these files supports the investigator in maintaining an accurate method of record-keeping. It also provides easy access to all documentation required by the sponsor and by governmental authorities on how the clinical trial was conducted. During monitoring visits the project notebook/study files can be quickly reviewed for completeness and the focus of the visit can be on review of the CRFs with the source documents.

Items that should be included in the project notebook/study files include the following:

1   Personnel sheet: listing of the name, address, work and home telephone number for the CRA, medical monitor and appropriate department director for the therapeutic area. If there are any changes during the study, then this information should be updated. The purpose of this sheet is to give the investigator a source of information that will be accessible in case of questions or emergencies that may develop during the trial.
2   Investigator brochure.
3   Protocol.
4   Protocol modifications: any modifications to the original protocol should be filed in this section.
5   Statement of investigator form (FDA-1572): The *Statement of Investigator Form*, along with a current curriculum vitae for the clinical investigator, is filed in this section.
6   IRB approval/IRB correspondence: Filed in this section is all correspondence between the investigator and the IRB. Documents that would be retained are comments on the consent form and the protocol, the letter of IRB approval, annual updates, reporting of any significant risks to the IRB, and a letter notifying the IRB of the conclusion of the study.
7   Informed consents/approved signed: In this section would be filed the IRB approved consent form and a completed signed and dated consent form for each subject in the study. It is a good idea to number each consent with the subjects' entry or randomization number.

8   Sponsor correspondence: All correspondence between the investigator and the sponsor is filed in this section. The only exception would be monetary matters, which would be filed separately.
9   Drug experience reports: Copies of completed serious adverse events would be filed here.
10   Drug accountability: Items included would be:
     (a)   copy of the shipping order listing what the investigator received;
     (b)   individual subject distribution sheet (what the subject received/returned);
     (c)   clinical supply return form/destruction record.
11   Laboratory normals: A copy of the laboratory normals will be filed in this section. If the normals change during the study then a new set will be added with the effective date of change.
12   Monitoring log: A log sheet is in this section and will be signed and dated at each visit by the medical monitor and/or the CRA/clinical scientist. The purpose is to document monitoring of the study by the sponsor and ensure that the project notebook/study files are up to date.

Freedom of information

All information with the exception of information under litigation and proprietary information, is available to the public under the Freedom of Information Act.

It is a good way to access information to determine what the current thinking is at the FDA regarding enforcement activities.

To access this information send a letter with your request to: FOI Staff, Food and Drug Administration, HFI-35, 5600 Fishers Lane, Rockville, MD 20857, USA. To expedite your request include the following statement: 'this request can be filled though HFD-344', which is the Department of Scientific Investigations.

FDA clinical investigator information sheets

The FDA, also as a service, provides information sheets that were generated in response to inquiries they had received at workshops and conferences. For clinical investigators the following topics are available:

1   Frequently asked questions concerning the identification of persons involved in a study and their responsibilities.
2   Required record-keeping in clinical investigations.
3   Informed consent and the clinical investigator.
4   FDA inspection of clinical investigators.
5   Clinical investigator regulatory sanctions.

6   Treatment use of investigational drugs.
7   Placebo-controlled and active controlled drug study designs.

IRB information sheets are also available from the FDA. There are 22 in this series. Examples are:

1   Acceptance of foreign data and IRB and informed consent requirements.
2   Advertising for study subjects.
3   Continuing review.
4   Emergency use of an investigational drug.
5   Non-local IRB review.
6   Payment for investigational products.
7   Payment to research subjects.
8   Sponsor–clinical investigator–IRB interrelationship.
9   Waiver of IRB requirements.

Both the clinical investigator and IRB information sheets can be obtained from the Office of Health Affairs. The address and phone number are: Health Assessment Policy Staff, Office of Health Affairs (HFY-20), Food and Drug Administration, 5600 Fisher Lane, Room 15–22, Rockville, MD 20857, USA. Telephone: 1-301-443-1382.

Conclusion

As stated at the beginning of this chapter, the best time to prepare for an FDA inspection is before you start the study. By reviewing the items that have been listed, implementing procedures and record-keeping systems, and ensuring that personnel understand the good clinical practice and the protocol requirements, you will be successful not only working under an IND but also in being audited by the FDA.

Acknowledgements

I would like to thank Ms Mary B. Ott for her technical review and Ms Diane Damiano for administrative support for this chapter.

9 Aspects of total quality in clinical trials

B Moore and P L Worthington

Introduction

We see Total Quality as being about creating the right environment and leadership to allow a company's processes to be continually improved by the people who work in them with the help of their managers. Naturally, this involves understanding your customers' (both internal and external) wants and needs – how do they use your service or product and how you can help them use it better. Of course, every company has constraints, but with a systematic approach to Total Quality these should not be seen as reasons for inaction.

How does this apply to Clinical Trials?

Drug development is a system of interrelated processes as in any other business, where what happens in one process affects another and all contribute to the total development time from laboratory to factory to customer. One such process which is prone to delay (frequently caused by queries) is the Clinical Trial process. It is unlikely that the target date for completion can be achieved without awareness of the whole system and the interaction between processes, understanding the variation between people who work with the processes, and leadership within a culture where cross-functional cooperation can exist without fear. Attention to constraints such as government legislation, regulatory bodies and parent companies must be part of the Total Quality initiative of course. However, Total Quality properly and sensitively carried out can be used to reduce the number of time-consuming queries in clinical trials and the time taken to process them, which can arise from inadequate Case Record Form (CRF) design or in the data-gathering/monitoring process. Every pharmaceutical company needs to know where it is going – a view to the future, and the benefits of implementing Total Quality in clinical trials and throughout the organization will be to improve its long-term prospects to be first in the market.

Basic principles of Total Quality

First, a few words about this popular phrase, 'Total Quality'. Many organizations see quality as something to be achieved. These organizations spend much time and effort on activities such as:

- Establishing and maintaining standards.
- Conforming to requirements.
- Meeting targets.
- Eliminating errors and defects.

More visionary organizations adopt a dynamic view by seeing that:

- Quality has to be a way of life.
- Conforming to current standards is the minimum achievement.
- Checking and correcting are both expensive and time-consuming.
- Short-term expediences can no longer take priority over innovation and continual improvement
- Their leadership style needs to allow all the above to happen.

A view of the transformation towards Total Quality

Figure 9.1 shows typical progressive stages of transformation towards the dynamic view of total quality.

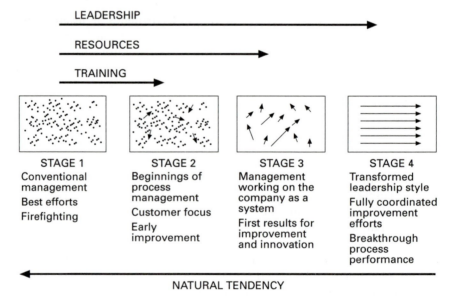

Figure 9.1   *Stages of transformation towards the dynamic view of Total Quality.*

Typically, the usual state of companies embarking on the Total Quality journey is a mixture of stages 1 and 2. There is a lack of a system approach to the company and certainly no alignment to a constant aim. Interestingly, we also find there is a tendency for organizations (and individuals) to regress towards the left side of the diagram – it takes leadership to maintain the momentum for ever. Also, no transformation can be achieved without providing the resources and training that the company's strategy for transformation demands. It is worth a few moments for readers to reflect on this diagram and assess how their company fits into the model.

Applying Total Quality principles to Clinical Trials

Now we see how some of the principles we mentioned above apply to clinical trials. First, let us portray the situation we have found in many pharmaceutical companies with regard to clinical trials.

All pharmaceutical companies are subject to constraints such as regulatory bodies and government legislation and many have parent companies. Although we have found there is a certain amount of cross-functional cooperation through project meetings, often unrealistic targets are set which take little account of the available resources. The result is increased pressure on the work force and low morale among department supervisors who know they cannot meet their target dates. People in one department often blame delays on other departments – league tables on departmental processing times only seem to fuel the blame. In the meanwhile, senior management are faced with making decisions with inadequate management data – inadequate in both style of presentation and in content.

The start of applying Total Quality to pharmaceutical companies (and clinical trials, in particular) is with viewing the organization as a *system*. That is:

- Recognizing that the organization is a network of interrelated sub-systems and not a number of loosely related departments such as Data Management, Statistics, Medical, Research and Development (R&D), Marketing, Consumer and Finance.
- Working on getting the best out of the system for the benefit of customers (internal and external).
- Instituting people-oriented leadership based on systems thinking.
- Recognizing that the system can only deliver what resources and training in every subsystem can provide.

But why should we view the organization in this way? It all stems from Dr Deming's* system view of an organization. In fact, there are two views of an organization (Fig. 9.2):

1   The old or traditional view.
2   Deming's view of the organization as a system.

VIEWS OF AN ORGANIZATION

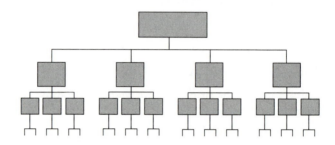

The old way to view an organization

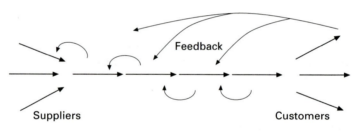

The new way to view an organization

Figure 9.2   *(Top) Traditional view of an organization; (bottom) new system view of an organization.*

The traditional view emphasizes several factors:

- Who is in charge?
- Who is accountable to whom?
- The functional divisions of the organization (each middle-management position represents division, line, operation or professional speciality).

---

*Dr W Edwards Deming (1900–94) was an American statistician responsible for introducing these ideas to the Japanese in 1950. We refer the reader to two of Deming's books: *Out of the Crisis* (1986) ISBN 0-911379-01-0 and *The New Economics* (1993) ISBN 0-911379-05-3, both published by Massachusetts Institute of Technology.

It has shortcomings. For example:

- It does not portray the interdependence of the various functional areas.
- It does not describe the organization as a work flow.
- It portrays individual accountability, rather than the group, the process or the output of the group and process.
- There are no references to services provided or customers (either external or internal) in this view.

The purpose of the organization as suggested by this traditional view is accountability and control – all paths lead to and from the top. To view the organization as a hierarchy of command and accountability will restrict people's ability to visualize the company as being customer and quality-oriented. This will inevitably limit their constancy of purpose in pursuit of quality improvement.

In 1950 Dr Deming proposed the system view of an organization to the Japanese – it is this that was at the heart of the transformation he wanted. The system concept depicts the following:

1   The interdependence of organizational processes.
2   The primacy of the customer (both internal and external).
3   The impact of customer feedback (e.g consumer research).
4   Continual improvement, based on customer feedback.
5   The importance of suppliers.
6   The network of internal customer/supplier relationships.

The important difference between these two concepts is not just theoretical. It is more than a difference in diagrams – they symbolize different ways of *thinking* that result in differences in priorities. Relating this concept of a system to a pharmaceutical company typically produces the following (simplified) diagram (Fig. 9.3) which shows the interfaces with various key components in the core process of drug development.

Straightaway, we see that Clinical Trials (the part on which we are focusing for the purpose of this chapter) is not an independent entity but interfaces directly with Medical Sciences, Clinical Investigations, R&D, customers and regulatory bodies. Also, there are the indirect interfaces through these direct ones. The importance of this is twofold:

1   On internal customer–supplier relationships.
2   On system data to enable better decisions and actions to be made (and to remove blame).

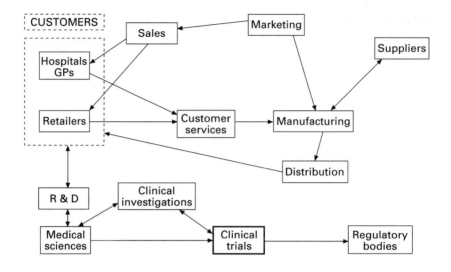

Figure 9.3   *Interfaces between key components in the core process of drug development.*

Internal customer–supplier relationships

Each interface indicated by an arrow on Figure 9.3 points to where suppliers (internal and external) can tap into the system to seek information from their customers – i.e. they are what we call '*Listening Posts*'. They should ask simple questions such as:

1 What do they want?
2 What is my service to them?
3 What are the customers' expectations of my service?
4 Is my service meeting these expectations?
5 What is the process for providing this service?
6 What action is required to improve the service?

They should also ask the most important question of all:

What does my customer do with the service and how can I help him/her to use it better?

Simple as they are, we have found these questions to be a most effective method of establishing meaningful dialogues with customers and encouraging early improvements. As a consequence, delays in the clinical trial process caused by the number of queries, for example, can be reduced by mutual understanding of each function within that process.

Better system data

Also, importantly, this system diagram indicates which Key Measures management and department heads *should* be using to lead the organization forward. For the management of a pharmaceuticals organization, typical system measures might be:

1   Drug development time.
2   Time to submission for product licence.
3   R&D costs.
4   Manufacturing lead time.

Figure 9.4 shows a typical system diagram for the Clinical Trial activity where incidentally we have also indicated points we regard as 'Listening Posts' for customers. Again, across each interface one can ask the same questions as previously suggested.

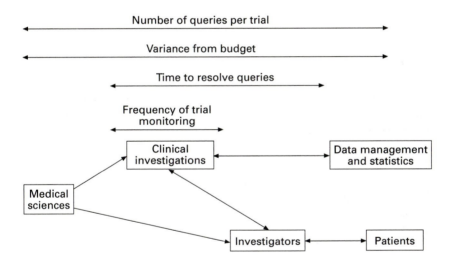

Figure 9.4   *System diagram for Clinical Trial activity.*

For this Clinical Trial system, examples of system measures are:

1   Number of queries per trial.
2   Time to resolve queries.
3   Frequency of trial monitoring.
4   Variance from budget.

These measures are drawn on the system diagram showing which part of the system impacts on them. This is crucial when deciding *who* should work on improvements on issues around these measures. This avoids the traditional tactic of apportioning blame to one part of the system. For example, in the clinical trials activity, working to reduce the number of queries per trial and the time taken to process them should involve a multidisciplinary team consisting of Clinical Research Associates (CRAs) and other personnel from Clinical Investigations, Data Processing, Medical Services, Statistics etc. rather than just CRAs, as can often be the case!

Better management of data

At this point, it is worth exploring in more detail the principles of how data are used and misused by many people (especially management – 'Better Data used in a Better Way'. This is crucial within the concept of Total Quality because it provides increased knowledge of:

1   Understanding the organization as a system of interrelated processes.
2   Statistical variation in processes and systems.
3   The interactions of people who work in those systems and processes.

It also helps to remove cross-functional 'blame' and barriers that serve only to hinder progress with improvements and innovation. We are not just looking at better ways of presenting existing data (although there is usually plenty of scope for this!). In many pharmaceutical companies, we have seen lots of data generated that are often not being correctly used and interpreted. Sometimes this is because the data are being presented in a form in which they cannot be exploited to their fullest – so much is hidden and/or lost by data presented solely in tabular form and computer-generated graphs such as bar charts. Unfortunately, such practices not only deter the data user from establishing a mental link with the messages the data are trying to convey, but messages are either missed or misconstrued. For example, trends (real ones) are missed, special occurrences missed or perceived where none exist and so on.

As an example, Figure 9.5 provides a short extract of 'Notes to the Accounts' from a UK pharmaceutical company. Like many companies, each month they commented on the sales volume and gross value variances.

(*Note*: For Budget, one can easily substitute Target, Plan or Profile, all of which imply something to be aimed at, whether or not the processes and system are capable of achieving it.)

Data presented in such tabular form may have a role in summarizing the performance for a particular time period, as in an end-of-year report.

Month of September 1992

	September 1992				Year to date		
	ACTUAL	BUDGET	VARIANCE		ACTUAL	BUDGET	VARIANCE
Sales volume (m³)	13,877	13,934	(57)		128,295	113,684	14,611
Gross value (£K)	4,464	4,474	(10)		41,973	36,510	5,463
Production costs							
Profit before tax							

Figure 9.5 *Sample extract from Notes to the Accounts of a UK pharmaceutical company.*

However, much harm can be done by misusing this format for making decisions for which it was never intended, such as:

● Predicting future sales.
● Taking decisions about the current or future state of a system or process.
● Identifying changes in the system or process.
● Identifying trends.

For these important decisions, we need the more effective concepts related to variation that were devised by Dr Walter Shewhart in the 1920s. It was he who pioneered and developed the statistical control of processes which was subsequently developed for management use by Dr Deming.

A better way of viewing data comes from the use of control charts – a technique which traditionally had been reserved for manufacturing operations. However, this technique is being increasingly used with management data to provide the correct guidance for better decisions. So now let us examine this alternative and more fruitful way of using and interpreting data. The secret behind this lies in understanding variation and controlling processes (administrative as well as production). This, in turn, comes from understanding the distinction between what Shewhart called *assignable* causes and *chance* causes of variation. In the 1950s, Dr Deming adopted the terms *special* and *common causes of variation* to emphasize who or what is responsible for working on the two causes of variation. The important distinction between special and common causes is summarized as follows.

Special (assignable) causes of variation

These are causes that are localized in nature and generate excessive variation that has nothing to do with the way the process was intended to operate. They are *not* part of the process and therefore should be considered abnormalities.

Thus, being exceptions to the system or process, they deserve special treatment.

Common (chance) causes of variation

These are causes of variation that are *inherent* in the process. They arise out of the process or out of the way the process is organized and operated.

This type of variation can only be effectively reduced by changing the process through management-led teams and the adoption of a systematic approach to improvement.

To help people distinguish between these two causes of variation, Shewhart devised what is known as the 'control chart'. The idea is that points within certain (calculated) control limits are due to common cause variation, i.e. part of the process. On the other hand, points outside the limits are regarded as being due to causes outside the process, i.e. special causes to which we can assign a reason. To illustrate the application of

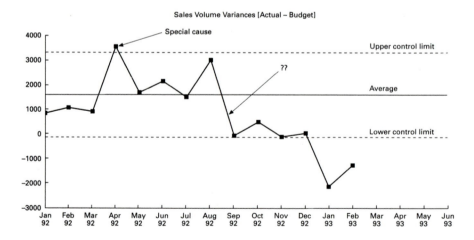

Figure 9.6   Control chart showing sales volume variances.

control charts to management data, we look again at the data from the 'Notes to accounts': when we display the variances (= actual – budget) as a control chart (i.e. in a better way, Fig. 9.6) we see quite a different view from that using the data in snapshot form.

Here we see an exception to the'norm' (i.e. a special cause) in April 1992 that warranted investigation in the sense of 'what could be learnt for the future from that extraordinary good month'. No other points until September 1992 are cause for investigation as the variation (undesirable though it may be from the production planning's view) is part of the forecasting process – in fact, to discuss each such monthly variance in detail would be like discussing random numbers, i.e. chance variation.

Then in September 1992, we have a point on the lower control limit – a special cause that warranted investigation which would have revealed a system change in September. However, because the senior managers were viewing their data in tabular form, it was not until some time later that this change was realized by the company; yet the comment recorded for that month was 'Sales volumes were in line with plan'. When managers do not have knowledge of such variation, we find monthly management meetings turning into discussions about chance variation – during which they discuss common and special causes with equal gusto (e.g. as with monthly or weekly sales). What is required is the longer-term view that control charts provide, together with a different set of questions that they prompt. Indeed, the managers of the above company are now viewing its management data in this new way and are asking a different set of questions related to improving processes rather than providing excuses. Questions such as:

- How did we expect the chart to look?
- Are we surprised by the amount of common cause variation?
- What is the impact of this variation on the system and its customers?
- What action should we be taking on the common cause variation?
- What about the special causes that are present? What action is being taken to error-proof against future occurrences?
- What is the preferred state of the chart? What needs to be done to achieve this state?
- What are the opportunities for improvement?

Using data in this better way is obviously of prime importance. However, the key to success is 'Better Management Data' that stem from a customer-focused view of the systems and processes. Such data will enable there to be:

- A better understanding and improvement of existing processes.
- More effective planning and forecasting.

● Managers and their staff controlling the processes, rather than the processes controlling them.

Also, at this stage it may not yet be fully appreciated that with a growing understanding of variation in processes and systems, leadership at all levels will develop further.

Control charts in Clinical Trials

Often in the area of Clinical Trials, management data are kept on the number of hours spent on each current project by each function (data entry, validation, coding, queries, statistical analysis, etc.) and used as Performance Measures. The data may be presented monthly in tabular form as previously shown and passed to the finance department. Sometimes data presented in this way are used to forecast the time likely to be taken for future projects in a particular therapeutic area. However, a much clearer picture on which to base decisions may be obtained using control charts, as illustrated here. In addition, more information may be gained on special causes which will need further investigation to eliminate an identified cause. Another main benefit will be for management to realize that they must work together to improve that system and hence reduce common cause variation. The reader is referred to the section on internal customer–supplier relationships (above) for initial ideas on how this may be achieved.

In addition to reducing the time to process queries, another improvement issue was to reduce the actual number of queries. The control chart (Fig. 9.7) shows the proportion of queries per project over a certain period. For this particular pharmaceutical company, proportion was defined as the number of queries out of the total number of pages (case record forms) to be completed in the patient booklet or workbook. As can be seen, a 'special cause' seems to have affected Project Number 16 and when this was investigated, it was found that the high proportion of queries was due to the introduction of new adverse event forms. Investigators and monitoring personnel were unfamiliar with the procedure for completing these new forms, and further training and guidelines were introduced to eliminate this particular special cause variation.

To reduce 'common cause' variation, a small team which included an experienced CRA, a data entry clerk and a data management supervisor was formed to identify ways in which the number of queries could be reduced. This team was led by a senior person from Clinical Investigations and given time from their normal duties to meet regularly. One or two changes were identified which the team believe will reduce the number of queries. These proposed improvements have now been implemented for certain projects and the next step is to collect data on the proportion of

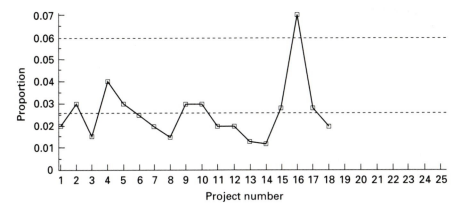

Figure 9.7   Control chart showing proportion of queries per project

queries arising from these projects to study the results of these changes to the process.

Key improvement issues

Although this chapter concentrates on Clinical Trials, the system as a whole is pivotal in any quality improvement initiative. Using information gained from listening to customers (internal and external), from key business measures and from the use of control charts as already illustrated, a number of improvement issues can be identified.

One of the most pressing from both business and customers' point of view is related to the time to process clinical trials. The management team should begin to deploy this improvement issue through their system – using an approach we call the Strategic Deployment of Improvement. Why? This enables them to demonstrate their commitment to leadership by working on the system with their people. Thus we see that this Strategic Deployment of Improvement ensures that each level of manager under-stands how his or her improvement activity will have an impact on Key Strategic Issues. Furthermore it helps to avoid people:

- Going into detail that belongs to the next layer down – yet their leader's role as a coach and mentor is clearly defined.
- Living in a world of their own – they are encouraged into cooperation both horizontally and vertically in the organization.

Applying the principles of Strategic Deployment of Improvement to clinical trials in one pharmaceutical company produced the schematic view of the improvement effort shown in Figure 9.8. Here, in drug development, a key measure was the time to develop drugs which in turn had an impact on the time to obtain a product licence. Figure 9.8 shows three levels of involvement (there could be more or fewer levels). At the more senior level, their improvement issue was 'Reduce Drug Development Time' and the systems view shows that they needed a team from Labs, Medical, Clinical Investigations, Data Processing (DP), etc. This team, led by a member of the senior management team, constructed a deployment flowchart and this, in addition to data collected, showed that the completion of clinical trials was one cause of delay. Within this, a number of contributing factors to this delay were identified, one of which was the time to process queries. To tackle this, a team of people led by a senior member from Data Management was formed and the issue was stated as 'Reduce Time to

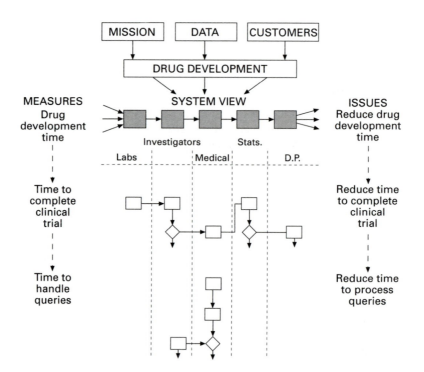

Figure 9.8 *Schematic view of improvement effort towards reducing drug development time in a pharmaceutical company.*

Process Queries'. Notice that at each level not only is there a clear statement of intent (the issue on the right-hand side) but also associated with
each statement is a measure to indicate progress with the improvement.

During their work on the improvement, each team was guided by three
simple basic principles – the three Ds.

1   **D**iscipline of approach, provided by the Plan–Do–Study–Act cycle of
    Dr Deming (Fig. 9.9).

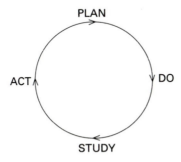

Figure 9.9   *Deming's plan-do-study-act cycle.*

(a)   *Plan*
   (i)   change aimed at improvement:
   (ii)   Firm up on the broad idea.
   (iii)   Articulate the statement of intent.
   (iv)   Assess the current situation by listening to customers and
           reviewing the existing data.
   (v)   Formulate initial change.
(b)   *Do:*
   (i)   Carry out initial change (preferably on a small scale).
   (ii)   Encourage experimentation of ideas.
(c)   *Study:*
   (i)   The results from the pilot.
   (ii)   What can be learnt.
   (iii)   What should be changed.
(d)   *Act:*
   (i)   Carry out the change(s) to the system or
   (ii)   Go through the cycle again using the new knowledge gained
           in the study phase or
   (iii)   Abandon the idea.

2   **D**ata from the process that helps everyone understand the process more fully, take the most appropriate action according to the presence or otherwise of special causes and helps to avoid action by 'gut feel'.
3   **D**etermination – that is, self-determination to pursue the improvement issue to achieve success.

Of course, an underlying assumption we make for this approach to succeed is that the culture allows all this to happen. By this, we mean:

- *Leadership* – Are the managers prepared to give the right leadership (see 'Attributes of a leader' below) and are the people prepared to accept change?
- *Teamwork* – people working on improvements and innovation, eventually generating a sense of all-one-team in the organization.
- *Attitudes* – of every one towards each other and trust in everyday relationships (which may take a long time to grow!)

Leadership

As we all know, there are many aspects of leadership – there is political, military, directive, reassuring (and so on) modes of leadership. However, there are a number of leadership characteristics which are particularly vital within the context of establishing a better environment for change. These characteristics, summarized below, are based on Dr Deming's attributes of a leader.

1   They understand how the work of their group fits into the aims of the company.
2   They work with the preceding stages and the following stages by understanding the needs of their internal supplies and customers.
3   They try to create joy in work and try to optimize the education, skills and abilities of everyone, and help them to improve.
4   They are a coach and counsel, not a judge but a colleague and part of the team working to improve the system.
5   They use process data to help understand the variation in people which in turn removes the fear and blame caused by misuse of data and by wrong data (e.g. league tables).
6   They work on improving the system in which they and their people work.
7   They create trust and are aware that the creation of trust requires taking a risk. (Remember that trust cannot be bought with artificial awards and merit pay!)
8   They do not expect perfection.

9   They listen and learn without passing judgement on those to whom they listen.
10   They improve continually their own education.

Adopting these attributes may come easier to some people than others. What is important is to 'have a go' at applying these attributes – this will begin to start the change in culture, in attitudes and in the ways people relate to each other and to the organization. Then the common cries of 'they don't listen' and 'we don't communicate' (and so on) begin to be resolved in a natural way through *everyone* changing their behaviour.

Conclusion

In this chapter we have attempted to outline the principles and practical steps involved in transforming your organization towards Total Quality. The Clinical Trial process is an important part of the whole system of drug development and, as such, is a logical area on which to concentrate. Applying the ideas of this chapter may reduce the time taken to obtain a product licence, and to be first in the marketplace is surely the aim of all pharmaceutical companies. Although the practical steps are straight-forward, they are not easy in practice. Your organization will probably be faced with the old proverb of the immovable object and the irresistible force. The immovable object factors may include:

● Your company's current working and managerial practices.
● Your level of belief in your current working and managerial practices.
● Lack of knowledge of a better way of doing things at all levels.

These factors may be countered by two things – a willingness to learn and a willingness to challenge and change.

The irresistible forces in your company will include

1   Your (developing) vision for the people and the business.
2   Your enthusiasm and excitement.
3   A belief that you can differentiate yourselves in the marketplace.

However, as a final thought it is worth recalling Newton's first law of motion:

'You cannot have change without doing something different!'

His second law says that you can only have as much change as the effort you are prepared to put into it.

10 Medical ethics and good clinical practice

C Jenkins

Medical practitioners enjoy a unique position in society; by the nature of their profession and duties they have the right physically and mentally to injure their patients in order to affect resolutions of their ailments. Thus doctors of medicine can legally use the scalpel, administer noxious substances and influence thought processes of patients who put their trust in them. Given such power and privilege it is not surprising that society expects protection from unscrupulous physicians.

Hippocrates, the 'father of medicine' (c.460 to c.375 BC) is credited with producing not only the earliest, but also the most impressive statement on medical ethics, the Hippocratic Oath, which even to this day is sworn by newly qualified physicians throughout the world. Nevertheless, over the centuries, the urge to advance medical knowledge has led to medical practitioners disregarding ethical considerations when conducting experiments on human subjects. During the Second World War, appalling experiments were conducted on imprisoned ethnic groups by physicians. These actions led to the issuance in 1947 of the Nuremberg Code, the first declaration of medical ethics requiring voluntary consent to be given by subjects invited to participate in medical research.

Abuses of subjects involved in medical research were not limited to war time; as recently as 1971 the *Lancet* published criticism of a study conducted in New York in which mentally defective children were infected with hepatitis for experimental purposes without obtaining informed consent.

A major advance in international medical ethics occurred in 1964 when the first Declaration of Helsinki was published by the World Medical Assembly. Since that time a number of amendments have been made to the document, the current version being adopted in September 1989 at the 41st World Medical Assembly in Hong Kong. This document offers guidance to medical doctors undertaking biomedical research involving human subjects. Acceptance of the provisions of the Declaration of Helsinki forms the basis of medical ethics and is incorporated in every guideline and regulation issued by national drug regulatory authorities concerned with ensuring that studies of new medicines are conducted in accordance with good clinical practice (GCP).

As the Declaration of Helsinki may be considered to be the lowest common denominator of ethical considerations relating to the testing of new medicines referred to in all GCP regulations and guidelines, it is important to comply with its recommendations. First of all, does the Declaration of Helsinki have legal power? The answer is no – indeed, the declaration itself states 'it must be stressed that the standards as drafted are only a guide to physicians all over the world. Physicians are not relieved from criminal, civil and ethics responsibilities under the laws of their own countries'. Thus, when considering any review of medical ethics and GCP, the appropriate local laws and regulations must always be taken into account.

Medical ethics, as related to GCP and the evaluation of new medicines, may be split into two distinct components: independent review of the study protocol and the subject's informed consent. The objective of this chapter is to compare the requirements of regulatory guidelines and regulations with the Declaration of Helsinki and offer advice to clinical researchers of new medicines to ensure that their research complies with GCP.

It is recognized that there are numerous GCP guidelines issued by drug regulatory authorities; they share the same basic objective, which is to ensure that clinical research of new medicines is conducted to the highest standards and that the rights of the individual are protected. For the purposes of this chapter, three different GCP guidelines and/or regulations are considered. They are those issued by the Food and Drugs Administration (FDA) of the USA, the European Community (EC) *Guidelines for GCP* and the International Conference for Harmonization (ICH) *Guidelines for GCP*. At the time of writing the latter are still in draft and are expected to be published in 1995.

Independent review of research proposals

The Declaration of Helsinki states that the design and performance of each experimental procedure involving human subjects should be clearly formulated in an experimental protocol which should be transmitted for consideration, comment and guidance to a specially appointed committee independent of the investigator and the sponsor, provided that this independent committee is in conformity with the laws and regulations of the country in which the research experiment is performed.

As with many advisory statements, it is the 'missing' information which can lead to problems when ensuring research projects are conducted in accordance with GCP. Thus, the Declaration gives no advice on the provision of independent committees, their constitution or composition. This is left to local law and practice; as there are few national laws covering research ethics committees, drug regulatory officials have addressed the question in the various guidelines for GCP.

It may be appropriate to clarify some terms; as noted above, the Declaration of Helsinki refers to 'specially appointed committees'. The title 'ethics committee' has been adopted by most countries to describe these independent committees, with the exception of the USA, which refers to Institutional Review Boards (IRBs).

FDA regulations and guidelines

The FDA of the USA was the first national drug regulatory authority to address the question of formal review of study protocols by independent committees. Since 1971 FDA regulations have required studies involving investigational new drugs performed on human subjects in institutions to be approved by an IRB and to be subject to continuing review by the approving IRB. In addition, in 1981 the FDA published regulations governing the composition, operation and responsibility of IRBs which review studies on products regulated by FDA (i.e. studies conducted under the 'notice of claimed investigational exemption for a new drug' or IND). These revised regulations were applicable to all studies of new drugs, not just those conducted in institutions. Since 1977 the FDA has also conducted its own review of IRBs in the USA as part of its bioresearch monitoring programme; these reviews are conducted by FDA inspectors during on-site inspections, similar to study investigator audits. Thus, for studies conducted in the USA under an IND, the message is loud and clear – FDA regulations must be followed.

In 1983 the FDA stated that it will accept clinical data derived from studies conducted in foreign countries to meet FDA requirements in support of marketing applications for drugs in the USA. These fall into two main categories; those conducted under an IND and those which are not. For studies conducted under an IND the clinical investigations must undergo IRB review and the informed consent process must conform to those FDA regulations in effect for studies conducted in the USA. Under exceptional circumstances, the FDA will consider requests to waive its regulations for foreign studies conducted under an IND.

For those studies not conducted under an IND, the FDA is much more flexible and recognizes that the US government should not impose its standards on other countries. For such studies the FDA requires that they must be conducted in conformance with the principles of the Declaration of Helsinki or with the laws and regulations of that country, whichever represents the greater protection of the individual. As there are very few laws and regulations concerning ethics committees in countries other than the USA, researchers are advised to adopt the requirements of GCP guidelines issues by the various drug regulatory authorities.

The FDA also expects the sponsor to provide detailed information of the ethical procedures used; the sponsor should explain how the research conformed to the ethical principles contained in the Declaration of Helsinki or the foreign country's standards, whichever were used. If the foreign country's standards were used, the sponsor should explain in detail how those standards differ from the Declaration of Helsinki and how they offer *greater* protection to the subjects.

When the research has been approved by an independent review committee the sponsor should submit to the FDA documentation of such review and approval, including the names and qualifications of the members of the committee. In this regard, a 'review committee' means a committee composed of scientists and, where practicable, individuals who are otherwise qualified (e.g. other health professionals or laypersons). The investigator may not vote on any aspect of the review of his or her protocol by a review committee.

Although it is recognized that there are a number of national guidelines throughout the world, there is little difference between them when considering ethical review.

EC *GCP guidelines* and independent review

The rules governing medicinal products in the EC Directive 91/507/EEC provide the legal basis for the *GCP Guidelines* issued in 1990. As with all such guidelines, the Declaration of Helsinki is the accepted basis for clinical trials ethics.

The investigator and/or sponsor must request the opinion of a relevant ethics committee regarding the suitability of clinical trial protocols and the method and material to be used for obtaining informed consent. The ethics committee must be informed of all subsequent protocol amendments and of serious or unexpected adverse events occurring during the trial which are likely to affect the safety of subjects. If appropriate, the committee should be asked to reconsider its opinion if the re-evaulation of the ethical aspects appears to be called for.

Subjects must not be entered into the trial until the relevant ethics committee has issued its favourable opinion on the procedures and documentation. The sponsor and/or investigator should consider recommendations made by the EC.

The guidelines give advice to ethics committees concerning their responsibilities and conclude by stating that the committee should give its opinion and advice in writing within a reasonable time limit, clearly identifying the trial, the documents studied and date of review.

The major difference, between an IRB and a European ethics committee is the level of government control exerted on the committees. In the USA the composition and constitution of IRBs are regulated by law and committees are subject to formal audit by regulatory inspectors. In Europe there is no equivalent central government control and the standards vary significantly from country to country. Taking the UK and France as examples of two members of the EC, there are major differences in national guidelines regarding ethical review of multicentre clinical trials. The Department of Health in the UK has published guidelines covering the provision of local research ethics committees, their constitution, composition and recommendations for review of research protocols. These require all clinical investigators to obtain approval from their local research ethics committee, thus a large multicentre study may require upwards of 50 ethics committee reviews for the same protocol. In France the recommendation is for a principal investigator to be identified who assumes responsibility for the study to obtain ethical approval; this single approval is normally acceptable to all investigators, although they may be asked to provide evidence of the approval to their local ethics committee. The EC *GCP Guidelines* give general advice on the composition and constitution of ethics committees and state that these details should be publicly available.

ICH GCP guidelines

The ICH guidelines are intended to cover the needs of all national regulatory authorities so they refer to both ethics committees and IRBs. In line with other similar documents, the Declaration of Helsinki is the baseline standard for independent ethical review. The ICH guidelines require the ethics committee not only to write giving its advice but also to detail by name and professional status those members attending the meeting, complying with FDA requirements. In other respects the ICH guidelines are very similar to the EC guidelines.

Informed consent

Under no circumstances should anyone be exposed to a medical experiment without consenting to the procedure, either personally or, under special circumstances, by proxy.

Regulatory authorities must be assured that studies of new medicines are conducted in compliance with GCP to ensure integrity of the data, the highest standards of research have been followed, that the study has been reviewed by an independent ethics committee and that the subject has been given full information concerning the study and has consented to participate. Once again, the lowest common denominator for standards of informed consent is documented in the Declaration of Helsinki which states:

> In any research on human beings, each potential subject must be adequately informed of the aims, methods, anticipated benefits and potential hazards of the study and any discomfort it may entail. He or she should be informed that he or she is at liberty to abstain from participation in the study and that he or she is free to withdraw his or her consent to participation at any time. The physician should then obtain the subject's freely-given informed consent, preferably in writing.

FDA guidelines and regulations

Studies conducted under an IND are subject to stringent controls and must conform with the FDA regulations concerning informed consent (Code of Federal Regulations 50.20, 50.23 and 50.25). These state that no investigator may involve a human being as a subject in research unless the investigator has obtained the legally effective informed consent of the subject or the subject's legally authorized representative. To ensure this requirement is met, it is important that all patients sign *and date* their consent. CFR 50.27 states that the consent shall be documented by the use of a written consent form approved by the IRB and signed by the subject or representative; a copy shall be given to the person signing the form. There are some exceptions allowed, mainly covering administration of test medications in urgent situations (CFR 50.23). In addition to the elements of informed consent noted in the Declaration of Helsinki, the FDA has a number of extra requirements.

1   There should be a statement confirming that the study involves research, an explanation of the purposes of the research and the expected duration of the subject's participation, a description of procedures to be followed and identification of any procedures which are experimental.
2   A description of any reasonably foreseeable risks or discomforts to the subject.
3   A description of any benefits to the subject or to others which may reasonably be expected from the research.
4   A disclosure of appropriate alternative procedures or course of treatment if any, that might be advantageous to the subject.
5   A statement describing the extent, if any, to which confidentiality of records identifying the subject will be maintained and that notes the possibility that the FDA may inspect the records.

6 For research involving more than minimal risk, an explanation as to whether any compensation and medical treatments are available if injury occurs and, if so, what they consist of or where further information may be obtained.

7 An explanation of whom to contact for answers to pertinent questions about the research and research subject's rights, and whom to contact in the event of a research-related injury to the subject.

The FDA also provides a list of additional elements of consent which may be appropriate for special studies. For studies not conducted under an IND, the FDA expects the consent procedure to comply with the Declaration of Helsinki or the local laws and regulations, whichever offer greater protection to the subject.

The EC *GCP Guidelines* are less stringent than FDA regulations. Consent should be given in both oral and written form *whenever possible*. The possibility of external review of confidential patient records is extended by stating: 'the subject must be made aware and consent that personal information may be scrutinised during audit by competent authorities and properly authorised persons but that personal information will be treated as strictly confidential and not be publicly available'.

Consent must be documented either by the subject's dated signature or by the signature of an independent witness who records the subject's assent. There is a special provision made for subjects in non-therapeutic research; their consent must always be given by the signature of the subject.

Finally, the ICH GCP guideline conforms with the EC guidelines with the following differences:

1 Information should be given to the subject by a medically qualified person. Although this is not clearly specified in the EC guidelines, the Declaration of Helsinki states that 'the *physician* should obtain the subject's freely-given informed consent'.

2 Access to the patient's personal information is extended to monitoring procedures as well as audit.

3 There is a requirement for the subject *personally* to date his or her signature confirming consent; also the witness must personally date his or her signature.

4 There is clarification within the guidelines of what is acceptable as an independent witness: 'one who can not be unfairly influenced by those involved in the clinical trial; and one who attends the informed consent process'.

5 There is a statement concerning members of hierarchial structures such as medical, pharmacy and nursing students, subordinate hospital and laboratory personnel, employees of the pharmaceutical industry and

members of the armed forces. This is to ensure that the willingness to volunteer is not unduly influenced by external pressure.

It should always be remembered that subjects are the most important people in any clinical research project; without their support there would be no research. It is imperative that their rights are respected by all those concerned with the evaluation of new medicines. A relatively high proportion of the content of every GCP guideline or regulation is concerned with ensuring that the rights of the individual are respected both in terms of ensuring that independent ethical review of the proposal is conducted and the subject information and consent process reviewed. The Declaration of Helsinki continues to form the bedrock of statements on medical ethics; however, the prudent clinical researcher will ensure that all projects are conducted to the highest standard required by any regulatory body or local law.

Regardless of where clinical research is conducted, it is the responsibility of the sponsor to ensure that the study has been submitted to the appropriate ethics committee/IRB for review and advice; documented confirmation of such approval must be provided to the sponsor regardless of whoever liaises with the ethics committee. With the cost of drug development increasing expotentially, pharmaceutical companies are increasingly conducting their phase III programmes on an international scale. It makes sense to ensure that all study documentation and procedures meet the standards expected by the regulatory authorities with responsibility of approving the drug for all potential markets. Until such time as the ICH guidelines for GCP are universally accepted, all national GCP requirements should be considered. As a minimum standard the sponsor should ensure that the following information is documented and filed to support future regulatory audits:

1   Written confirmation of submission of the protocol for review. This should clearly identify the protocol by full name, number, date and status (i.e. final). There should also be a statement confirming that the informed consent/patient information sheet has been included or appended plus any other documents, especially amendments. This letter should be dated.
2   Written confirmation of ethical review. This should confirm the name of the ethics committee or IRB and the address and be dated. The full title and identifying code number of the study protocol should be recorded. The committee should confirm its approval of the informed consent.
3   Constitution and composition of ethics committee/IRB. The committee should provide details of its constitution (working practices) and composition. In addition, details of those members attending the

meeting should be provided. The list of members should contain the names and professions of all members. If a member of the investigational team is listed then assurance must be obtained that he or she did not vote on the proposal.

4 Study protocol amendments. All protocol amendments must be submitted to the approving EC/IRB, at least for their information. If an amendment is likely to affect the safety of subjects, the committee must give its opinion in writing. Such amendments should not be implemented until the required approval has been received unless the delay caused by this process exposes subjects to immediate hazard or danger.

5 Safety issues. The approving committee must be informed of all serious and/or unexpected adverse events occurring during the course of the study. The FDA requires IRBs to be given annual reports of studies they have approved.

Multinational clinical research

It is common practice for pharmaceutical companies to conduct their large phase III studies on a multinational basis; as time is of the essence for these programmes, knowledge of the local ethical review procedures is essential. To review all the different procedures, even within Europe, is outside the scope of this chapter; nevertheless the following suggestions may be helpful.

The majority of ethics committees are comprised of volunteers giving freely of their time to ensure that medical research projects are reviewed and to confirm that ethical requirements are met and that subjects are protected. Ethics committees are often poorly resourced in terms of secretarial support; it is in the interests of the sponsor and investigator to help by providing essential documents promptly. Always provide exactly what the committee expects in terms of information and document what is provided. If information concerning the constitution, membership, etc. is required, request it at the time of submission, not later. Always explain why such information is needed; ethics committees often do not appreciate the regulatory constraints applied to sponsors of research.

For studies conducted in hospitals, the usual practice is to obtain approval from the ethics committee for each institution. There are some differences. For example, as noted previously, in France it is normally enough to have approval from one central committee with that approval being submitted to other participating institutions for information.

If there is no local ethics committee available for consultation, especially for studies conducted in general practice, it may be acceptable to use the services of a central ethics committee. There are a number of commercial ethics committees offering this service in Europe. Before commencing a study with a central ethics committee approval, always check that the procedure is acceptable to the appropriate regulatory bodies.

Conclusion

Medical research, regardless of where it is conducted, must always be subject to formal review by a correctly constituted independent ethics committee or IRB. To comply with GCP such reviews must be documented. No study should commence without written confirmation of a favourable response from the appropriate ethics committee or IRB.

References

Food and Drug Administration, Federal Register ZI CFR 10.90.
Guidelines for GCP. The Rules Governing Medicinal Products in the European Community, Vol. III (Addendum) July 1990.
Guidelines for Good Clinical Practice, European Community Directive 91/507/EEC.
Guideline for Good Clinical Practice (ICH), Step 5, May 1996.

PART FOUR

Multinational studies – pitfalls and benefits

11 Practical problems of auditing multinational trials

R Corrigan and G J Marsat

Introduction

The ideal clinical author would be one who was so well-trained that he or she was able to conduct audits all over the world. For an auditor to do this he/she would need to be aware of all regulations, guidelines, local laws, standard operating procedures (SOPs), medical practices and cultural differences. A further characteristic would be to be multilingual and knowledgeable of all therapeutic areas. Unfortunately such persons seldom exist and, if they were to, would be considered to be too experienced and for it to be a misuse of their talents to be merely contributing to a multinational site audit programme. Even if such an auditor existed, many of the problems that are encountered in auditing multinational trials would still remain, as only some of the variables will be limited. In many respects the problems encountered in auditing multinational trials are comparable to those faced by clinical research personnel when conducting such trials.

This chapter will address some of the problems faced and variables that can exist when auditing multinational trials. Attention will also be given to issues which arise when trials are inspected by a regulatory authority, in particular the Food and Drug Administration (FDA).

The rationale for initiating and conducting multinational trials varies and is dependent upon the individual pharmaceutical company. An argument often presented by the companies is that they wish to introduce the product into the market continent-wide rather than into a single country. The multinational trial will also have the effect of reducing the time between development and enable one product licence application to be made in Europe. To maximize this process it has become increasingly more important and routine for companies to conduct trials multinationally with prominent investigators.

Why audit?

The purpose of a quality assurance (QA) department is to determine if recognized standards are being achieved and therefore to be able to give assurance that the quality of the trial is being maintained. Audits are conducted of the trials to assess consistency with the protocol, accuracy and completeness of the data reported in relation to the requirements and the actual trial conduct. In addition, the compliance with SOPs and company policies, applicable regulations, guidelines and local laws must also be considered as well as the current and local medical practices. All of these variables can affect a trial in each individual country where it is being conducted but when the trial is being conducted in a number of countries, then the number of variables can increase dramatically and standards may become affected. However, there should be consistency in auditing procedures, whether the trial is a local one or conducted on an international basis.

General practical problems

A first consideration in initiating a programme of audits on multinational trials will be that of cost. In most companies the QA department is situated primarily in Europe, USA and/or Asia although there may be departments in all of these locations. The cost of sending auditors to the various countries will of necessity be expensive. In some cases it will be necessary for the auditor to require assistance in translating documents. If the monitor is not capable of performing this task then a translator will have to be employed, which will increase the cost.

The audit process

1   Selection of investigator site.
2   Schedule audit appointment.
3   Preparation.
4   In-house audit.
5   Site audit.
6   Report findings.
7   Follow-up.
8   Close audit file.

Planning stage

Investigator site audit selection

Multinational trials tend to be carried out in a core of countries, the selection of which is based upon the size of the pharmaceutical organization in that country or the possible patient population for a specific disease area. Clearly there are particular countries where there is a greater experience in conducting clinical research. Allied to this, the depth of understanding of good clinical practice (GCP) can vary greatly across countries. In Europe, Central Europe and Australia, the USA and Canada there are established regulations and guidelines with which doctors involved with clinical research should be well-acquainted. This may not be the case in less developed countries and those of the former Soviet bloc.

In selecting which countries to audit, which will require more attention, the auditor will inevitably be biased by the perception of standards in that country. In part this will also be influenced by what it is felt would be the attitude of a regulatory agency, such as the FDA, should they be presented with a trial from that country. Therefore it may be expected that auditors will devote more attention to those countries where previous problems have been shown or where there is a lack of clinical trial experience. It has been known for senior management in companies to request that all sites for a particular country be audited until reassurance may be given that the quality of work produced is of an acceptable standard.

The selection of trials for auditing will depend on the type and importance of the trial. In many cases multinational studies are commonly termed 'pivotal' since they will be used to demonstrate efficacy in the registration application. Although not always the case, pivotal studies are usually given immense resource support which will also include an auditing programme. Those trials conducted under a US investigational exemption for a new drug (IND) will also normally require auditing, as they will be open to inspection by the FDA. If there is a likelihood that the FDA will inspect a trial then it makes good sense for the company to audit it to ensure that it complies with the IND requirements. In some countries these are difficult to comply with, as many European ethics committees will approve a trial protocol but will not be involved further. Ethics committees are not currently undertaking their responsibilities with regard to an annual update review or even the 10-day alert.

The obtaining of written informed consent is another source of non-compliance with IND requirements. In some European countries it is still difficult to acquire a signature from patients.

The next problem to be confronted is the selection of the sites for audit. Seldom does the situation arise where a QA department is in the position to audit all investigator sites.

The criteria for selection of an investigator site may be quite diverse, depending on specific company requirements. Features that are often used to prioritize and help in the selection of sites for audit are:

1   Specific percentage (15–35% depending on company policy or priorities).
2   Percentage high patient recruiters across all countries.
3   Problem sites.
4   Percentage selection of sites from each country.
5   Percentage selection of sites for each monitor.

There are no definite rules on the number or which sites should be audited but it is advisable, if possible, to conduct audits in each country, with each monitor and to incorporate the high-recruiting investigators. This may result in more sites needing auditing than would normally be the case, but this will ensure consistency and identify possible differences in trial conduct between countries and monitors. The differences which are often identified relate to interpretation and cultural practices but when found in sufficient numbers will greatly affect the trial results. Where resources do not permit auditing in each country then a first priority should be to audit the high recruiters. Another method would be to review the data in-house to discover if anomalies exist. If distinct areas do exist then they can be followed up at the relevant investigator site. An example of this might be variation in the type and number of adverse events between countries' specific investigator sites or monitors.

If the focus is only on the highest recruiters across all countries then inevitably the low recruiters will be excluded from the audit programme. However, low recruitment rates are often associated with sites and countries that are inexperienced in GCP. It is important therefore that the auditor considers all the available information before selection of sites for audit. Either way the selection is fairly often random or arbitrary and there will always be 'hit-and-miss' errors or opportunities, depending on how one views it!

Timing of site audits

In considering when an audit should be carried out it is critical that for it to be meaningful the audit must be completed before the trial database is frozen. This will allow potential corrections to the database before analysis of the data commences. If the audits are carried out after the database has been locked then corrections which were needed to be made could compound any problems. The merits of timing site audits at different stages during a trial have been considered by many in the industry. There are benefits to conducting audits early, during and at the end of recruitment as it provides the auditor with insight to potential problems at each stage. Practical considerations make this very difficult to plan. Ideally the auditor would wish to conduct a number of trial audits in each country at one time.

The rationale behind this is that it reduces costs and limits the amount of travel that the auditor has to undertake. Too much forward planning of audits is difficult as it is impossible for the auditor to predict the future enrolment rate at each centre. Some guidance on the enrolment rate may be obtained from the monitor, but it will be an arbitrary figure.

Another problem associated with the planning and timing of audit is the availability of site personnel. There are many national holidays which differ from country to country which need to be considered when scheduling. In Europe it is often very difficult to plan an audit during the summer months. For example, many hospitals in Norway and the Scandinavian countries close wards for a month to allow the staff to go on summer vacation and patients are transferred to rehabilitation units for care. Likewise, a similar situation occurs in Italy and Spain where the whole country appears to go on vacation in August. In general it is difficult to get appointments for audits close to other holidays such as Christmas or Easter. When considering an auditing programme of a multinational trial across several continents then there is the added complication of seasonal differences, especially if the disease is of a seasonal nature. All of the above must be taken into consideration but equally the holiday and seasonal circumstances where the auditor resides and works may also affect his or her availability.

Not only has the availability of the trial site staff to be considered but also that of the monitors. It is preferable for monitors to be present at the time of the audit, therefore their schedule must also be accommodated. It is usually better for the auditor to request the monitor to arrange the dates for the audit. This not only lightens the workload for the auditor but it is also easier for the monitor since he or she will be aware of local details. The coordination of a large number of people is very difficult when one is permanently located in one place and it is difficult for the auditor to take responsibility for it if travelling across many countries or even continents.

Medical practices

Differences in medical practices invariably exist in relation to a multinational trial. Although potential areas of concern should be addressed and resolved where possible, it is not always the case that all these differences are known at the start of a trial. It is also the intention to conduct trials on a homogeneous population, but where it can be expected there will be heterogeneity in medical practices.

Before embarking on an audit it is advisable for the auditor to review the protocol in detail but also to help anticipate the potential variation that may be a result of medical practices. An example of this might be where patients in a British hospital would have blood taken at the outpatient department but frequently in the Netherlands and in Italy for example the patient would go to a specific commercial laboratory to have a blood sample taken. A consequence of this type of practice is that patients in the Netherlands often do not have their blood taken on the same day as the trial visit.

The generation and retention of medical documents may also be affected. In Germany patients may choose the doctor they wish to have treat them. It is possible for a patient to visit a different physician for treatment of each disease episode. This will present a problem for the auditor as there will be little, or almost no, medical history available for the patient. The patient may provide some medical history but this cannot always be relied upon to be accurate or complete. It is also impossible to establish accurately whether the patient is being treated by another doctor while in a trial.

A further example relates to the medical records, which in the UK are the property of the Department of Health, while in France and Italy patients own their personal records. In the latter case the retention of some documents for the purposes of clinical trials can become a serious issue. Scan reports, X-rays or blood sample results belong to the patient and if the audit has not been well-planned, this could present a problem in that these records will not be available for the audit.

There may be occasions for a multinational trial to be audited some years after the trial was completed, although this should occur very rarely. If this were to happen then there may be some difficulty gaining access and obtaining the source documents at the trial sites as there exist major differences not only relating to the documents that are archived by a hospital but also the retention time. More hospitals are now microfilming documents but this is far from the norm. There are no set standards covering this area; both intra and intercountry differences are apparent.

Cultural differences

The auditor must be able to adapt to various situations and understanding of cultural habits. Many differences will be encountered in cultures when auditing multinational trials but these differences tend not to be so great between Europe and North America or Canada. However, before the auditor works in a different country, especially if this is in East Asia, Japan or the Middle East, preparatory work needs to be done and information acquired. In doing so the auditor will become aware of how the local population work and behave. Complying with local customs, habits and practices will create a more professional image and lead to better cooperation.

Cultural differences can have an impact upon the days in the week in which hospitals operate for routine work. The normal practice in the UK or USA is Monday to Friday but this may not be routine in other countries.

For example, in Israel it is not uncommon for an audit to be conducted on a Sunday.

The hours of work also vary with the culture. In many Mediterranean countries it is common for the locals to have a siesta in the afternoon as it is too hot to work during the summer months. This will result in hospital clinics being held early in the morning, allowing staff and patients to be at home for the siesta in the afternoon.

It is also important that the auditor is aware of cultural differences in relation to social issues. In Spain it will be difficult for an auditor to find a restaurant open for dinner much before 9.30 p.m., which contrasts greatly with the USA where restaurants are open for dinner from 5.00 p.m. Also the auditor needs to be able to adapt to different food and diets when travelling.

As clinical trials start up in less developed countries, auditors should be aware of local health requirements. This could require immunization or vaccination prior to visiting the country. Specific prophylactic medication may also be advisable. Some companies now provide routine medical packs for auditors working abroad. Visas and travel documents may be required when visiting some countries.

Access to source documents

In many countries access to patient records must follow a strict process. As stated earlier, the ownership of patient medical records varies depending on the country. In most cases it is now accepted practice that the auditors of the sponsor company may have access to the medical notes of a patient as long as that patient has consented to it. However, this may not always be sufficient in every country. In Germany and Scandinavia the patients sign and consent separately to give permission for access to their medical notes. It may also be necessary for auditors to sign a document for the hospital staff stating who they are, their reason for reviewing the notes and confirming that they will maintain confidentiality. Likewise, in France it appears to be necessary for the sponsor's French medical director to sign a document which states that the auditor is employed by the company and will require access to patients' medical records for the purposes of the trial.

In general, in those countries where GCP is established, it is expected that an auditor will have direct access to source documents. This is the standard that the sponsor company should require from the onset of the trial. However, there may be occasions where indirect access may only be permitted to patients' source documents. It should be borne in mind that such access is not acceptable to the FDA and if they cannot have direct access there remains the danger that the data from that centre will be disallowed, which could compromise the whole trial.

Additionally, the Dutch inspectorate has recently stated that in the event of a patient not consenting to give direct access to the medical records, the trial would not be eligible for a GCP compliance statement/certificate.

Regulations, guidelines and local laws

It is vital that an auditor taking part in an auditing programme of a multinational trial is experienced. A key component of the experience will be knowledge and interpretation of the regulations, guidelines and/or local laws under which the trial is being conducted. If, for example, a trial is being conducted under an IND these regulations will be applicable as well as local regulations of the country where the trial is being carried out. In general, GCP standards are fairly similar but the main differences pertain to interpretation. When auditing in France, for example, the auditor must be aware of local requirements such as the reporting of adverse events and check that there is adequate information documented.

Company standards

Different companies will have different standards as defined in their local and central SOPs, which will have to be considered when auditing. It may be the case that local offices in different countries will define different standards for similar tasks and the auditor must remain aware of these.

Audit stage

Internal audit

The internal audit of a multinational trial will be dependent upon how the study is organized and managed. The trial may be monitored directly from a central European office or corporate headquarters office. Indeed, either office may act as the coordinating centre with the monitoring being conducted by the medical departments in the local countries or by an appointed contract research organization (CRO).

Where a trial is managed from a central office then it is expected that there should be a central trial file in addition to the files that are held at the local office which is monitoring the trial. In this situation both sets of files must be audited before the site audit. These files must be reviewed for consistency and completeness, also checking that all relevant information has been communicated to both the local office and the trial site personnel. If a CRO is involved then the approach would be essentially similar. This will involve more time and may also increase the costs considerably. Before visiting the local office it will first be necessary to visit the central office for each site audit as the information can change considerably from week to week. Of course, if site audits are planned close together then it is possible to do the central internal audits at the same time.

It can be expected that there may be documents such as regulatory documents at the local office which will not be present in the central file. Many documents at the local office will be in the local language, which may cause the auditor some problems if he or she is unable to speak the language. These documents will need to be translated which may slow down the audit process and require the involvement of extra personnel. However, it is to be expected that all documents in the central trial file would be already translated. Where documents such as patient information leaflets have been translated into the local language, there should also be back-translation to ensure that no substantive changes or omissions have been made.

Ability of the auditor

As already stated, the auditor needs to be well-informed of local requirements and laws, regulations and guidelines for each country participating in a multinational trials. It is important that these are well-understood when planning a trials as the auditor may have to advise on areas that may affect the conduct of the trials. The understanding of the regulations and guidelines is of the greatest importance when carrying out the audit.

Diplomacy is an essential characteristic for an auditor who will have to work in numerous countries involved with the trial and with various levels of in-house trial site personnel. In some countries medical doctors may not fully understand the audit process and can appear antagonistic and uncooperative. The auditor requires diplomacy and patience to gain the confidence of doctors in these situations. The ability to speak the language of that country is a great advantage as it will allow the auditor to review source documents independently. This will enable the audit to proceed smoothly and quickly without the need for the help of a nurse or monitor to act as translator.

In some societies there is a reluctance for the site staff to converse in English, even if they are capable of doing so. Again the cooperation of these staff may be gained if the auditor can be seen to be making an effort to converse in the local language. It is always advantageous to have the monitor present during the audit as he or she may be able to assist and explain issues and thus avoid any misunderstandings taking place. The monitor may also act as a mediator and facilitator during the audit process.

It may not always be possible for a QA department to carry out all the audits for a multinational trial due to limited staff resources. More demands are being placed upon QA departments, which invariably results in stretching the available resources. In some companies, in order to audit effectively worldwide the QA workload is being contracted out to a CRO. A check should be made on this CRO to ensure that it will conduct the audits to the same standards required by the company.

There is no clear way for management to decide which auditor is right to do specific audits. Some companies divide the workload by country for multinational trials. Other companies may decide that specific auditors will audit specific therapeutic areas, compounds or trials, regardless of the geographic location. The way in which the workload for multinational trials is distributed is dependent upon the individual company and the QA department resources available.

Conduct of the site audit

The conduct of the site audit for a multinational trial should be to the same standards as any other one. The auditor should, where possible, request that the monitor responsible for the trial is present during the audit to assist when necessary. The monitor may assist in many ways, by acting as translator, providing and explaining information in relation to the trial, allaying any fears that the site staff may have and in general smoothing the process. It is recommended that the sole purpose for the monitor being present during the audit is to assist the auditor and site staff and not to perform monitoring duties.

Audits other than investigator site

The auditing programme for a multinational trial should not be limited to investigator sites. If a central laboratory has been used for the analysis of blood samples then this should be checked to review, for example, how the samples have been handled and if there are any inconsistencies in the results across the various countries. QA may be requested to advise on the suitability of local versus central laboratories for analysis of blood samples; where there is a need to have results quickly to change the dose of medication or selection of therapy then it may be necessary to use local laboratories. Alternatively, if it is necessary to check the blood levels of the trial drug for toxicity or compliance then these tests may need to be carried out centrally, especially when the trial is a blinded one. It would be advisable for the auditing programme of a multinational trial to include such laboratories.

Frequently various parts of the trial are contracted out. This may include the monitoring in some countries, data entry or even in some cases the packaging of the clinical trial supplies. In some large multinational trials this may result in various CROs being involved, although where possible this should be avoided. Preferred CROs are now becoming common for some pharmaceutical companies, which limits such involvement of multiple CROs. However in this chapter space does not permit a full analysis of those problems encountered when auditing laboratories and CROs for multinational trials.

Findings and reporting

After completion of the audit it will be necessary to report the findings and to ensure that adequate follow-up to any findings ensues. Format of the audit report and its subsequent distribution will be company-specific. In some companies it is the policy for the QA department to release just one controlled copy of the audit report, which must be circulated to those on the distribution list. It is almost always the policy for all companies to prohibit the photocopying of audit reports. The most important issue in relation to the audit report is to ensure that all those involved with the trial in management and monitoring should be made aware of the findings. This must be achieved on a worldwide basis. It is also vital that the auditors on a worldwide basis are informed of the findings and outcome of the audit, especially if they are responsible for auditing the trial in their part of the world.

In relation to the follow-up to the audit findings, it is not usually necessary for the auditor to travel back to the site to check if the issues have been addressed or resolved. There may be occasions where major problems have been identified, when a site may require to be re-audited, which will require an auditor to return to reassess the situation. Ultimately it must be the responsibility of the monitor to respond in writing to the audit report, detailing his or her responses as to how issues will be addressed. The monitor must be trusted and accountable for this and may be requested to supply documentation to support the response. It is also important that all actions that the monitor has agreed to implement are followed up to completion. It is the trial management team's responsibility to check if the monitor is doing his or her job.

If an audit finding is detected or suspected fraud then this will require appropriate follow-up which will be dependent on the country in which it is found and also the company policy. Space does not permit a full discussion of this matter in this chapter.

Auditing consistency

As stated, in most companies QA departments are situated in one or all of the following locations – Europe, the USA and/or Asia. One obvious problem encountered when there are several departments sharing the responsibility of auditing a multinational trial is consistency. This consistency should exist in the broadest sense, beginning with how the sites are selected and audited, then afterwards with how the findings are reported, followed up and communicated. Worldwide QA SOPs will help to ensure that there is a consistent auditing process. Cross-training of the auditors will provide members in each department with the opportunity to share experiences, discuss opinions on processes, and to confirm and clarify interpretation of standards. Such activities will help to reduce the subjectivity of individual auditors but will not eliminate it. As QA is really the key element in clinical research for providing an objective view, the management must continuously strive to ensure objectivity exists. Auditing in pairs with members from each department will help ensure that there is good understanding and awareness of country-specific issues.

The FDA inspection (outside the USA)

The FDA role is to ensure that clinical trials are conducted in compliance with GCP and that the data submitted in a new drug application (NDA) are reliable.

The FDA will conduct foreign inspections when US trials will not provide the basis for approval and non-US trials will provide most of the data presented in a submission. Although in the USA the FDA has the right to inspect investigators' facilities, outside the North American continent the approach is slightly different. However, it is in the sponsor's interest to cooperate, as without inspection the product cannot be approved on the US market. The preparation of an FDA inspection necessitates commitment from the sponsor (monitoring team and compliance group) and also forward planning.

Pre-inspection activities

Notification of inspection
If the sponsor company has offices and a regulatory affairs department in the USA, the FDA will contact them directly. This is mainly due to the fact that the US Regulatory Affairs will process and submit the NDA.

The notification is in most cases a phone call from the Scientific Investigations Division of the office of compliance. At that time the protocols to be reviewed are identified as well as the sites to be visited. The FDA investigator will also propose a time frame for the inspection.

At this point the sponsor's US Regulatory Affairs should hand over the task for the practical aspects of the preparation to the responsible compliance person for the identified country.

Inspection dates
The FDA will propose a time frame, but this will have to be discussed with the relevant clinicians. This is one of the most difficult tasks as the inspec-

tion can cover two or even three countries, taking into account individual national holidays and cultures.

The intention is for the inspection to flow from site to site, minimizing delays. The other important point is that only an approximate time frame can be given to the clinical investigators (usually 5 working days). The key issue is to convince clinicians that they will need to be flexible with regard to the start and finish dates.

The last point is to achieve a consensus between FDA, sponsor and clinician.

Preparation of the inspections
This is in two parts – first, the collection of documents to be forwarded to the FDA before this visit and second, the pre-inspection site visit.

Documentation
For each investigator a collection of documents has to be sent to the FDA, in duplicate, it is also worth noting that, data on CD Rom is also now acceptable.

1   Protocol, amendments (with translations).
2   Sample of a blank case report form (CRF).
3   Investigator's curriculum vitae.
4   Investigator's brochures and updates.
5   Copies of each patient CRF; originals to be available on site.
6   The list of the ethics committee members.
7   A Summary of all serious adverse events.
8   A list of patient names with treatment and trial identification numbers.

This last item, depending on the country, can be difficult to acquire since, for confidentiality reasons, clinicians are not prepared to reveal patients' names.

The reason for this request is that, if the CRF calls for the patient's initials, confusion can occur as at times, the first-name initials are first and at other times last. Here again it depends very much on the country involved.

On a more practical aspect, the sponsor or in some cases the investigator has to ensure the FDA in writing of the following:

1   All records exist on site.
2   The FDA inspector will have access to all original documents.
3   For the duration of the inspection at each site, a photocopier, slide/microfiche reader and a view box for X-rays will be available on site.

4   An independent translator, approved by the FDA, will be present for the duration of the inspection.
5   All dates have been confirmed and agreed by all patients involved.

Pre-inspection visit to the sites
The main purpose of this visit is for the sponsor to assess the availability of all trial records, explain the inspection process and agree on the review of the records by the FDA inspectors.

The inspection

This is conducted in a very similar way to a sponsor audit:

1   Initial interview with the clinical investigator.
2   Review of source documents.
3   Visit of facilities.
4   Exit interview with clinical investigators.

The practical problems associated with the inspection are numerous and also unpredictable. The aim of the compliance person representing the sponsor is to facilitate the process.

The initial interview is usually difficult as the clinician is very nervous about the inspection. Also, in the case of non-English-speaking investigators, all communications have to be translated into the local language and then back into English. This process, if not managed properly, can create multiple obstacles such as misunderstanding or misinterpretation of what is required. At times people try to use their own initiative and perform their own translations; this again can lead to all kinds of misinterpretations and frustrations.

The inspection is a 'fact-finding mission' and during the initial interview numerous questions are asked by the inspectors, helping them to appreciate the trial conduct better.

The investigator is advised to answer questions as asked, rather than offering additional information which may lead to misunderstandings. Good management of this initial step by the sponsor is essential as it sets the foundations for the rest of the inspection.

At the review of the source documents stage, the sponsor needs to use tact and diplomacy to ensure that the clinician is prepared to let the FDA inspectors review the documents. In many cases a couple of files will be missing, as maybe the patient is still treated at the hospital and a visit day happens to fall at the same time as the inspection. The sponsor's role is to convince not only the clinician but also the secretaries that the missing files need to be brought back to the investigator.

The review process is tedious and interruptions should be avoided. It can be tempting for the clinician or the nurse involved in the trial to try to influence the inspectors in the approach to the data review. This, if not requested, creates confusion and frustrations and lengthens the process.

In the case of non-English-speaking countries, the medical information in the hospital records is in the local language. This can slow down the inspection as documents have to be translated and sometimes clarifications are required. Another point is that each country has its own way of abbreviating medical terminology.

The choice of interpreter is critical, as that person must be fluent in the local language as well as well-acquainted with hospital practices and record-keeping. An interpreter who is a native medical doctor will enhance trust with the clinical investigators and also facilitate the review of the medical records.

The visit of facilities such as ward, pharmacy or other departments can present challenges as patients are treated differently in certain parts of the world to how it is done in the USA. We all know that the patient population is more homogeneous than doctors and that one of the challenges of doing clinical trials is to use a single treatment in a large patient population with multiple clinical practices.

As the inspection progresses all involved parties become conscious of the time. Clinicians anxious to go back to these patients and inspectors to complete their review and move on to the next site.

The sponsor, who is the link between both FDA inspectors and clinical investigators, always needs to anticipate potential problems and is also the person to whom both the inspector and the clinician will look for help and assistance.

Summary

There are many lessons that have been learnt over the years in auditing multinational trials which should be considered when embarking on an audit programme.

Audits are becoming easier to perform, mainly due to the fact that now both sponsor and investigator view the audit process as an integral part of a clinical programme.

Harmonization will facilitate the process further but for many years to come the auditor will continue to be confronted with challenges such as language, culture differences and even medical practices.

PART FIVE

Animal health industries and good clinical practice

12   Good clinical practice in veterinary clinical trials

J Walters and S Hughes

Background

The late 1980s and early 1990s will remembered in the animal health industry as a period of intense turmoil in the marketplace, highlighted by numerous take-overs and mergers, and significant raising of the hurdles to registration, particularly in the veterinary product field. At all points in the research pipeline, additional requirements had led to escalation of out-of-pocket costs, regulatory review time and human resource costs, inevitably promoting constant reappraisal of cost–benefit evaluations of developing new products and maintaining old ones on the market.

Not surprisingly, the majority of these changes have surrounded the legislation that governs veterinary medicines, mirroring to a large extent the changes that have taken place in human pharmaceutical research and registration. Both types of products are governed by the same Directorate General – DG VI – and both have been subjected to varying degrees of harmonization as the single market took shape.

The veterinary products in question in this chapter come under the base legislation laid out in Council Directive 81/851/EEC (1981) and the related Directive 81/852/EEC (1981). Both were introduced for community-wide adoption at the end of 1981, although in reality it is only since the early 1990s that all member states have brought their local legislation into line. The 81/851 Directive was upgraded twice in 1990, first by amending directive 90/676/EEC (1990) and then 90/677/EEC (1990), which brought immunological products into the frame. Homeopathic veterinary products were incorporated by means of a further amendment in 1992 and then the attention turned to the 81/852 Directive, which was the origin of all subsequent standards and guidelines. The publication of its major amendment – Commission Directive 92/18/EEC (1992) – provided the first concrete signs of hard-and-fast standards for running clinical trials in veterinary products.

In the years leading up to the publication of 92/18, the Commission's scientific group, the Committee for Veterinary Medicinal Products

(CVMP), comprising regulatory and scientific experts from all member states, had produced a whole raft of guidelines describing in some detail the design features desired in efficacy trials on all manner of products and animal types. The broadest of these guidelines was the note for guidance on the conduct of clinical trials for veterinary medicinal products (1990), which was approved in May 1991 but has subsequently been superseded. It dealt with the definition and rationale for clinical trial design and gave a detailed account of the desired elements of the study protocol. The study report, clinical trial material labelling and clinical trial approval requirements all received brief coverage as well.

This document was complemented by Directive 92/18/EEC which dealt primarily with the requirements for reporting trial data in applications for marketing authorization. However, neither one gave much practical guidance on the conduct of studies.

It is beyond the scope of this chapter to describe in detail the content of other individual guidelines but what is deserving of comment is the process of consultation through which they passed. In addition to the many reviews that took place within the Commission, the documents were put out to industry for its comment and input. This enabled a range of experts to add elements of practicality to the final product and, although by no means perfect, it provided a basis for much useful dialogue.

The main channel through which these guidelines reached industry was via the European Association of Animal Health companies, the Fédération Européenne de la Santé Animale (FEDESA), based in Brussels. It was a subgroup within the federation, the Efficacy Working Party, made up of industry experts in clinical trials and regulatory affairs, which handled the lion's share of the work. The individuals in turn were able to call upon the wealth of expertise in their own companies, many of whom operated in the USA where a similar process was already well-advanced, with the result that an effective and highly constructive iteration ensued.

At the same time as these guidelines on trial design were emerging, the issue of *standards* was beginning to take shape. Probably the major stimulus was the issuing of the guideline on good clinical practice (GCP) for human pharmaceutical products, adopted by the Committee for Proprietary Medicinal Products (CPMP) in July 1990 and brought into operation in July 1991. This laid down, in some detail, the procedural steps that were expected, as well as emphasizing the ethical and data integrity considerations that would become so important in the running of clinical trials on human pharmaceuticals.

The animal health industry, already believing itself to be operating to fairly high standards, recognized that here was the next likely development for its own industry to face. Any lingering doubts were removed when the first draft of Directive 92/18/EEC was delivered for consultation to the FEDESA offices. At a certain point in the text, the words 'good clinical practice' were included (later to be removed), as was the following paragraph:

> Pre-established, systematic, written procedures for the organisation, conduct, data collection, documentation and verification of clinical trials are necessary to establish the validity of data and to improve ethical, scientific and technical quality of trials.

This, and the stimulus offered up by the GCP for human trials, persuaded the FEDESA group that they should take the initiative and establish a set of standards for the European animal health industry for the conduct of clinical trials on veterinary products. The process was started in the late 1980s, using the human GCPs as a framework, and a document finally emerged which combined the elements of the May 1991 CVMP guideline and the 92/18 Directive with significantly increased guidance on the conduct of studies. The gestation was long and the birth a difficult one, partly because terminology was often awkward in a multilingual environment and partly because, as the text emerged for consultation, everyone realized (especially those smaller European companies without the US experiences to draw upon) the enormity of the task ahead. The animal health industry was still getting to grips with good laboratory practice (GLP) and good manufacturing practice (GMP) and here was another apparent mountain to climb.

Nevertheless, born it was, in the form of a *Code of Practice for the Conduct of Clinical Trials on Veterinary Medicinal Products in the European Community*, issued by FEDESA in 1993. European industry, despite its reservations, was, by acceding to this adoption, unanimously agreeing to work towards the standards.

In a process that mirrored the earlier exchanges, FEDESA offered its code to the CVMP working party which by now was gearing up to generate its own document. It is a tribute to the efforts of the industry contributors that the text was firstly accepted and then adopted almost in its entirety as the essence of the EU Note for Guidance – *Good Clinical Practice for the Conduct of Clinical Trials for Veterinary Medicinal Products (GCPV)* – that was formally adopted by the CVMP in July 1994.

If industry felt justifiably proud of the outcome, the time frame for implementation was a source of major disappointment. The guideline called for the trials initiated after 1 July 1995 to be carried out in accordance with its recommendations. This virtual lack of a transition period left industry feeling unreasonably imposed upon, with minimal allowance being made for the extended time frames on which product development programmes inevitably operate.

The scope

Focusing specifically on the good clinical practice for veterinary medicine (GCPV) guidelines, it is worth defining the types of studies embraced. The prime target is clinical field trials on veterinary medicinal products in both companion animals and agricultural livestock. These are the types of studies that can be subject to the most variation and individual interpretation since often natural infections are involved as well as clinical judgements.

In reality, of course, the scope of GCPV is wider, embracing dose titration trials, designed to set a single dose or an effective range, and dose confirmation studies which take that single dose or dose range and confirm, in a larger number of animals, that the doses and use programmes are appropriate. The field efficacy studies really come at the end of the line, usually as larger-scale studies designed to confirm that the product will do what is claimed under practical conditions of use and to confirm that there are no adverse effects from using the compound as prescribed.

It is also important to emphasize that all the legislation and guidelines in place as this book goes to press relate only to veterinary medicinal products. So far, productivity enhancers and other substances coming under the banner 'feed additives' and handled by DG III under Directive 70/524/EC remain unaffected by the developments described.

Also specifically excluded from the scope of GCPVs are safety and preclinical studies and pharmaocokinetic studies. These are all subject to alternative, very specific guidelines which were part of the group of documents released by the CVMP working party before GCPV was in place. And in general, preclinical work may be governed by GLP requirements.

Main elements of the GCPV

Responsibilities

Critical to the success of any clinical trial is the assurance that responsibilities of the various parties are well-defined. This is why the opening section of the guidelines focuses on the specific roles and duties of the sponsor, monitor and investigator or site supervisor. It is a well-recognized trend that more and more companies are forced to seek third-party operations to conduct clinical trials. When these are established contract laboratories, used to handling GLP and GMP, then the task of implementing GCP requirements is a relatively simple one. The case is very different, however, with other types of institutions, universities, veterinary surgeons and the like who have not previously been exposed to such standards.

Inevitably, this state of affairs puts a great deal of onus on the sponsor to appoint well-educated and well-trained monitors who in turn play a major role in helping the investigator understand the importance of all elements of GCPV. They have to ensure that, before any contracts are signed, there is a high likelihood that all steps will be followed.

But it is also well-recognized that individual company approaches to this education problem are unlikely to solve the main issue – the lack of widespread awareness that the world has moved on and that much higher standards of validation and transparency are required. Recognizing this as an industry problem, FEDESA has again spearheaded an initiative to put in place training sessions for investigators and related disciplines. Its first step has been the publication of an *Investigator's Handbook* (1994), intended to offer a basis for a modular training programme to be run by the national associations and companies. It is encouraging to note that CVMP members and other regulatory officials have actively supported this training initiative and in many instances have expressed a desire to be part of the process both to learn and teach.

Whilst the definitions of the sponsor, monitor and investigator roles are self-evident, it is worth highlighting from the various documents what are seen as primary responsibilities of these parties.

The main *sponsor* responsibilities, many of which will be carried out through the appointed monitor, are relatively straightforward, relating to agreeing protocol, supplying appropriate safety information, obtaining appropriate trial clearances, establishing in-house standard operating procedures (SOPs) and generally keeping appropriate controls on and records of the test. As part of the ongoing, legal obligations, sponsors must also ensure that suspected adverse drug reactions (ADRs) are reported to the competent authority and they must provide adequate indemnity for the monitor and investigator and compensation for animal owners in the event of death or injury to an animal or loss of productivity.

Monitors, as extensions of the sponsor, have a key role since it is they (often in consultation with their research management) who could be involved in assessing that sites have appropriate facilities, equipment, expertise and time to conduct a study. They will invariably become involved in training the cooperating personnel, both in the details of the study and the main elements of GCPV, and they should become the main interface between the company and the investigator site personnel. Good record-keeping of all conversations, contacts and visits is essential and 24-hour availability is a virtual must!

This leads on to the *investigator*. This role is far more demanding than ever before, for not only does it take on the practical performance of the trial and responsibility for the health and welfare of the animals, there is also the added burden of being responsible for the validity of the data. It is sometimes a hard message to convey, but in agreeing, usually by formal contract, to run a clinical trial according to GCPV standards, the investigator is also contracting to take responsibility for the validity of the data generated. In the USA, this has reached the extreme where the investigator is personally liable in law for the accuracy and validity and indeed a number have been prosecuted for apparent falsification or lack of rigour in their control of studies. Hopefully, things will never reach that level of mistrust in Europe.

Animal welfare and the investigator

Although there is no formal requirement for ethical committee approval in the development of protocols (in contrast to human pharmaceutical research), there is a strongly implied requirement for veterinary surgeon supervision of trial animals. Indeed, the preamble of the GCPV guideline clearly states:

> The welfare of the trial animals is the responsibility of the investigator for all matters concerning the trial. All investigators must demonstrate the highest possible degree of professionalism in the observation of the animals in the trials and the reporting of such observations. Independent assurance that the trial animals and the human food chain are protected should be provided by the authorization procedure of the competent authority and the procedure for informed consent of the owner of the animals.

This latter point – informed consent – deserves some expansion since it can be one of the more challenging elements of GCPV, considering the wide range of studies and conditions embraced. The guideline calls for the investigator to provide animal owners with information *in writing* about their rights and responsibilities, including risks or inconveniences, objectives and possible benefits from the study and instructions for the subsequent handling of animals and animal produce. These latter points are especially critical where withdrawal periods are involved in animals destined for the human food chain. All this needs to be tied in with the owner's consent and a copy signed and dated by the owner for inclusion in the trial documentation. With companion animal studies, this is reasonably practical but with some trials in livestock, involving individual case recruits from a widespread locations, there can be major difficulties.

In the broad sense, the investigator takes full responsibility for all other trial personnel involved at a particular site or location and for its day-to-day running. In other words, it is necessary for them to be closely involved in a study rather than merely providing academic oversight.

Data handling and the investigator

Investigators, in agreeing to sign and date all record sheets, *guarantee* the correctness of the data and guarantee that it has been collected according to the protocol. This is where the monitor should be of great assistance in clarifying that data are being handled, recorded and managed in the correct way.

Chapters 3–5 of the guidelines give extensive recommendations for the proper handling of data, management and validation of electronic systems and expectations in terms of facilitating a complete data trail. In the end, all original raw data need to be included in the trial master file and held in archive, under the supervision of the sponsor, for at least 5 years after the product is no longer on the market. This demand is far more onerous than that for human pharmaceuticals.

Written procedures

As with GLP and GMP, the essence of the veterinary clinical standard is to encourage, wherever relevant, all parties to commit all procedures, agreements, amendments, analytical steps, sampling steps, data handling and verification tests, animal management – in fact everything that can be committed – to paper. The animal health clinical trial world has come to understand what is meant by 'if it's not written down, it did not happen'. Along similar lines, the Food and Drug Administration phrase 'trust but validate' has also gained in notoriety as many individuals being faced with GCPV for the first time wondered if their personal integrity was being challenged!

Clearly, SOPs and protocols form the backbone of any study, and the latter is heavily emphasized in the guideline. Key elements include the obvious need for clear objectives, good selection criteria for animals entering the trial, clarity in treatment schedules, blinding of studies were possible, definitive and realistic criteria for assessing clinical outcomes and efficacy – all decided *before* study start. One often forgotten part is a detailed schedule of events – a 'who is doing what to whom and when?' type document for the control and monitoring. This can be the most useful outcome of the dialogue between monitor and investigator since it shows how well the protocol has been digested and understood.

The final report

Extensive guidance is offered on what should constitute a final trial report (FTR). The responsibility is given to the sponsor company to ensure that there is one and that it conforms to a standard lay-out – essentially the format of the trial protocol, which also forms part of the report. What happens in practice is variable – between the report actually being written by a member of the sponsor company (usually the monitor) and the total document being prepared by the investigator. In either case, the investigator will be asked to sign the document as proof that he or she considers it a complete and accurate record (even though this is not specifically asked for in the guidelines).

One relatively new development that emerges from all this is the requirement to prepare an FTR for regulatory purposes, whether or not the study has been completed as planned. With naturally occurring disease studies, this can lead to a situation of numerous summary reports of uncompleted studies where the disease did not occur as anticipated, or a different or complicating condition arose. These reports may, however, be brief.

An industry perspective

It would be presumptuous to suggest that there is a single industry perspective on the impact and value of the veterinary GCPV guidelines. Certainly, those closely involved with their preparation in FEDESA recognized how complex they could have been had industry itself not had the opportunity to lay the foundations. It is generally felt by responsible members of the industry that there was scope for improving standards. The very nature of clinical trials, dealing as they do with sick animals, variable pathogens and subjective clinical assessment, makes them open to tremendous variation, complexity and misinterpretation. Over the years, as has often been reported, the quality of many so-called clinical trials that have found their way into the literature has been open to criticism because of bad design, lack of control groups, poor clinical inclusion/exclusion criteria and so on. So it was appropriate that attempts should be made to upgrade these types of studies and that steps should be taken to build in processes for verifying, tracking and storing source data.

A concern that has arisen is the potential for confusion between GLP and GCP. The plea of most involved in clinical field trials is to keep them separate! Even human clinical trials are not required to be run to GLP so neither should animal trials. The very nature of the conditions under which much of the clinical field work is conducted predicates against the installation of GLP procedures. The latter can be applied to permanent, frequently used facilities where consistent events are the norm, and routine practices are easily repeated. In the farm or domestic pet situation, often with farm or lay staff and animal owners involved and with the normal biological events that occur, much more flexibility is needed. As long as the EU Directives require field studies to be carried out under practical conditions prevailing in Europe, GLP will remain inappropriate.

The trends that have taken place in the USA have indicated that the FDA may see it differently. Certainly, there is an unwritten rule that studies will be audited against GLP standards and, unlike Europe, there is a large official inspectorate to 'police' the situation. The net result of this approach has been to force industry to use a growing band of specialist investigators, researchers and veterinarians who have developed facilities for clinical trials that can be set up to run to GLP standards. The danger with this approach is that studies can become too artificial, too removed from natural disease aetiology, so that it is only in the post-marketing situation that a product is tested in a real-life situation.

The future

There are signs, as global harmonization talks get underway in the veterinary regulatory field, that the USA may modify its approach and adopt the more appropriate GCPV-type guidelines to which Europe has moved. Meanwhile, Europe will not stand still. One can assume that sometime in the future, some form of inspectorate will be established to give accreditation to sites and studies and conduct live audits. Once this was in place, one could envisage more reciprocal recognition of European clinical studies as pivotal parts of US submissions, as happens already on the human side.

Equally, on the legislative front, we may well see the GCP guidelines being enacted as part of a directive, rather than being 'voluntary', as they are today. As this book goes to press, it still remains to be seen how regulators will assess, judge and comment on studies that have been run to the guidelines as they stand in 1995. It is to be hoped that they recognize the tremendous effort that the industry has brought to bear to reach this new level of trial quality. There has been much pain, massive additional expenditure and a great deal of energy expended in the process of matching the regulator's demands. And the only certainty is that it is not finished yet!

References

Clinical Trials for Veterinary Medicinal Products in the European Union – an Investigator's Handbook (1994). Brussels: FEDESA.
Code of Practice for the Conduct of Clinical Trials on Veterinary Medicinal Products in the European Community (1993). Brussels: FEDESA.
Commission Directive 92/18/EEC (1992) modifying the annex to council directive 81/852/EEC. *Official Journal* L 97, 10.4:1.
Conduct of Clinical Trials of Veterinary Medicinal Substances. CVMP Note for Guidance III/3775/90–EN.
Council Directive 81/851/EEC (1981) on the approximation of laws of the member states relating to veterinary medicinal products. *Official Journal* L 317 6.11:1.

Council Directive 81/852/EEC (1981) on the approximation of laws of the member states relating to the analytical, pharmaco-toxicological and clinical standards and protocols in respect of the testing of veterinary medicinal products. *Official Journal* L 317, 6.11:16.

Council Directive 90/676/EEC amending Directive 81/851/EEC (1990). *Official Journal* L 373 31.12:15.

Council Directive 90/677/EEC (1990) amending the scope of directive 81/851/EEC on the approximation of the laws of the member states relating to veterinary medicinal products and laying down additional provisions for veterinary medicinal products. *Official Journal* L 373, 31.12:26.

Good Clinical Practice for the Conduct of Clinical Trials for Veterinary Medicinal Products. The Rules Governing Medicinal Products in the European Union, Vol. III, pp. 3–20.

13 Practical aspects of monitoring and setting up animal health clinical trials in the European Union

C N Dent

Introduction

With the introduction and acceptance of the European Federation of Animal Health (Fédération Européenne de la Santé Animale; FEDESA) Code of Practice for the Conduct of Clinical Trials in 1993, many animal health companies within Europe started to review some of their existing practices and resources relative to clinical trials. The FEDESA code of practice was followed by the Committee for Veterinary Medicinal Products (CVMP) European Union (EU) Good Clinical Practice in Veterinary Medicine (GCPV) guidelines in July 1994. These guidelines require all clinical trials initiated after July 1995 to be carried out in accordance with GCPV. The differences in content between the FEDESA and CVMP documents are very little and therefore if the former was adopted by companies in 1993 the implementation of the latter required minimal further effort.

Companies also had to decide whether they would only conduct trials on medicinal products to GCPV standards or if they were going to include non-medicinal products such as feed additives and avoid dual standards, when conducting clinical trials.

Prior to the introduction of the FEDESA code of practice, in general, clinical trials were being conducted according to GCPV but without some of the paperwork requirements formally in place. For example, study investigators would have been selected for their experience and qualifications relative to the trial requirements, but this may not have been documented in the form of a curriculum vitae and retained in the trial master file. Also the conducting of clinical trials was very often a secondary, if not tertiary, place role for a member of staff. This may have therefore not allowed the required time to fulfil monitor responsibilities as outlined in the FEDESA code and CVMP guidelines. A trials monitor may obviously have more than one role within a company, but the role of the monitor had to move more into the forefront.

These are two examples of areas which may have had to be reviewed by companies initially relative to the FEDESA code and then the CVMP guidelines. These areas will be covered in detail in this chapter with suggestions on how to set up and monitor clinical trials and fulfil the requirements of the CVMP guidelines. Whether a company decides to conduct trials to GCPV standards for all products or only those for medicinal products is their choice, but the suggested systems and procedures will be the same for all products and all types of trial.

Project planning

For the smooth running of a clinical trial, initial project planning is required.

Identify the product

The product which is to be investigated in the clinical trial will have been identified as a new product, a line extension, or an existing product for further indications. Whichever category the product is in will affect the local regulatory requirements which allow the trial to take place.

Outline the study

Identify the type of trial, for example whether it is an efficacy or safety study.

What species of animal are to be used? Will single or multicentre locations be required?

Identify the personnel who are to be involved in the trial, both in-house and externally. Possible trial sites may be suggested at this time point.

Make a timeplan

Before proceeding further, a useful exercise is the preparation of a timeplan outlining the timescale for each critical phase of the trial.

A detailed timeplan may already be in existence for the development of the test product covering areas from research and development up to the market launch. An example of such a plan is presented in Figure 13.1. This type of plan can avoid ambiguities and misinterpretations and presents a clear picture of the predicted and expected completion of each phase to all parties involved.

From the overall product timeplan a detailed plan can be prepared for the clinical trial segment (Fig. 13.2). All the activities from the preparation of the draft protocol through to the production of the final report are included in the timeplan.

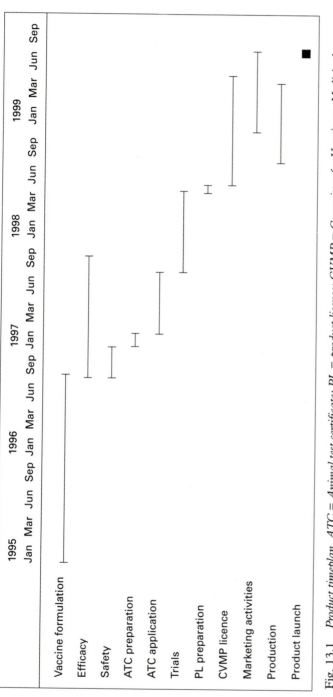

Fig. 13.1 *Product timeplan. ATC = Animal test certificate; PL = product licence; CVMP = Committee for Veterinary Medicinal Products.*

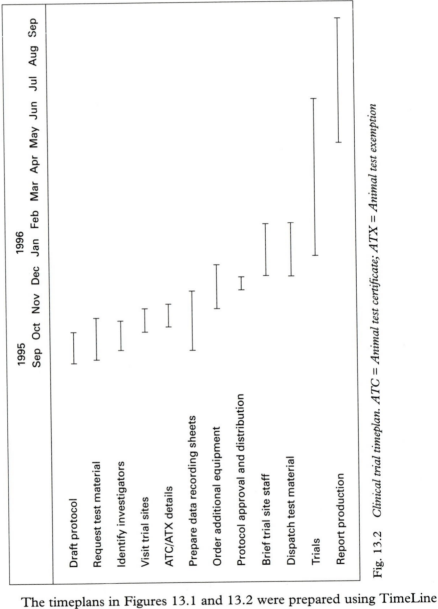

Fig. 13.2   *Clinical trial timeplan. ATC = Animal test certificate; ATX = Animal test exemption*

The timeplans in Figures 13.1 and 13.2 were prepared using TimeLine computer software.

Investigator product profile

The guidelines require the sponsor to 'inform the investigator/site supervisor of the relevant chemical/pharmaceutical, toxicological and clinical details as a prerequisite in planning the trial'. An area omitted in the list is immunological, which would be an important feature of vaccines.

A method of informing the investigator or supervisor of these details is by the sponsor providing them with a product profile containing all the relevant details. The information contained in such a document would obviously be of a confidential nature. Each copy of the document could therefore be supplied with a front page containing the following information:

> This investigator product profile is the property of *(sponsor name)* and as such must be kept in a confidential manner and may only be used in connection with the clinical trial. Information supplied within the product profile may not be reproduced or transmitted in any form without written consent from *(sponsor name)*.
>
> The product profile shall be returned to *(sponsor name)* upon request.

A record of product profile recipients, when they were issued and when they were collected or returned can be maintained using a form as presented in Appendix 1.

Obtain approval

Ensure that approval to perform the clinical trial has been obtained relative to the local legislative authority.

Budget

Within most companies a budget is allocated annually for conducting clinical trials. It is therefore advisable at the planning stage to ascertain estimated costs for a trial. The costs can be calculated more accurately during the project design stage following enrolment of the investigators and finalization of the protocol.

Project design

During the design stage of a project it is essential to have teamwork. There must be interaction between all parties, both within the company and with external contracted bodies. Use all the available expertise.

Protocol preparation

In forming the project team to prepare a protocol there are various disciplines and parts of the organization which need to be represented. Details on protocol production will be discussed separately in this chapter.

The sponsor

The sponsor company may be represented by an individual who is often referred to as the project leader. This individual will hold a position of authority within the company which will allow him or her to fulfil sponsor responsibilities regarding financial matters relative to the clinical trial. As project leader he or she will usually also have an in-depth knowledge of the test product and/or the clinical disease to be investigated.

Clinical Development

Clinical Development will usually assume responsibility for the compilation of the protocol, monitoring the clinical trial and report production. They will be able to give advice on the practicalities of the trial and suggest possible study investigators and trial sites.

There will usually be a clinician as a member of Clinical Development. They will therefore have knowledge of the clinical disease, to assist in protocol and trial design.

Regulatory

Advice may be required from registration to ensure that legal requirements are considered to achieve the licensing of the test product and to enable the trial to proceed.

Quality Assurance

Another area of expertise which may be called upon is Quality Assurance. If the sponsor company requires Good Laboratory Practice (GLP) compliance or work to the principles of GLP it may require or expect similar standards of external laboratories where samples from the clinical trial may be sent for processing. Quality Assurance may therefore be required to perform audits of these facilities. Also, if work is to be done for submission to the USA, quality assurance advice may be required as auditing of clinical trials is mandatory.

Marketing

Conducting clinical trials can be expensive and therefore where possible it makes sense to obtain as much information from them as possible. In addition to the information and results required for regulatory purposes to allow the product to be licensed, it may be possible to obtain information which may be used after licensing for marketing purposes. For example, where a positive control is required there may be a preferred choice relative to competitor products which marketing may be more aware of. Generally, data generated by clinical trials subsequently become most useful to marketing.

Test product supplies

If the test product is being manufactured within-house then a staff member will be able to indicate availability of product, as regards both time and quantity. If the product is manufactured by a third party there should be someone to act as a liaison person who can present details regarding availability.

It also needs to be decided at this time point whether the test product and control, either placebo or positive control, are to be blind-coded.

Statistical analysis

Access to biostatistical competence is mandatory. Some sponsor companies may have access to a statistician within the company or an external expert may be used.

The initial input of a statistician will be with reference to the number of animals required, randomization methods and other bias-reducing factors. It is for them to suggest requirements to ensure that usable data are generated for statistical analysis.

The previous seven areas, which should be represented at the draft protocol preparation stage, may in some companies form a project team of seven or more persons, each area represented by one or, in some cases, more than one person. In other companies the project team may only consist of two or three persons, each one representing two or three disciplines. Whichever is the situation is not important, but that all areas are covered at an early preparation stage is important.

Selection of investigators

Investigators may be identified in various ways. They may have been successfully involved in previous trials for the sponsor company. This is obviously an excellent recommendation. Investigators may be recommended by colleagues within the company and in some cases by the company sales force. Approaching the sales force in some companies for investigators may have to be done with care as with a new product they may have a tendency to sell the product as soon as trials are mentioned. Clinical trials are not a guarantee that the product will reach the marketplace, and therefore the sales force may be more suited to suggestions of investigators for line extensions or additional indications to products.

New investigators can be approached in particular areas of expertise either associated with academia or geographical location relative to disease, farming practices or social criteria, e.g. horse-racing stables, city locations for small animal trials.

An investigator may be a veterinarian in practice, small or large animal, and he or she may be in academia, ministry departments, either service or research. A manager of an establishment such as a farm, riding stables or kennels may also be an investigator. The choice is generally dictated by the study requirements and location.

An initial phone call to enquire whether the investigator may be interested in participating in the trial is followed by a copy of the draft protocol and product profile. The investigator is then given sufficient time to read the protocol and product profile to allow him or her to decide if he or she is interested in proceeding further.

A visit by the monitor would then be appropriate to discuss the details of the protocol, the timescale, trial sites and financial costs. At this time the monitor can establish whether the investigator is committed to the proposed trial and whether he or she is appropriately qualified and experienced in areas pertinent to the trial. Commitment to the trial is essential to the sponsor to ensure protocol adherence and appropriately qualified and experienced investigators are a requirement of the guidelines. Investigators must show that they are suitably qualified by submission of an up-to-date curriculum vitae and other credentials. A suggested format for this purpose is presented in Appendix 2. The investigator qualification form can then be filed in the trial master file.

Finalize protocol

The discussions between the investigator and monitor will allow details of trial sites to be included into the protocol and any additional useful comments which the investigator may have made on the protocol content and the trial.

There may be slight changes required to the protocol relative to individual trial sites. In such cases, depending on the changes, additional input may be required by the statistician, the clinician or any one of the areas represented at the draft protocol stage.

Protocol approval and distribution

The protocol must be signed by the sponsor and the investigator in agreement of the details of the clinical trial.

Other signatures may also be required depending on company requirements, e.g. regulatory manager, the head of department. An example of a signature page is presented in Appendix 3. A distribution list is also included on the signature page to record where protocols have been sent so that in the event of amendment to protocol, each person on the distribution list will receive a copy of the amendment.

Agreement and approval of the final protocol should be straightforward as all parties who are likely to be required to sign it have been involved from the draft protocol stage.

Activities concurrent with protocol finalization

Record sheets

Pro forma record sheets generated and supplied by the sponsor need to be clear in requesting all information which must be recorded. Where possible, loose-leaved sheets are to be avoided, particularly in a farm situation where they are more easily mislaid. Provide bound sheets of paper if feasible.

The record sheets must request only the data as required by the protocol.

In some situations farm pro forma sheets can be utilized and the required clinical trial data can be extracted from it. The poultry and pig production industries in particular are very good record-keepers, whether they are computer-generated or hand-written.

Whatever formats are used, check that the data recording sheets meet the protocol requirements and that there is provision to record all data requested.

Test product

The availability of the test product must be confirmed and the quantity required for each trial site ascertained. Identify whether packaging differentiation is applicable or possible between treatment groups. Colour coding is an excellent method of distinguishing between treatments either by using coloured labels or receptacles.

The test product may be required to be dispatched in one consignment to the trial site or in batches for each treatment time point. If the latter is required then provision must be made for a dispatch timetable to be prepared.

Carriage of the test product may be by hand, with the monitor making the delivery. In the event of use of a carrier, special arrangements may be necessary as delivery may be to a farm which is not routinely staffed all the time, and wheel-washing or other sanitizing measures could be required. Therefore have the test product delivered to an office or site where it is known that someone will be there to accept delivery. In the event of wheel-washing, ensure the carrier is made fully aware of such requirements. These are just two examples of special considerations.

Before dispatch of the test product, ensure there is sufficient storage space available of the required specification. For example, if the material must be stored at +5°C ±3°C, ascertain that there is refrigerated storage space available which conforms to these limits.

Additional materials and equipment

For some clinical trials the sponsor may be required to supply some materials and equipment to the investigator. These supplies may be disposables such as ear tags, syringes, hypodermic needles, blood sampling tubes, sample pots and bags and labels to be used to identify collected samples. Non-disposable items may include ear tattooing equipment, clinical thermometers and drenching guns.

Larger pieces of equipment may be required such as weigh crates, balances or creep feeders. The larger items may at the end of the trial be used to contribute towards any compensation due to the owner of the animals in the event of productivity losses.

Ensure that all materials and equipment are ordered or provided to be available when required during the clinical trial period.

Confirm regulatory authorization

Details of the trial site, the number of animals at each site and the supervising veterinary surgeon may have to be supplied to the regulatory authority, depending on local requirement, requesting authorization to carry out the trials. Confirm that the authorization has been granted for the site.

Protocol production

Information which should be considered for inclusion into a protocol is included in Chapter 2 of the CVMP guidelines.

Protocols for trials were obviously being produced by companies long before the CVMP guidelines came into existence and as such companies had their own in-house format and phraseology in place. For example, the headings justification and objectives in the guidelines may read as introduction and aim, respectively, in an already existing format, which is perfectly acceptable.

Although the chapter on the protocol is a comprehensive guide, there are specific sections which can be enlarged upon as follows.

Section 2.3 (schedule) suggests the expected start and finish dates of the trial but a timetable or flow diagram could also be included in the protocol, as shown in Figure 13.3. This provides an easy reference for the investigator and site supervisor of the critical time points during the trial period.

Section 2.4 (design) will include all details of randomization methods, which may be allocation to groups and to housing to eliminate house differ-

Group 1: Canine Anthelmintic	
Day after whelping	Action
14–16	Collect faecal samples or swabs from bitch and pups (on day 14 only) *Treat bitch* *Treat pups*
21	Collect faecal samples or swabs from bitch and pups
28	Collect faecal samples or swabs from bitch and pups
35–37	Collect faecal samples or swabs from bitch and pups (on day 35 only) *Treat bitch* *Treat pups*
42	Collect faecal samples or swabs from bitch and pups
49	Collect faecal samples or swabs from bitch and pups
56	Collect faecal samples or swabs from bitch and pups

Fig. 13.3   *Treatment timetable.*

ences, which is particularly pertinent to farm production systems. The statistician will very often have a primary input into these details.

Other bias-reducing factors which may be considered are treatment groups within one litter. This could be achieved within litters of puppies, kittens and piglets, where half the litter receive the test material and the other half act as the control group.

Section 2.7 (treatments) includes details for the control group. Where possible, use a positive control as opposed to placebo or no treatment. This is viewed far more sympathetically when dealing with commercial production farming, companion animal owners and by veterinarians on welfare grounds. In some instances, use of a positive control is not possible, but where possible it is worth considering as it will make animal inclusion into the trial speedier.

Rules for use of concomitant treatment must be made clear in the protocol. For example, routine use of a growth enhancer may be counterproductive if the objective of the test product is to control disease, where weight gain may be a critical observation of the trial.

Section 2.8 (assessment of efficacy) will usually be derived by the clinician, monitor and statistician. Between these parties an agreement will be reached as to what must be observed and recorded, and what can be practically observed and recorded to provide usable data.

Section 2.9 (adverse events) must be reported to the sponsor, usually via the monitor by the investigator. Details of the reporting procedure are to be included in the protocol, but can also be included in an informed consent form: an example is presented in Appendix 4. The owner would report such events usually via the investigator and not directly to the sponsor.

Section 2.10 (operational matters) is a section which may be lost in the main body of a protocol and should therefore possibly be placed at the beginning for easy reference to the investigator.

Although the subject of confidentiality is not mentioned in the CVMP guidelines, it is obviously a very important area for the sponsor. The following statement when used in the protocol is agreed upon by the investigator by signing the protocol. The signing of the protocol is an agreement to its contents.

Important notice to investigators. Confidentiality statement

The information contained in this protocol is intended solely for veterinary surgeons and trialists who have contracted with (*sponsor company name*) to conduct studies using (*sponsor company name*) preparations. The information must not be given to third parties or used in publications or lectures without the written consent of (*sponsor company name*).

Confidentiality regarding results produced from the trial can be covered in the informed consent form, ensuring that investigators or owners do not divulge the results to a third party.

Changes to the protocol may be in the form of an amendment or deviation. The difference between the two may have to be explained to the investigator to ensure that he or she appreciates that an amendment must be produced prior to the operation taking place and a deviation is a record of an unforeseen event. Examples of other operational matters such as data recording, signing of an informed consent form, test product accountability and invoicing are presented in Appendix 5.

As regards section 2.12 (evaluation), if a scoring system is to be used as a measure of the test animals' response a clear definition must be provided. This is an area which may require discussion with the investigator at the draft protocol stage as to whether the proposed definitions are appropriate in the practical situation.

Section 2.14 (supplements) can include specific procedures in detail, which will be particularly relevant for trial sites such as veterinary surgeries and farms, where there are no standard operating procedures (SOPs) in place. For example, where samples of any description are to be collected, details of the collection of the sample, labelling, packaging and postage should be provided.

The final protocol, as mentioned in the section on finalizing protocol earlier in this chapter, is signed by the sponsor and investigator and other persons as required by the company. The protocol is then distributed to all relevant parties prior to the start date of the trial.

The test product

Availability, packaging and shipment requirements have been discussed early in this chapter. This section will therefore concentrate on the request, manufacture, analysis, labelling and accountability of the test product.

Request

The request for test product is to be made as early as possible to allow for manufacturing. An example of a request form is presented in Appendix 6.

Manufacture

If the test product is being manufactured by a third party, an audit visit may be required of the manufacturing facility. The visit should be made to ensure that the sponsor is confident in the production process. This may be done by the monitor, either on his or her own if he or she is familiar with the processes involved, or accompanied by either a specialist in the discipline or someone with Good Manufacturing Practice (GMP) knowledge.

Analysis

Analysis of the test product must be completed prior to the start of the trial. Again, if the analysis is performed by a third party, an audit of the laboratories may be required by the sponsor company. The certificates of analysis are maintained in the trial master file.

Labelling

Labelling of the test product must conform to regulatory requirements and should include the words 'For veterinary clinical trial only'. The following is an example of a label used for a blind-coded trial in cats.

---

100 Tablets **Test Compound A**

For Veterinary Cat Clinical Trial Only

Dose to be divided into two and administered orally 12 hours apart in accordance with trial protocol.
  Do not administer to pregnant queens or breeding animals.
  Store in a dry place below 25°C   Expiry date: Sept. 96

Keep out of reach of children

For animal test purposes only   ATC _____ / _____

Accountability

Dispatch

An account is to be maintained of the quantity of the test product dispatched to each investigator. A dispatch form (see Appendix 7) is sent with the product and on receipt of the product the investigator signs the form and returns it to the monitor as an acknowledgement.

Dispense

The quantity of product dispensed is to be recorded by the investigator. This is particularly relevant in the case of a small animal trial where a veterinarian may be required to dispense product over a period of time to more than one pet owner. Provision for the amount of test product dispensed can be made in the data-recording sheets provided by the sponsor. If this cannot be done, a record form specifically for the purpose should be provided.

Return

All unused product must be returned to the sponsor by the investigator; where practical, empty containers should also be returned. An example of a returns form is presented in Appendix 8.

With the record of the quantity of test product dispatched to the investigator, the dispensing records maintained by the investigator and the amount of unused product returned, a final audit can be performed to ensure complete accountability.

A sample of each batch must be retained for reference for 1 year after the end of shelf-life. All unused product should be destroyed in a manner appropriate to the type of product.

Responsibilities

The responsibilities of the sponsor, monitor and investigator are comprehensively outlined in Chapter 1 of the CVMP guidelines.

As mentioned in the introduction to this chapter, the role of the monitor is possibly a function to which sponsor companies now have to dedicate more time.

The monitoring of a trial requires visits before, during and after its completion to ensure adherence to the protocol. These visits to a trial site, are also a positive aid in promoting good communication and cooperation with the trial site staff. The staff at the trial site, whether it is a farm manager or a veterinary nurse, are very often the personnel who are relied upon on a day-to-day basis for the smooth running of the trial. The investigator may be responsible overall, but may not actually be involved in observations and data entry. Monitoring visits may also provide the opportunity to identify problems which can be solved before they have a detrimental effect on the trial, particularly if visits can be made at critical time points such as sample collection, vaccination, or movement of stock from one housing system to another. Problems which may arise during these activities can then be solved as they occur.

The investigator's responsibilities are in general a mirror image of those of the sponsor and monitor. Although both the investigator and monitor have responsibilities regarding informed consent, ensuring trial site staff are fully informed of the trial details, test product storage and accountability and data recording, the monitor will very often take the lead role.

However, in time, as investigators become more aware of GCPV requirements and of their responsibilities they may require less assistance from the monitor who will be able to take on a supportive role in these areas. The publication of the FEDESA *Investigator's Handbook* is a useful aid in training and informing investigators in their responsibilities.

'In life' activities

During the life of a clinical trial there are activities which need to be fulfilled to ensure adherence to the protocol and the smooth running of the trial.

Monitoring

The most effective way of monitoring a trial is by visits to the trial site. The frequency of the visits will depend upon the duration of the trial and the number of critical timepoints which can be visited by the monitor.

If the trial is being conducted at more than one trial site, it may seem obvious to visit two sites in a day but it may not be possible if they are farms. Some pig and poultry establishments, in particular, will request that visits to other farms with similar stock are not made within 48 hours of their visit. Check before arranging two visits in one day. Also, in a farm situation, enquire whether protective clothing is provided by the farm or if the monitor needs to provide his or her own. Disposable coveralls are practical for this purpose as there is then less possibility of cross-contamination between farms. Visits to veterinary surgeries do not generally require protective clothing.

During the monitoring visit the objective is to check adherence to the trial protocol. The test animals should be seen and the number on test, their housing status and requirements, group identification and individual identification confirmed as outlined in the protocol. This can be done quite easily for housed farm animals but in a veterinary practice situation the animal records are relied upon to confirm inclusion and status in the trial.

Protocol requirements which can be checked, whether the trial site is a farm or a veterinary practice, are adverse events, test product storage and usage, data recording and ensuring that any points identified for action during the previous visit have been completed. All adverse events should have been reported as they occurred but ensure that they have been appropriately recorded in the data-recording system. Also ensure that all deviations have been recorded. The storage of the test product must be checked with reference to environmental conditions and that only product within its expiry date is in store; this is applicable for long-term studies. The product usage records must be cross-checked with the quantity recorded as used. All data-recording entries will be looked at and confirmed as up-to-date, legible, in ink, signed and dated with no use of correction fluid.

Time should be allocated for discussion of how the trial is progressing, any problems which may have been identified and suggested solutions. Also, ensure that everyone involved in the trial is content with how the trial is progressing and with operational matters.

Upon completion of the visit a monitoring visit report (see Appendix 9 for an example) can be completed, circulated to the sponsor and the report maintained in the trial master file.

Supply of test product

During a trial, a supply of test product must be ensured by request and dispatch of product at various intervals. The collection of used, and more importantly, part-used packs allows the monitor to account for usage of test product as the trial progresses. This can be easier than leaving the entire accountability until the study close-out.

Report to sponsor

The monitor is required to keep the sponsor informed of the trial progress. This includes all communications, letters, faxes and telephone conversations, results as they become available and trial monitoring visits.

A separate report on all communications can be made to the sponsor by the monitor in writing or the trial master file section containing these details can be circulated. The frequency of reporting to the sponsor should be agreed upon prior to the start of the trial.

Study close-out

At the end of the clinical trial period, known as the study close-out, all the data recording for all aspects of the trial is required by the sponsor for processing. This is usually done by the monitor.

Test product accountability

A final account of the quantity of test product supplied, used and returned is required. This can be done quite efficiently with the use of the request, dispatch and return forms, previously mentioned in the test product section in this chapter.

Ensure that a reference sample of the test product is retained. The reference sample is to be kept for 1 year after the shelf-life expiry date. All other unused product may then be destroyed. The destruction method will be appropriate to the test product. An example of a form recording the destruction of unused material is presented in Appendix 10.

Final trial report

Information which is to be included into the final trial report is detailed in Chapter 6 of the CVMP guidelines. A report is required for all clinical trials conducted, irrespective of whether they are completed as planned or not and whether the results are favourable or unfavourable.

The data collected during the clinical trial period require verification, which is done by the sponsor/monitor. All discrepancies which are found during data verification are to be included in the report.

All statistical methods and calculations employed to analyse the data require validation. The use of validated computer software packages removes the need for validation, but the methods and results of the validation must be available if required by a third party. Any missing, unused and spurious data during statistical analysis must be accounted for.

The final trial report must reflect the methods and SOPs in accordance with the trial protocol, the data recorded during the trial, all the results and adverse events. The report is signed by the sponsor and monitor to indicate that it represents a complete and accurate record of the clinical trials.

Archives

The sponsor should be supplied with all raw data from a trial for archiving. If this is not possible and the raw data have to remain at the investigational site, copies must be provided for the sponsor. In such situations the sponsor must ensure that the archive facility at the investigational site is adequate and details of the location of raw data are to be recorded in the trial master file.

The trial master file containing all documentation and data relevant to the trial must be retained for 5 years after the product ceases to have a market authorization (Directive 92/18/EEC).

All documentation and data must be made available for inspection if requested by relevant authorities and for audit by an independent body if required.

Financial payments

Financial payments should be settled to compensate the investigators or site supervisors and owners of trial animals for expenses incurred in the conduct of the clinical trial.

Costs involved in the trial and compensation agreements will obviously have been discussed and agreed at the time of investigator selection but compensation where loss of productivity has occurred will require to be finalized.

Final Comment

When conducting clinical trials to GCPV standards there can be an assurance of generating quality data for regulatory and marketing purposes. The suggestions in this chapter are one way of implementing GCPV, but as we are all aware there is more than one way to achieve the aim.

References

Clinical Trials for Veterinary Medicinal Products in the European Union. An Investigator's Handbook. (1994) Brussels: FEDESA.

Commission Directive 92/18/EEC (1992) Modifying Annex to Council Directive 81/852/EEC. Office Journal of European Community, L97, 10.4:1.

FEDESA (1993) *Code of Practice for the Conduct of Clinical Trials on Veterinary Medicinal Products in the European Community.* Brussels: FEDESA.

Good Clinical Practice for the Conduct of Clinical Trials for Veterinary Medicinal Products. (1993) Brussels: FEDESA.

TimeLine (1991). TimeLine Version 5.0. Cupertino CA: Symantec Corporation.

Acknowledgement

Thank you to Nicola Heron for the typing of the original manuscript.

Appendix 1:   Record of investigator product profile recipients

Test product:			Protocol no.:		
Investigator product profile issue date:					
Investigator product profiles were distributed to/collected from the following individuals:					
Name	Address	Distributed		Collected/returned	
		Signature	Date	Signature	Date

Appendix 2: Investigator qualifications form

Test product: Protocol no.:
Investigator name: Investigator address:
Curriculum vitae/résumé date:
Qualifications:
Experience in relevant areas:
Adequate time for this protocol:
Availability of trial sites:
Willing to permit an audit of all documentation. Willing to perform the trial according to the protocol and the CVMP *Guidelines on Good Clinical Practice* (1994).
Investigator: Signature: Date:
Name (monitor): Signature: Date:

Appendix 3:   Protocol approval signature page

Sponsor Name	Distribution list
Study Investigator Date	Archives (original protocol)
Monitor Date	
Vaccine Research and Development Manager Date	
Feed Additives Manager Date	
Clinical Development Manager Date	
Regulatory Manager Date	
Head of Technical Date	

Appendix 4:   Informed consent form

Study title ....
ATC no.................. Protocol no........................
Name ....
Address ....
        ....
Details of animals ....
        ....

I hereby certify that:

1   I have given consent for the animals in my care, as detailed above, to be involved in the above-mentioned trial.
2   I understand the objectives of the trial and agree to be bound by the trial design as described in the trial protocol, including details of payments and compensation.
3   I agree to comply with all instructions on the administration of the product, and health and safety data provided in respect of the use, handling, storage and disposal of the product. This includes information on the subsequent disposal of treated animals or the taking of food-stuffs from treated animals.
4   I will report to (*sponsor name*) all suspected adverse drug reactions considered to be related to the use of the test product, in line with the guidelines included in the protocol.
5   Information supplied in order for the trial to be performed should not be duplicated or passed on to a third party. The trial results produced will become the property of (*sponsor name*) and may be used by (*sponsor name*) in published literature and in reports to regulatory authorities for veterinary products in the UK or elsewhere. Representatives of (*sponsor name*) may review, or request, copies of any data derived from this study at any time, giving reasonable prior notice.

6   If any loss is suffered as a result of the participation of the animals in the trial, including their death (*sponsor name*), only liability will be to pay the compensation as set out in the trial protocol. In no circumstances will (*sponsor name*) be liable for any indirect or consequential losses or damages of any kind howsoever arising.

7   If I am unclear on any health and safety aspect of the product, or other query relating to the trial, guidance and advice can be sought from the trial supervisor or (*sponsor name*) monitor.

Signed .... Date ....

Appendix 5: Examples of operational matters

Protocol changes

Amendments to this protocol shall be justified, signed and dated by the Investigator/study supervisor and approved by (*sponsor name*) prior to implementation. All deviations from the protocol shall be explained, documented, signed and dated by the study supervisor.

Test product accountability/medication

Records must be kept of product usage and unused test product to be retained for collection by the monitor, also all medications given to any animal participating in the trial during the course of the study.

Data recording

Recording books will be supplied by (*sponsor name*). These must be maintained by the supervising veterinarian and will be inspected on a regular basis by the monitor. All corrections to data must be made with a single line through the error, dated, signed and a brief explanation for the error given. *Typist's correction fluid or similar materials must never be used for the purpose of correcting data entries.*

Trial costs

The sponsor will cover the following costs:

1 Free of charge, supply of test product including positive control test product and concomitant medication for the treatment of participating animals.
2 Veterinary fees relating to examinations and consultations of participating animals for the duration of the trial.

3 Administration costs of the supervising veterinarian in monitoring the trial and recording data.
4 Veterinary pathology and clinical pathology costs incurred due to requirements of this protocol. These will include practice laboratory work as specified.

Compensation

Compensation will be paid for any animal dying or requiring treatment as the result of administration of the test product, provided that it is administered according to the instructions contained in this protocol.

NB: All correspondence and invoices should be sent for the attention of (*name*) at the address shown above, and must be identified by the relevant protocol and trial site number and labelled cost centre 12345. Failure to do so may result in a delay in processing.

Informed consent

It is a requirement of the protocol that the supervising veterinarian and the owner of individual animals sign an informed consent form as supplied with this protocol.

Appendix 6: Test product request form

Test product:	Protocol no.:
Investigator name: Trial site address:	
Requisition number:	
Product required: Quantity required: Labelling instructions: Blinding instructions:	
Delivery address:	
Date required:	
Authorized by:	
Name (monitor): Signature:	Date:
Dispatched by (name): Carrier method: Signature:	Date:

Appendix 7:   Test product dispatch form

Test product:	Protocol no.:
Investigator name: Trial site address: Tel:	
Delivery address:	
Dispatch date: Details of carrier method: Special instructions for handling/storage:	
Description of items dispatched: Batch/lot number: Expiry date: Number of packages dispatched:	
To investigators: Please sign and return a copy of this form to the sponsor acknowledging receipt. This information is important so that an up-to-date record of supplies issued can be maintained.	
Investigator signature:	Date:
Name (monitor): Signature:	Date:

Appendix 8:   Return of test product form

Test product:	Protocol no.:

Investigator name: Trial site address: Tel:

Address for return of unused product:

Return date: Details of return carrier method: Special instructions for handling:

Description of items dispatched: Batch/lot number: Expiry date: Number/quantity returned: Number of empty containers or quantity of partially used product returned:

Investigator signature:	Date:

Returned items received by: Name: Signature:	 Date:

Appendix 9:   Clinical trial monitoring visit report

Trial site: Protocol number: Study: Visit by:	Visit on:
Trial stage:	pre-placement in-life close-out
Staff present:	supervising vet site supervisor others
Trial product:	storage usage records adverse reactions details
Trial animal:	group ID individual ID number on trial details
Housing status:	
Sample collection:	type details
Deaths:	

Non-protocol events:

Data recording: site file
                                 product administration
                                            animal ID
                                      sample collection
                                              housing
                                          body weights
                                           medication
                             other (give details below)

Details:

Additional comments:

Monitor: Signed:
                                              Date:

Clinical Development   Signed:
Manager: Date:

Circulation:

Appendix 10:   Test product destruction form

Test product:	Protocol no.:

Product returned:
Investigator name:
Trial site address:

Quantity returned:
Batch no.:
Quantity destroyed/sent for destruction:
Place of destruction:
Method of destruction:

Date of destruction/sent for destruction:

Signature: Date:
(monitor)

14 Assuring quality in European clinical field and laboratory studies carried out by the animal health industry

N J Dent

We are currently facing an increasing round of legislation in the animal health industry which, in may ways, has been mirrored by the earlier standards set for the pharmaceutical, agrochemical and allied industries. Legislation for the industry in general has been drawn up in these areas covering the testing of new chemical entities (NCEs) by Good Laboratory Practice (GLP); Good Clinical Practice (GCP) and Good Manufacturing Practice (GMP). For many years the animal health industry has been subjected to GLP when carrying out safety and residue studies in animals where the residues, such as meat, eggs or milk, will be subjected to human consumption, or enter the food chain. More recently, we have seen the advent of good clinical practice in veterinary medicine (GCPV) and the most noticeable documentation is that produced by the Fédération Européenne de la Santé Animale (FEDESA) and the Committee for Veterinary Medicinal Products (CVMP). This document is entitled *Good Clinical Practice for the Conduct of Clinical Trials for Veterinary Medicinal Products* (1994).

The document, which has been described in detail by other authors in this section (and is attached as an appendix to this book), is largely taken from the European GCP document which was referred to above and was designed by the EC for the conduct of clinical trials in human subjects. The key players in this animal health document have been FEDESA and CVMP. These organizations selected key people from industry and academia whose aim was to produce documentation to aid the implementation of testing NCEs, generic and existing products in the animal health industry.

This was to ensure the safety and efficacy but, moreover, to ensure that the data are internationally acceptable. As the reader will have noted from the other chapters, the key players are the sponsor, the investigator and the monitor. Those persons who are familiar with GCP in human volunteers and subjects will notice that there is no formal mention in the GCPV document of a quality assurance unit (QAU) or aspects of auditing the study. The main references in the CVMP document are:

1   Responsibilities.
2   Guide for conduct.
3   Data handling and statistics.
4   Data verification and the final report.

It was a deliberate aim of the persons concerned in drawing up these guidelines to ensure that the industry was not, at this time, restrained by the formal requirement of an audit by independent persons as is quite common in GLP and GCP within the human and agrochemicals areas.

However, this does not detract from the fact that, although the GCPVs are regarded as a guidance document, where applicable and appropriate, independent auditing should be carried out but, more importantly, a high level of quality control (QC) should be implemented at all stages of the clinical trial.

The animal health industry should by this very nature assure the quality of their clinical studies with exceptionally good selection of investigator sites and clear training for the monitors and the investigators. Above all, ascertaining that an appropriate and well-detailed study design has been produced ensures that the objective of the study is met with the maximum credibility of science and integrity of data. Most of all, this should be subjected to QC at every stage of the study.

To these ends, the industry should learn from its counterparts in the pharmaceutical, chemical and agrochemical areas and the author suggests, therefore, that the animal health industry does not reinvent the wheel. We have had GLP since 1976, GMP in excess of that and GCP in the formal sense in Europe since 1990. A large majority of companies therefore have extensive standard operating procedures (SOPs), clear protocol design and an audit unit set up specifically for these areas or activities. It is important that training records and all ancillary documentation mentioned in the GCPVs, which have been proven over a long period of time, are rapidly put into place. The animal health industry should therefore utilize the expertise within its own companies where these systems exist or talk to other colleagues who have already placed these items under the formalization process. We should learn from their expertise, problem areas and resolutions.

Although there is no formal requirement for audit and the document at present is a guidance document, the main difference is that there is no mandatory QA as for the human arena. This however does not mean that many companies do not have this in place and, in certain companies, the QAU responsible for the human testing and audit is now carrying out that function for the animal health products.

It is very important at this stage to define quality, quality assurance and quality control.

Quality control

QC is basically a voluntary measure put in place by operatives at all levels of science. QC guarantees that the scientific design, data generation and reporting as well as the work have been carried out to the highest quality; the integrity of the data is preserved; traceability and reproducibility are also covered and have received review by several persons. The QC aspect can be put into place in all areas by all people and should ensure that, at the end of the study, the protocol is accurately reflected in the final report, the data are available and archived and, more importantly, the standard procedures have been followed to generate these data.

Quality assurance

This, in terms of GLP, is an *independent* unit whose sole function is to review the data to ensure that the objectives stated in the protocol have been met and are accurately reflected in the final report and SOPs have been followed. Again the integrity of the data is preserved, and the overall results, conclusions and extrapolations are reflected in the final report in an accurate manner. The main difference between this and QC is that frequently only a snapshot picture is taken by the QAU. They may perform random checks of the data and subsequent calculations and be present at only certain of the critical operations that have occurred in the in-life phase of the study. This could be considered as additional QC but the QAUs would primarily involve themselves with checking that the QC systems that the company has instigated are in place and, more importantly, are being followed. The overriding difference of this unit is that it has *total indepen-dence* from those involved in the actual study. QC, however, is carried out *by the persons conducting the study*.

quality assurance vs QUALITY ASSURANCE

The author is suggesting that, until a formal request is made of the industry to perform QA by an independent unit, it is ethically and morally the responsibility of the animal health industry to assure the quality of the data produced. This, at the moment, can be done by regular QC checking; some aspect of auditing is carried out by persons who are not independent from the study. Hopefully, as time goes on and expertise is gained, a formal QAU should be built into the guidelines and, more importantly, this system oper-ated by all animal health companies involving themselves in clinical trials.

The objective, therefore, of this chapter is to continue to cover QA but to indicate to the reader areas where their company can assure quality either by the utilization of extensive QC systems or, where the company feels it applicable and appropriate, to have an independent QAU. It is not the author's intention to indicate that QA carried out by independent unit is mandatory or essential, but it certainly should be desirable. This independent unit, however, must be set up on a cost-effective basis and if small companies who are already extended in terms of staffing levels and budgets wish to implement such a system then, looking at past experience in GLP from the industry's point of view, it can only be seen as an additional layer of benefit. Studies will be conducted to a higher standard of science, work will be less likely to be repeated, the numbers of animals utilized will be reduced. More importantly, data, when generated as a submission document will be readily accepted by the reviewer and, most importantly, will allow multiple submissions to be made across EU countries and other major international countries without needing to repeat the studies or carrying out additional tests.

Where then can quality be assured?

If we look at a typical study, there are at least eight main areas where quality can be built in, checked and the assurance of this data or task maintained by QC systems.

1. Study design

To say that GLP and GCP are something new is an overstatement. The main aspects of GLP and GCP are basic common sense. If we examine in detail GLP and GCP we will find that these are techniques that have been carried out by the scientist, field and laboratory workers for many years. Now these activities require a more formal approach, perhaps with more signatures, perhaps with overviews by line managers but, more importantly, to ensure that the study can be reconstructed from data held in a secure archive for the required period of time.

With this in mind, study design should receive paramount attention as this is the overall starting block for any study. It is at this stage that all the appropriate tests, both scientific and statistical, must be considered and built in. A clear objective of the study is required and these objectives should be met by well-designed protocols, well-thought-out study designs and attention to the science. If these facets are covered, then GLP and GCP can be built in at a later date.

The whole aspect of study design is to bring together persons whose expertise will allow a study to be built up covering the science, covering the veterinary aspects, covering the husbandry, covering the statistics, covering the ancillary analytical and biochemical or laboratory assays and, finally, enabling these points to be brought together under a well-designed protocol.

The QC aspects for study design, therefore, should be to ensure that all persons likely to be involved in the study are brought together to discuss the study. The laboratory tests that will be involved should again be the subject of consultation to ensure that the tests that are required are not only applicable from the expertise known within the laboratory, but that they are also possible to be performed. More importantly, there are QC parameters that can be built into the tests in the laboratory to ensure the validity of the data.

Other aspects regarding study design would be to ensure that the feasibility of the study allows it to take place in a credible manner. The weather conditions, the availability of the host species, the viability of the animal, the availability of investigators and monitors, the selection of appropriate sites are all important considerations. The ability for the monitor to achieve the tasks laid down in the guidelines and that these can be carried out in a timely fashion with sufficient allocations made for travel and budgetary resources must be appreciated by senior management.

The final layer of QC is for the management of the facility to ensure that adequate resources are made available to allow the study design to proceed. Resources naturally immediately spring to mind, such as money, but also should cover animals, study sites, personnel, the supply of the vaccine or new drug substance and that all of these should take place in a timely manner to allow the study design to proceed in line with the project plan.

Having therefore addressed the general concepts of study design, the next logical phase would be to take this and put it on to paper. This then would become the formal study plan or protocol, as described in the CVMP guidelines. The author does not propose to cover this in detail as other chapters in this section have addressed protocol design and compilation. Reference to the appropriate section in the CVMP guidelines will give the reader the minimum information necessary to incorporate into the protocol and this naturally will be extended according to the study in question, the expertise of the persons involved and the overall study objectives to be met.

However, there are certain aspects of assuring quality in the protocol which must be addressed.

2. *The protocol or study plan*

This document is the prime document that concerns all contracts taken out with other laboratories, sites, investigators but, equally important, it is the detailed description and objective of the study that will be carried out in the company's own facilities.

It is of prime concern that good study design takes place, based on the scientific knowledge of the personnel involved in the study. The worries about GCP compliance should be secondary to the good scientific content and design of the protocol.

It is quite easy to amend protocols and this is one facility that the scientist and contract laboratory have to ensure so that the study progresses in the correct manner. However, one should not see amendments as a quick and easy way of getting a study underway without detailed thought about study design. The fewer amendments that are seen, the better. Too frequently one sees at least six amendments before the study has even started. This certainly leads to a general indication that no thought has been given to the planning and design of the study in the early stages.

The QC aspect of protocols rests firmly with the study director and the investigator. These two persons should liaise to make sure that the full objectives required by the sponsor are met at the investigator site. Where deviations are brought about, these should be minimal and, as far as possible, have little or no scientific impact on the study.

There needs to be a clear understanding as to the difference between deviations and protocol amendments. An amendment can be written to prevent a problem and should be prepared in advance of the new event taking place. A deviation is a result that has been unavoidable and is a complete documented set of notes relating to how and why this protocol deviation occurred.

The QC aspect of these two documents is of paramount importance. It should be quite clear why these were drawn up, the areas that they covered in the original protocol but, more importantly, to ensure that these documents go to all the relevant persons receiving the initial protocol and have gone through the review process internally.

The selection of the investigator and the advice of that expert person must be taken on board by the sponsor. In several instances I have seen companies approach an eminent investigator with a draft protocol seeking his or her advice on where to proceed from that moment. This advice is then unheeded. Despite exhaustive discussions and several good points raised by the investigator, the sponsor is adamant that the protocol will remain unchanged. The design aspect in this area is therefore completely lost as the investigator, having been asked in the initial instance to participate and provide advice, sees his or her efforts and advice to no avail. Yet the sponsor will then proceed with this investigator, expecting him or her to do a high-quality scientific study, whilst indicating that they are not really interested in his or her overall general comments.

In general, there should be standard protocols. Once these are set up and quality-controlled, this will enable studies to proceed rapidly and in a format that will be acceptable both to the sponsor and the investigator. Less thought will be required in the short-term standard studies, but a word of caution is relevant here. Standard protocols cannot always be brought into play when specific aspects of experimentation are required. In many instances standard protocols suppress scientific innovation and, with the advent of word processors, standard protocols held on file frequently begin by mentioning one species, only to move on to a second species within that study, mainly because somebody has forgotten to overtype or accurately proof the protocol. How frequently we see protocols discussing exploratory studies in pigs, when halfway through these animals change to cows and, more miraculously, at the end of the protocol revert to pigs.

In the protocol production phase, the paramount good practice is QC. Certain companies are involving QA in reviewing protocols; other companies feel that this is not currently required. The general consensus is, however, that when you involve QC, QA or assure the quality of the protocol, this very important document must receive extensive reviews by all parties involved in the study and the objective of the study must be clearly defined in this document. For further information regarding the content of these protocols, the reader should refer to the CVMP guidelines.

The protocol is certainly the forerunner of or, in many instances, the legal contract taken out between the investigator or contract laboratories. It must clearly therefore spell out retention of samples, responsibilities and, more importantly, clauses where, if necessary, the study can be terminated early or alternative aspects covered should things go wrong.

The protocol itself should clearly state that the ownership of samples is either that of the sponsor or the contract laboratory. The protocol should state the possibility for the sponsor to send in his or her own monitors or, if necessary, QA, for reviewing the study as it goes on or at termination. The QC of this document therefore is to ensure that all points are dealt with in writing at the beginning of the study rather than trying to put into place additional work or additional monitoring during the study.

This document, which as has already been noted is most important, should finally be distributed to all workers. This involves the main personnel – naturally, the investigator, but, more importantly, the workers at the 'sharp end' of the study, for example: the stockman, the person in charge of milking, the person in charge of feeding the pigs, etc. This protocol is a very detailed document explaining how the study will be carried out on a day-to-day basis giving finite detail. It is essential that everybody involved in the study sees either the document or the relevant sections to make sure that they can carry out the study according to GCP/ GLP and to the requirements of the sponsor.

One should not consider that the protocol is merely a document drawn up to satisfy bureaucracy but it should be utilized to ease the situation regarding variations in procedures. Key elements, operations and data can be extracted and made into a laminated diary format and placed in all critical locations in the farm, office or commercial stock areas. As we will hear later, all of the operations should be covered by an SOP but, in the clinical arena, often many situations arise where a test or an observation will be carried out only once during that period of experimentation. It is certainly not necessary in this instance to produce a formal SOP detailing what, when, why and how and have this formally signed off and issued. The protocol in this instance can clearly indicate what the procedure will be. Where minor variances of techniques are involved, these can clearly be described in the protocol and therefore the protocol not only becomes a set of objectives, but it will enable the operative to build in certain aspects of procedures into this document, thereby making it doubly useful.

3. Team approach

It cannot be overemphasized that, in GCP, multiple spheres of knowledge and team approach are essential for a good study and its design.

Likewise, to assure the quality of these studies, there should be several levels of QC. These aspects of QC primarily concern the checking of data, the checking of operations, the checking of test material and the final report.

Each member of the team must be responsible for checking his or her own specific area.

It must be clearly understood that signatures are required on documents and at all stages of the study. These should not be placed into empty boxes, just because the GCPs require identification of the operative.

One of the best procedures to draw up initially in any company is that detailing why people sign and for what purpose they are signing; in other words, their responsibility.

For example, the investigator naturally signs all documents to assume responsibility for the scientific conduct of that study and the accuracy and integrity of the data.

The monitor, by signing documents, confirms that he or she has visited, checked and approved the overall progress and acceptability of the study.

Technical and scientific staff sign documents to guarantee the accuracy and control that they have carried out in performing those aspects of the study.

The sponsor's representatives also sign the documents to state that they are happy with the progress of the study, its compliance with the protocol and associated procedures plus GCP compliance.

One of the final signatures is that of QA and these signatures on various documents comply with the requirement to carry out an independent review of the data and, most importantly, the only authorization that the signature carries is one for compliance with GCP. There is no indication from this signature relating to the accuracy, or otherwise, of the science.

Following on from the team approach, it is at this point that the circulation of all the relevant documents must be checked. For example, the protocol should be sent to all relevant parties and most especially to those support laboratories who may not be in the immediate forefront of the analyses but need to know exactly what to do and what the time frame is.

When new, exotic or different tests are carried out, these require to be validated and QC, both physical and theoretical, needs to be built into the testing systems. It is with the team approach again that we can ensure that the sponsor requirements are met but, more importantly, the capabilities of the laboratory can be reviewed and discussed to ensure that all of the data are generated as required and as accurately as possible.

The final aspect of the team approach is necessary to make sure that discussions are held with regard to resources.

These resources come in many guises. The prime resources are people, test species and equipment. It may be necessary to move these around to fit particular peaks and troughs. Another resource is the test substance – will this be made on time and are the appropriate QC paperwork and certificates of analysis available before shipment to the investigator?

Time is all-important and frequently sufficient time is given for the study to be just completed, but insufficient time is allowed for QC and the assurance of quality. All of these facets must be built into the overall timeplan when the project is first conceived.

One of the main resources that is often overlooked is money. Sufficient thought must be given to insurance, recompense in case of problems occurring, overtime and drafting in additional people to help out in times of overload. All of these thoughts need to be explored and many of these will involve extra expenditure. In these days of financial constraints, budgets are very tight and midway through a study extra financial resources are not always easily obtained.

4. Investigator

Several of the other authors have addressed investigator selection.

One of the prime concerns is preselection. This should be based on training and expertise, publications, the availability of the investigator and his or her willingness to participate in a GCP trial. It is not sufficient just to go to an eminent professor who will eventually pass the work down to a junior veterinarian, nor to elect somebody whose prime concern is to publish papers. The overall selection of the investigator must cover all of the facets detailed above.

Investigator meetings should be set up and it is here that the QC aspect of the study must be stressed. The investigator must be acutely aware of the study, and his or her role and the QC checking that must be carried out at all levels during the study. The investigator should be involved in draft protocol discussions and, as has been described above, his or her comments taken into account with production of the final protocol.

In any control system, it is essential to brief the investigator at all times. Information may come to the sponsor's knowledge from other clinical trial sites which will be relevant to the particular study carried out at a particular site. There must be clear lines of communication and an indication as to how this information should be transmitted to all investigators.

SOPs should be drawn up for or by the investigator, clearly indicating how the study will be carried out. These must reflect what will be done. These procedures will be the basis of checking by the monitor and, where applicable, QA. This again is an aspect of QC and assurance of quality.

Data-recording forms should be discussed with the investigator, both in production and completion. The time frame must be dealt with and strictly adhered to and – of prime importance – the sponsor should not discuss the expected outcome of the study. It is all too often the case that the sponsor indicates what has happened at other sites or what he or she expects to see. Even the most well-trained and well-disciplined investigator can, if given this information, make the study slant towards the sponsor's requirements.

Having selected the investigator, the overall theme is to build in quality. The investigator should be trained in the company's procedures, as well as trained in producing or using his or her own procedures where applicable. He or she should be well-versed in the equipment and its calibration and maintenance. On a regular basis, internal controls should be built in by the investigator, the staff and the sponsor's monitor to ensure that data-recording forms are accurately and completely filled out. Additional data are generated in a clear and concise manner and kept in a safe place. Storage of the test material and any samples should be reviewed and checked to make sure that these are in compliance with GCP/GLP, available for review by all parties but, most importantly, to ensure that the material is kept in the best and most viable situation.

The last aspect of assuring quality of the investigator is to make sure that the responsibilities are clearly defined in the protocol. Define in site documents where the sponsor's activities start and finish and the investigator's take over, where the site personnel must assume responsibility and report back to the investigator and where, if applicable, any independent monitoring or auditing will take place and to whom these reports will be sent.

One of the most important aspects of any study is to extract the major action points from the protocol, use an appendix in the form of a study plan and then produce a one- or two-page summary or listings of these action points. The summary should then be laminated and strategically placed around the site and laboratories, so instructions as to what to do at all times can be clearly seen. If applicable, an indelible marker should be attached to this laminated plan by a piece of string. The operative should tick off actions on the outside of the laminated plastic to indicate that these have been done. This would not be regarded as raw data but merely the satisfactory completion of action points. These action points should then appear on a formal checklist contained in the raw data file in the immediate environment of the animal or experimental area where they would be signed and dated. The laminated card is just an *aide-mémoire* so that the operative can immediately see what needs to be done and indicate that this operation has been carried out satisfactorily.

5. Monitoring

A programme should be designed to encompass several layers of QC, by the study staff, the investigator, the monitor at the site and on return to the sponsor location.

If data have been manipulated locally, at the investigator site, then this should be completely checked. Errors can then be verified and rectified. Ensure that regular monitoring is carried out and keep a good and detailed record of the visits. Phone calls should be logged together with a description of the call to allow complete reconstruction of the outcome and agreements.

A good correspondence file should be set up to cover letters, faxes and memos so that, again, in a controlled environment, this can be utilized by any third party to reconstruct the study.

The reader should realize that not all companies have the luxury of an independent QAU. Often the monitor will be responsible for on-site monitoring, as far as possible for independent reviewing and to ensure that all aspects comply with the protocol and GCP.

Where companies have a QAU, then naturally this can be undertaken by this independent body.

Irrespective of whether there is QA or the assurance of quality, it must be seen that all actions are discussed with the appropriate person, resolved and, where applicable, followed up.

6. Documentation

If we are looking to produce a quality study, all documentation must be easy to use. It must reflect the protocol, especially in the data-recording forms. Everything that is asked for in the protocol must have a relevant section in the data-recording form to enter the answers. The data-recording form should not be ambiguous, should not necessarily always ask for yes or no responses and where descriptive text is required there should be sufficient space to write this information, or use standard coded responses.

To comply with GLP, the material used for recording information should be ink. At all times staff should be discouraged from using pencil.

Attempts, however, must be made to ensure that where 'damp recording environments are prominent – filling out forms in the rain, in a milking parlour where liquids are about etc. – attempts are made to preserve the original entry.

There are not too many no carbon required (NCR) multipart data-recording forms in use in the animal health industry and therefore the types of forms and the media for filling these forms out should be very carefully thought out at the beginning of the study.

The QC checking of these documents is of paramount importance and often the original, which should be preserved at all times, suffers some minor mishap. There should be an attempt, wherever possible, to have the original document but in the case of pigs chewing part of the identification card on the cage, documents being eaten by cows or, unfortunately, excreta severely contaminating the original paperwork, then these may need to be amended or photocopied as authenticated copies. It may be that photocopies have to be taken or secondary documentation generated. Providing this is noted in the study file and a photocopy or other documentation is annotated as authenticated copy, signed and dated by the responsible person, then these data will be acceptable to a regulatory authority when contained in the original study file.

Whatever the situation is regarding documentation, this is one of the prime areas where strict and accurate quality control is necessary to ensure accuracy, continuity and completeness of data.

7. *Overall quality control systems*

Having outlined six areas where internal QC should be put into place, this will stand the originator of a clinical trial in a very good position. It will ensure that, not only has he or she designed a good study, and selected a good investigator, but also will have extensive monitoring of the systems to produce data which will be acceptable to a regulatory authority.

The final aspects of QC should be to ensure that good study conduct has the ability for an independent third party to review all aspects of the study. This system should be able to determine the following:

1 Why was the task necessary?
2 Who performed the operation or the task?
3 When was this done?

4   How was the event recorded?

5   What actions were necessary and who is responsible as regards the problems encountered?

6   Have the original aims detailed in the study plan been achieved and are they reported?

7   Has a good report been produced reflecting the overall high-quality standards that the work has achieved? Has the original objective been achieved and is it completely obvious to the regulatory reviewer with the information supplied in the final report?

8   Has the final report been quality-controlled? Is it a true reflection of the data? Has the integrity of the data been maintained? The report should also be a 'stand-alone' document and does not need further supportive documentation or interpretation.

9   Have *all* raw data now been collected, filed in a logical and chronological sequence and placed in an archive?

10   Is the archive itself in a secure place that will allow the documentation to remain in that area for the required amount of time, dependent on the country concerned? Is any movement of this paper in and out of the archive accurately logged?

8. *Quality assurance systems*

As has been outlined, at the current time there is no requirement for a formal QAU to be set up to monitor the GCPVs as with GLP human and GCPs. It is, however, a system that is being implemented by many large companies and has shown positive benefits over the years in terms of cost saving and ensuring that high-quality data and reports are produced.

There are no problems with an independent person being involved in this action from the company provided that there is no actual involvement of this person in the trial that he or she is reviewing.

If the company has decided to set up a distinct QAU, then this person or group will undertake all the actions shown previously in this chapter and be able to give management assurance that the study not only meets the scientific standards by reference to SOPs and protocols (study plans), but that it is in compliance with GCPV.

This unit, however, must be acutely aware that its role is to review the compliance and not the science. The science is the responsibility of the scientific personnel performing the study and the independent reviewer merely looks to see consistency between study plan and report and to ensure that the work is carried out in conjunction with SOPs.

Common sense versus good science

In the early part of this chapter there was a discussion on QA versus QC.

Equally, one must look at GCPV as being effectively the compliance of common sense in a scientific arena.

There is nothing new about the implementations of this new good practice in the animal health industry. After 18 years of GLP in preclinical science and a similar period of time for GCP in the area of human pharmaceuticals, the overriding factor is that the good practice is merely a formal way of recording data and ensuring what has commonly been carried out in laboratories and field studies over a long period of time is traceable.

Common sense must prevail and good study design is of paramount importance. The finer points of GCPV will then be the formal recording and review.

Regulatory authorities

Until an inspectorate has been established to monitor GCPV effectively, it is up to the individual companies concerned to claim compliance and to ensure that these claims can be substantiated.

One must not overlook the fact that it is the regulatory authority, the Committee for Veterinary Medicine (CVM) or Veterinary Medicines Department (VMD), who will review the data for the science and ensure that a marketing application is granted. Eventually, when an inspectorate is set up, it is this group that will be responsible for reviewing the compliance.

GCPV can provide bad-quality data and it is not possible to audit in quality or compliance if the study plan has been poorly designed and the study carried out to a less than satisfactory standard of science. It is the regulator who will be reviewing the latter and, at that time, can only make recommendations for additional work or clarification. It is the inspectorate who will be performing the compliance and, to a large extent, this is the area that will be new to the veterinary industry.

Typical QA problems

Although GLP has been established for some time in the veterinary and animal health areas, it is of paramount importance to remember that there are specific difficulties and differences in ensuring quality for GCPV by an independent QAU or reviewer. Such things as the site, the availability of appropriate staff, the weather and the seasons must be borne in mind when the QA reviewer is aiming to go to the site to perform audits.

The locations must be borne in mind as several of these may be some distance from the sponsor company and will require well-planned audits to ensure that the reviewer arrives on site to see the critical actions and has the ability to go from site to site. The latter aspect may pose a problem if there are visiting restrictions and if the person assuring the quality has previously been on a farm or site which does not allow him or her access to a second similar location. For example, it is frequently not possible to go between sites where there have been pigs within a certain period of time. Although a full plan has been drawn up to carry out independent reviews, this is where the plan may fall down. When arriving at the site, the first question that is asked is: 'Have you recently been on another pig farm?' If the answer is yes, then you may be denied access and the whole of the audit plan now falls into disrepair.

Other areas that could well be seen as a problem for the review are the data availability, the untrained investigator and the reluctance of the company to spend more money on a formal QA area.

Many of these are often unsurmountable and relate to company policy.

Data availability may be due to the fact that the monitor has not indicated that a third-party review will take place, or that the data are contained at another location other than the trial site. In extreme cases, it may be that, due to carelessness, the 'patients' may have actually eaten part of the data if it has been left in the vicinity of the pens or the field situation.

Regarding the untrained investigator, this again refers to the company taking time to set aside training and explanation as to what is required from the investigator.

Finally, with regard to a fully fledged QAU, this must have the backing of management and should not be seen as merely a means of satisfying a regulatory authority and as an unnecessary administrative burden. It must be seen as an independent check to ensure that high quality data are produced and, more importantly, that they are active members of the team involved in producing the final quality product for review. This action must certainly not be seen as one to police the effectiveness of the monitor or the investigator.

The failure of quality control with or without QA

Even in the best study design and the most effective company, QC systems will fall down and it is not possible to ensure quality after the event. Such areas as the monitor not having time to perform the QC checks are frequently seen to lead to problems in the acceptance of the final data and report.

Poor study design, with many protocol amendments, are often the normal means of carrying out work, but again this points to the lack of thought at the initial planning stage. The investigator, despite having discussions with the sponsor and the monitor, may well not approve of the protocol or not know sufficient detail regarding the protocol to carry out a full study. This, coupled with a lack of monitoring, naturally leads to a very poor study.

The inability of the monitor or the investigator to brief the staff adequately, especially those junior and manual staff who are very important in the study but may be overlooked in being given sufficient information for them to carry out their duties accurately.

However conscientious study personnel are, data inevitably become lost during the study. There may be a variety of reasons such as the animal actually devouring the data, data-recording forms, pen cards and ear tags; poor filing systems at the sponsor site, the investigator site or in the main experimental areas; information not being accurately recorded, notes being made hurriedly on pieces of scrap paper, or data-recording forms not being sufficiently well-designed to allow for the information to be written down; the use of non-standard forms which, when brought back to the sponsor site, do not allow the data entry personnel to take the information in the required format and therefore may result in data not being entered into the system or a précis of this data not giving the full picture.

QA personnel can prevent some of these, although the main criteria are for the monitor to perform good QC and for the company to assure quality. Those points mentioned above frequently happen, even though good monitoring takes place and is usually as a result of the monitor not being at the site on a regular basis. Certainly, to rely on a QAU to pick these up would be very remiss of the sponsor as that unit would only be present on very limited visits and can only hope to obtain a snapshot view of the overall study.

The prime concern is to be at the right site at the right time. This information can only be gained from using investigators and sites frequently and putting together those two combinations which give the sponsor a comfortable feeling when carrying out repeat work.

Conclusion

It is hoped that, through this review of GCPV, areas and pitfalls have been pinpointed that can be avoided by the sponsor, the investigator and the monitor and that the overriding objective have been met. If the reader thinks back to the initial stages of this chapter, the prime concern was to assure quality in European clinical, field and laboratory studies carried out by the animal health industry.

Once again, the overriding points to be borne in mind are good study design, effective monitoring, well-trained and selected investigators and an independent reviewer who can assure the quality of the study without being actively involved.

References

Good Laboratory Practices for Non Clinical Laboratory Studies (1980) Code of Federal Regulations, Federal Register 45:24865.

Good Laboratory Practice, The UK Compliance Programme. (1989) London: Department of Health.

The OECD Principles of Good Laboratory Practice (1995) Environment monograph 45. Brussels: OECD.

EEC Note for Guidance: Good Clinical Practice for Trials on Medicinal Products in the European Community (1988) Luxembourg: Office for Official Publications of the European Community, III 3976/88.

The Rules Governing Medicinal Products in the European Community Vols 1–4 (1991)

Good Clinical Practice for the Conduct of Clinical Trials for Veterinary Medicinal Products (GCPV) (1994) Brussels: FEDESA.

15 A contract laboratory review of large animal studies performed to good clinical practice guidelines

O Svendsen

Introduction

Good clinical practice (GCP) is an instrument to control the credibility of clinical trials with new drugs. The European Union (EU) Committee for Proprietary Medicinal Products (European Community, 1990) and the Food and Drug Administration (FDA) in the USA (FDA compliance manuals, 1985, 1988a) have drawn up GCP guidelines for clinical trials with human drugs.

These guidelines describe the necessity for systematic and pre-established procedures for the conduct of clinical trials to ensure their ethical, scientific and technical quality as well as to protect the rights and integrity of the trial subjects (patients). These guidelines are primarily intended for clinical trials associated with the pharmaceutical industry since the trials are mainly directed towards drug licensing.

Recently the EU Committee for Veterinary Medicinal Products CVMP (European Community, 1994) has drawn up a *Note for Guidance* of good clinical practice for the conduct of clinical trials for veterinary medicinal products. The provisions of the *EU Note for Guidance* apply for clinical trials with veterinary medicinal products initiated after 1 July 1995.

The European Federation of Animal Health (Fédération Européenne de la Santé Animale; FEDESA) published in 1993 their *Code of Practice* for the conduct of clinical trials with veterinary medicinal products in the EU and the provisions of this code apply to clinical trials initiated after 1 January 1996. Although the *EU Note for Guidance* draws much of its essence from the FEDESA *Code of Practice*, the latter has been updated in accordance with the new dispositions (FEDESA, 1996a). Recently FEDESA (1996b) published a book on clinical trials for veterinary medicinal products in the European Union.

The *EU Note for Guidance* intends to ensure that clinical trials submitted for regulatory approval of new veterinary medicinal products are conducted and documented in accordance with the Annex to Directive 92/18/EEC.

For this purpose pre-established systematic written procedures for the organization, conduct, data collection, documentation and verification of clinical trials are necessary to establish the quality of trials and the validity of data obtained.

Both the *EU Note for Guidance* and the FEDESA *Code of Practice* include six chapters:

1   Responsibilities.
2   Guide for the conduct of clinical trials/trial protocol.
3   Data handling.
4   Statistics.
5   Data verification.
6   Final trial report.

The aim of the present chapter will be to give a contract research laboratory review of large animal studies performed in accordance with GCP guidelines. In particular, this chapter will review the aspect of who has most importance for a contract research laboratory: the investigator is immediately responsible for the execution of the trial, the trial site and facilities.

Responsibilities

Responsibilities for a clinical trial are specified for the sponsor, the monitor and the investigator. The sponsor is typically an organization which takes responsibility for the initiation, management and financing of a clinical trial. The monitor is a person appointed by the sponsor to be responsible to the sponsor for the monitoring of the trial and for verification of data. The investigator is immediately responsible for the execution of a trial and in case the investigator is a contract research laboratory, a great deal of the responsibilities specified for the sponsor and monitor can in practice be transferred to the contract research laboratory on their behalf. In order to avoid possible misunderstandings it is important for a contract research laboratory to outline to the sponsor its expertise for any specific study to be undertaken, and to specify to the sponsor and monitor its competence during study conduct.

Although each sponsor is responsible for establishment of standard operation procedures (SOPs) for the elements contained in the protocol, the contract research laboratory is expected to provide detailed SOPs for activities the laboratory has agreed to undertake. Unlike the good laboratory practice (GLP) regulations for safety studies with drugs and chemicals, the *EU Note for Guidance* or the FEDESA *Code of Practice* for clinical trials do not specifically require a separate quality assurance unit (QAU). The responsibilities of the monitor as specified in the *EU Note for Guidance* are very similar to those specified for a QAU and therefore may be transferred to the QAU in contract research laboratories which adopt a QAU system of monitoring. Before entering into a study this transfer should be detailed between the contract research laboratory and the sponsor plus monitor. Conflicts may arise between the contract research laboratory and a sponsor-appointed monitor who is unfamiliar with the QAU system. Such conflicts are difficult to manage to satisfy the customer and at the same time remain in compliance with GCP guidelines.

Standard operating procedures

SOPs are the instructions that govern all aspects of daily activities in a laboratory and animal facility. The Organization for Economic Cooperation and Development (OECD, 1982) principles define the function of SOPs as to 'describe how to perform certain routine laboratory tests or activities normally not specified in detail in study plans or test guidelines'; and the purposes as 'intended to ensure the quality and integrity of the data generated in the course of the study'.

The OECD principles state clearly that SOPs should be available for, but not limited to, the following categories of laboratory activities: test and reference substance, apparatus and reagents, record-keeping, reporting, storage and retrieval, test system, quality assurance procedures, and health and safety precautions.

Different individuals have different ways of performing the same or similar operations. SOPs are technical documents designed and written as instructions for the person carrying out an operation and they are intended to be readily available to personnel performing operations. Writing SOPs involves a critical examination of these operations either to define the optimum method or to allow options. SOPs are thus reference manuals to allow procedures to be checked before implementation and to ensure that all operators perform in the same way.

As mentioned above, the sponsor of a clinical trial is responsible for establishment of detailed SOPs for the elements contained in the protocol. This obligation may most practically be transferred to the contract research laboratory which in many cases already has SOPs for a great many of the activities involved in clinicial trials. At Scantox, working according to GLP regulations of the OECD the laboratory would be reluctant to work to the sponsor's SOPs, and the laboratory has never been asked to do so. It would, in many cases, necessitate translation, rewriting into the SOP style of Scantox and training staff in the sponsor's procedure.

For any new critical procedure by a protocol, it is important for the contract research laboratory to establish SOPs in the form of a rational standardized recording system of clinical data with a valid scoring system in particular for subjective clinical parameters. These and existing SOPs for other critical procedures should be discussed in detail with the sponsor.

Protocol

A well-designed trial relies predominantly on a thoroughly considered, well-structured and complete protocol. Both the sponsor and the investigator sign the protocol as an approval and agreement of the details of the clinical trial. This includes the investigator confirming that the work will be carried out according to the protocol and the GCP guidelines.

Since most clinical trials are complicated, expensive and based on non-routine design, it is always worthwhile considering a preceding pilot study including the most critical elements of the subsequent trial. A pilot study may provide the sponsor and the contract research laboratory with information important for protocol design, SOPs, record sheets, data handling, etc.

The protocol for the clinical trial must, where relevant, include the following information:

1   General information.
2   Justification and objectives.
3   Schedule.
4   Design.
5   Animal selection.
6   Inclusion/exclusion criteria.
7   Treatments.
8   Assessment and efficacy.
9   Adverse events.
10   Operational matter.
11   Handling of records.
12   Evaluation.
13   Statistics.
14   Supplements.
15   References.

Animal selection, inclusion/exclusion, criteria, treatments and assessment of efficacy are those points which should be given most attention since the aim of the study is to establish dosages and effectiveness. The usefulness of a trial depends primarily on thorough consideration of these points, first of all for the protocol, but also for the design of SOPs and record sheets in order to facilitate correct execution of the study and subsequent interpretation of the results obtained.

Not only the type of animal to be used, but also the housing and the management (feeding, etc.) have to be specified in the protocol and subsequently documented during the trial. The protocol should also give provision of a clear statement of diagnostic admission criteria and a detailed list of the criteria for inclusion, exclusion and post-admission withdrawals of animals from the study. Properly and pre-trial-designed record sheets for these aspects ensure protocol compliance and subsequent documentation.

In particular in clinical trials with pregnant animals, young animals or animals carrying an experimental disease, the contract research laboratory should inform the sponsor about difficulties that may arise as regards fulfilment of inclusion or exclusion criteria. This may include non-pregnancy, outbreak of spontaneous young animal disease or too little or too great efficacy of challenge dose.

As for the treatment, clear and precise descriptions in the protocol of dosing schedules, treatment periods and concomitant treatment are important together with establishment of measures to promote and control adherence to this part of the protocol. Such measures may again be pre-trial-designed record sheets.

The assessment of efficacy relies on the definition of the effects to be achieved before efficacy can be claimed, and on descriptions of how such effects are measured and recorded. They are consequently crucial elements of the protocol and thoroughly designed record sheets are useful for documentation of the effects obtained.

To be considered is also alternative therapy in the event of drug failure and subsequent recording of the response to the alternative therapy.

Record sheets

The importance of pre-established record sheets tailored to meet as many requirements of the protocol as possible cannot be overemphasized. Establishment of specific record sheets take a good deal of time but when the trial has been completed, this time is regained by making the interpretation of the data much easier.

Pre-established record sheets assist in ensuring compliance with the requirements of the protocol. Proper usage of record sheets is not only important for the documentation of data obtained. They can be equally important for documentation of adherence to the protocol. A few examples have already been given under the protocol section describing animal selection, inclusion criteria, treatment and measurement of effects.

Three examples of record sheets are given in Appendices 1–3.

Dispensary records

Drug accountability is an important part of the integrity of a clinical trial. Certificates of delivery of the drug, including quantities of drug supplied, must also detail the method and place of storage. It is important to establish that the correct amounts and dosage forms of the drug, as specified in the protocol, were received by the investigator. In addition, it is important to document that the drug has been accurately given to the patient, and for this purpose the investigator must keep accurate and up-to-date records to maintain a full inventory of receipt, usage and remaining stocks. An example is given in Appendix 4.

To assure integrity of the study, it must be possible at the end of the trial to reconcile delivery records with those of usage and returns, including accounts for discrepancies.

Information of trial staff

Adequate information of the trial staff about the details of the clinical trial is critical. This includes detailed information about the protocol, SOPs, observations to be made and related pre-established record sheets.

Since it is required that the sponsor maintain records of the quantities of drug supplied for a trial with batch number and that the contract research laboratory maintain a full inventory of receipt, usage and remaining stocks of each batch, the system established to fulfil this requirement is important to keep the staff informed.

The development of a new drug formulation requires identification of suitable methods for evaluating efficiency and safety. The methods of assessment of the response (endpoint) must be well-defined and reliable. This is considerably simpler to achieve with objective physiological parameters such as heart rate, body temperature or blood pressure. However, clinical parameters are subjective measurements and require rational standardized recording systems with valid scoring systems. Information about this is in particular important for the trial staff in order to obtain valid data for evaluation. In some cases even staff training in the scoring of subjective measurements may be required.

Data handling

Any observation being made during the conduct of a clinical trial has to be signed and dated in (water-resistant) ink or ballpoint pen by the person recording the observation. This applies to observations to be recorded in pre-established record sheets or additional observations considered significant. All corrections on a record sheet or elsewhere in the raw data must be made by drawing one straight line through the erroneous values, which should still be legible. The correct data must be inserted with date and signature and preferably with reasons for change.

Statistics

Where and by whom the statistical analyses are carried out is the responsibility of the sponsor. However, the sponsor may transfer some tasks and obligations to a contract research laboratory providing biostatistical competence.

The type of statistical analysis to be used is described in the protocol. Any subsequent deviations from the plan of the protocol have to be described and justified in the final report. It is required that calculations and analyses are confirmed by a named statistician. The statistician and the QAU (monitor) ensure that the data are of high quality at the point of collection and subsequent processing. An account has to be made of missing, unused and spurious data during statistical analysis. Finally the statistician is also expected to ensure the integrity of subsequent data processing by using proven and scientifically recognized statistical procedures.

Data verification

Data verification is the responsibility of the sponsor or monitor and includes a long list of functions to be performed. Since the activities expected in this respect are similar to those required by GLP principles, this task can practically be handled by the QAU in contract research laboratories with an established QA system.

Final trial report

It is the responsibility of the sponsor to prepare the final report for regulatory purposes. The final report must include a copy of the trial protocol. The *EU Note for Guidance* presents a long list of detailed information to be presented in the final protocol. In case the clinical trial is being conducted by a contract research laboratory, the final trial report is most practically written by the investigating laboratory and signed by the investigating laboratory and the QAU to indicate that it represents a complete and accurate record of the trial.

The final trial report also has to be signed by the sponsor.

References

European Community (1990) *Committee for Proprietary Medicinal Products Good Clinical Practice for Trials on Medicinal Products in the European Community*. III/3976/88-EN-Final, Brussels: European Community.

European Community (1994) *Committee for Veterinary Medicinal Products. Good Clinical Practice for the Conduct of Clinical Trials for Veterinary Medicinal Products*. III/3767/92 Final, Brussels: European Community.

FDA (1985) *Compliance Program Guidance Manual, 7348.001*, Biopharmaceutics.

FDA (1988a) *Compliance Program Guidance Manual, 7348.810, Sponsors, Contract Research Organizations and Monitors.*

FDA (1988b) *Compliance Program Guidance Manual, 7348.811, Clinical Investigators.*

FEDESA (1993) *Code of Practice for the Conduct of Clinical Trials on Veterinary Medicinal Products in the European Community*. Brussels: FEDESA.

FEDESA (1966a) *Good clinical practice for the conduct of clinical trials for veterinary medicinal products*. Brussels: FEDESA.

FEDESA (1996b) *Clinical trials for veterinary medicinal products in the European Union. An investigators handbook*. Brussels: FEDESA.

OECD (1982) *Principles of Good Laboratory Practice in the Testing of Chemicals*. Paris: OECD.

Appendix 1:   Dosing record

Study no.   _____

Dosing record			
Group no.:	Dose:	Mg/kg:	Ml/animal:

Animal no.	Weight	Ml/animal	Time
1			
2			
3			
4			
5			
6			
7			
8			
9			
10			
11			
12			
Day no.			
Date			
Initials			

Appendix 2:   Blood sampling record

Study no. _____

Blood sampling record								
	Animal no.:		Animal no.:		Animal no.:		Animal no.:	
Time	theor.	pract.	theor.	pract.	theor.	pract.	theor.	pract.
Before dosing								
Dosing								
15 min								
30 min								
45 min								
60 min								
120 min								
240 min								
480 min								
Date								
Initials								

theor. = Theoretical time; pract. = practical time.

Appendix 3:   Swelling and pain reaction around four injection sites

Study no. _____

Swelling and pain reaction around four injection sites					
Animal no.					

Day	Reaction				Comments	Date Initials
	Anterior left	Posterior left	Anterior right	Posterior right		
1						
2						
3						

Scoring: 0 = Normal; 1 = slight swelling, up to 3 cm in diameter; 2 = moderate swelling, between 3 and 6 cm in diameter; 3 = marked swelling, more than 6 cm in diameter.

Appendix 4:   Dispensary record

Study no. _____

Dispensary record
Test article name:_____ Batch no.: _____
Test description: _____
Description of packing: _____
Labelling:_____ No. of containers: _____

Date	Weight (g) or number of test article and container		Test article used for★	Initials
	Before removal	After removal		
			Arrival Scantox Arrival dispensary	

★1 = Preparation of test article in study; 2 = preliminary examinations; 3 = transfer to other study no. (state study no.); 4 = other (state reason).

Storage (underline)
Room temperature/refrigerator/freezer

Filed: _____
                    (date and signature)

Return to sponsor: _____
                    (date and signature)

Destroyed: _____
                    (date and signature)

16   The animal health industry – struggling to go global

G M Gawlik

Introduction

Striving for harmonization on a global level is the benchmark that the international business and scientific communities are struggling to attain in the 1990s. The animal health industry, representing a small but significant niche in the pharmaceutical industry, is currently doing double time to keep in step.

The lack of new animal drug availability due to rising research and development (R&D) and regulatory costs and the fact that the animal health field does not command the same status as its human health counterparts are creating worldwide concerns within the industry. This lack of availability is causing large-scale illegal drug use, counterfeiting of drugs, as well as illegal importation of drugs in many countries. Drug development for minor species is quickly disappearing merely because its economic impact is undervalued.

Through the concerted efforts of their respective animal health industry associations, the European Union (EU), the USA and Japan are the major players in the harmonization process, working hand in hand with the International Conference on Harmonization (ICH). Not to be overlooked, however, are a number of international treaties such as the General Agreement on Tariffs and Trade (GATT) and the North American Free Trade Agreement (NAFTA), which are also having a positive impact on worldwide veterinary drug harmonization. Latin America, while coping with its own political, economic and social upheavals, represents another significant animal health market which, because of its tremendous potential, demands to be included in this process.

The inherent problems of the animal health industry are universal in scope. Most nations, while struggling to maintain their own identities and standards, recognize that global harmonization is the key element to a prosperous economic future. The animal health industry, with proper guidance, will also profit from the harmonization experience.

The animal health industry – the state of affairs in the European Union

Lack of drug availability – a key issue

The lack of drug availability is also a crisis that faces the European community. At a 1994 general assembly of FEDESA, the European animal health industry association, Bruce Jones, a leading analyst warned: 'Unless there is resolution of the problems faced by the animal health industry in maintaining a full product range, there have to be serious doubts whether Europe will have enough products in future to sustain a healthy livestock industry, and to be ready to cope with any new disease situation that may arise' (FEDESA, 1994).

In Europe there is an increasing concern over the drastic reduction in the therapeutic arsenal of European veterinarians because the industry is faced with:

> political interference in the product authorization process, constantly changing regulations, lack of harmonization, unnecessary testing requirements, exorbitant fees and long assessment times. Because the political climate is more favorable in the USA there is a growing tendency for companies to conduct their business there. Due to the distinctly adverse operating climate and the diversion of funds to meet EU requirements R&D expenditures have been reduced and black market activity is encouraged (FEDESA, 1994).

Mr Jones (1994) noted that: 'Europe is in danger of becoming a backwater in animal health industry terms'.

New product development is now evaluated on its projected economics even before efficacy and safety data are collected, so that the real benefits of a new drug may not be realized if the product will not generate enough money. With rising development and regulatory costs companies will only register products for mainstream species with well-known diseases.

In Europe the animal health industry is considered a commodity business and with new product ventures looking less exciting as investments, the results will be price-cutting and general market devaluation. The USA and the Pacific Rim countries have already taken the lead in market development.

Lack of product availability will also hurt the practice of veterinary medicine. With fewer products and fewer approved species claims off-label use will undoubtedly increase. This will also affect the human health area causing illegal use of human drugs in animals which will, in turn, increase illegal counterfeiting and imports. Multinational businesses have expressed a concern that the declining availability of medicines is causing a decline in

European R&D spending. Biotechnology research is leaving Europe and it is no longer viewed as a global growth region. Many businesses are looking at their futures in terms of survival strategies. Many smaller businesses may be driven out of the animal health market, and the industry that does remain may develop and sell products in Europe with a different perspective (Medicines availability at risk? 1994). At a 1994 meeting of a FEDESA/AISA (Italy's industry association)-sponsored meeting on the harmonization of European drug legislation, Fernand Sauer, the director of the newly formed European Medicines Evaluation Agency (EMEA), stated that: 'The basic principles of quality, safety and efficacy will stay and the Agency will stick to these criteria' (EMEA, 1994). At that same meeting FEDESA's Secretary General Dr Johan Vanhemelrijck noted that regulatory authorities should move away from a zero-risk philosophy towards a risk management approach.

Another concern voiced at this meeting was that there is a real danger that drugs for minor species, including horses, could disappear from the market if licensing requirements became too rigid (EMEA Approvals, 1994).

There are various scenarios in the EU that have contributed to a significant decrease in the number of licensed products reaching the market. Cost and complexity of the former licensing procedures are part of the problem. Also, over the decades member states have adapted themselves to national cultures and tend to implement EU legislation in heterogeneous ways, which adds to the disharmony.

The EMEA is a working partnership with the industry to promote innovation. The new centralized system should encourage R&D-based companies to continue to invest in new products due to its expected efficiency and predictability. Also it should respect registration time limits.

The centralized system will be utilized by the industry if it is perceived that the risks are low and the benefits are high. Some of the benefits of the new system are as follows:

1 Speedy and full market access.
2 One master file.
3 One summary of product characteristics.
4 One assessment report.
5 10-year marketing exclusivity.
6 A common starting date in all EU countries for supplementary protection of patents on their expiry.

User fees for veterinary products are still considered to be too high. Products for minor species may be left out of the market in the wake of higher-selling product registrations.

What role the FEDESA will have in this new process is still unclear (FEDESA, 1995a).

The EMEA is also working with each member state to establish a pharmacovigilance system in which procedures are consistent between human and veterinary products, with some terminology specific to veterinary medicine (CVM, 1994).

One drawback of the EMEA as it is presently structured is that it is somewhat limited in its control over the drug approval process. Currently the agency allows local authorities – not the agency itself – to conduct good manufacturing practice (GMP) inspections. US officials would prefer to have GMP inspections performed under one centralized plan rather than inspections conducted by individual member states (Wechsler, 1995).

The GCPV guidelines

Further to the harmonization effort in the EU, in 1995 FEDESA issued two manuals, *Clinical Trials for Veterinary Medicinal Products in the European Union* and *Good Clinical Practice for the Conduct of Clinical Trials for Veterinary Medicinal Products* (the GCPV guidelines) (FEDESA, 1995b). These manuals provide guidance for investigators as to how to conduct clinical trials for veterinary products. The *Code of Practice for the Conduct of Clinical Trials on Veterinary Medicinal Products*, published by FEDESA in 1993, provides the fundamental procedures for the GCPV guidelines. The code was originally accepted by the EU Committee of Veterinary Medicinal Products in July 1994 (FEDESA, 1995b). The code imposes strict requirements on both sponsors and clinical investigators. The intent of the code is to promote high standards of integrity and increased public awareness and confidence in veterinary medicines and also to enhance transparency in the methods used to conduct clinical trials.

The implementation of these guidelines will have a significant impact on associated R&D costs. The cost of conducting individual clinical trials could increase by 50–100%, which would increase overall costs by approximately 20%. Also clinical development programmes will require major revamping and some investigators may face fundamental changes in the manner in which they conduct trials (FEDESA, 1993).

The GCPV guidelines are described in six chapters as follows:

1   *Chapter 1: Responsibilities:* This chapter describes sponsor, monitor and investigator/site supervisor responsibilities.
2   *Chapter 2: Guide for the conduct of clinical trials:* The general outline of the trial requirements is described through general information; justification and objectives; schedule; design; animal selection; inclusion/exclusion criteria; treatments; assessment of efficacy; adverse events; operation matters; handling of records; evaluation; statistics; supplements and references.

3   *Chapter 3: Data handling:* The method of data handling is described. This includes general data and record-keeping procedures; investigator and sponsor responsibilities; and archiving of data.
4   *Chapter 4: Statistics:* The sponsor is responsible for the overall bio-statistical competence; the method of statistical analysis must be specific in the protocol and a statistician must be identified who will ensure the integrity of the data and subsequent data processing.
5   *Chapter 5: Data verification:* Procedures for data verification are described as well as sponsor/monitor functions regarding data.
6   *Chapter 6: Final trial report:* The sponsor is responsible for the preparation of the final trial report (FTR); the FTR requirements are listed; the FTR must be signed by the sponsor and trial monitor.

The above guidelines became effective on 1 July 1995 and all studies initiated after that date should be conducted in accordance to these guidelines (GCPV, 1995).

The animal health industry – the state of affairs in the USA

Slowdown in the rate of new animal drug approvals

In 1993 the animal health industry in the USA had annual sales totalling only $2.3 billion, which included all the over-the-counter, prescription and feed-added drugs. Compared to the $51 billion in annual human prescription pharmaceutical sales, it is obvious that the animal health industry is not large, but it is still vitally important.

Ranchers and farmers rely on animal health products to keep their animals healthy, to control food costs for consumers and also to ensure that the USA has a safe and abundant supply of meat, milk products and eggs. Veterinarians also rely on these products to promote and ensure the health of pets and zoo animals. But a major crisis exists in the USA in the 1990s – the shortage of available animal drugs. The shortage of approved products to meet the needs of all species of animals has the industry in the midst of a drug availability crisis. This availability problem is compounded by the fact that there has been a slowdown in the rate of new product approvals from the Food and Drug Administration's (FDA) Center for Veterinary Medicine (CVM) which is the animal health product industry's chief regulator. From 1989 through to 1993 only six new chemical entities were approved for food-producing animals, in spite of the fact that there were numerous new animal drug applications submitted to the agency and that the industry doubled its research and development expenditures during that period.

The Animal Health Institute (AHI) represents animal health products manufacturers in the USA. Through several of its recent surveys the following facts were uncovered:

1   Animal pharmaceutical products do not generate large profits. Eighty-seven per cent of products had individual sales totally under $1 million. Only 1% of products had individual sales of more than $25 million.
2   In 1992 the animal health industry spent $400 million on research and development, which represented 18% of its total sales.
3   In the USA it takes approximately 11 years to bring an animal pharmaceutical product to market and only one in 7500 chemical compounds ever gets approved for commercial sale.
4   US federal law requires an approval decision in 6 months but it takes an average of 34 months for a food animal product approval.

The animal health product market is limited by US export law which states under sections 801 and 802 of the Federal Food, Drug and Cosmetic Act that the export of animal pharmaceuticals is limited to 21 foreign countries. If a US company wants to export to countries excluded from the list of 21, the company must manufacture its products outside the USA. Because of US export limitations the net result has been the loss of thousands of construction and manufacturing jobs, as well as the tax revenues.

The lack of animal drug availability has caused serious problems for livestock producers. Their frustrations are compounded by the fact that diseases exist for which no approved animal health products are available, Also, because the animal drug approval process is so time- and money-intensive, there is little incentive to develop drugs for the health needs of minor species.

Another far-reaching effect of decreasing animal drug availability is the extra-label use of products by veterinarians who use products outside their labelled specifications. Veterinarians are forced to continue this practice to meet growing animal health needs. The issue of illegal drug residues in food-producing animals is a major concern to consumer advocacy groups.

There are also economic concerns relating to the lack of animal drugs and the time-consuming approval process of animal drugs. Products are often available sooner in other countries. Also, many companies are experiencing downsizing of their domestic facilities and constructing facilities in other countries, whereby the US loses both manufacturing jobs and revenues (Animal Health Institute, 1994).

Introduction of user fees to speed the drug approval process

Both the animal health industry and the CVM agree that the drug approval process has slowed considerably and both the industry and government are to blame for this situation. Industry officials have conceded that drug applications sent to the CVM are often sloppy and incomplete, with the expectation that the CVM reviewers will somehow fix them. An industry representative noted that: 'The greatest thing the industry can do to speed the approval process is to submit high-quality applications that emphasize data integrity'.

One of the major problems facing the CVM is that the steadily increasing workload has overextended its resources, which remain the same. This overextension puts a heavy burden on the drug approval infrastructure whereby the CVM devotes insufficient attention to communicating application deficiencies and updating regulations. In 1993 the CVM presented an update on its study of the drug approval process at the Food and Drug Law Institute's (FDLI) 37th annual educational conference. The animal health industry praised the CVM's progress. There has been some improvement in the manner in which NADAs (new animal drug applications) and INADs (investigational new animal drugs) are being processed. A US congressional mandate was established to study the feasibility of industry covering some of the costs of the regulatory process. This would be accomplished by charging user fees. The human drug industry already has user fees in place.

The AHI officially opposes the collection of user fees. AHI representative Richard Ekfett noted that: 'Industry believes that if it must pay user fees, concurrent steps must be taken to improve the new animal drug approval system in a manner that will quickly alleviate the drug availability problem that currently prevails' (NADA/INAD, 1994). He goes on to say that a 'sunset provision' should be included in the user fee bill which would absolve the respective manufacturer from paying the fees if the CVM cannot meet its commitment to process timely reviews (NADA/INAD, 1994).

The CVM contends that the user fee requirement would almost halve the product approval time after 5 years of being operational. The CVM has identified three major problems which it says have 'slowed the approval process to a rate unacceptable to the industry'. They are as follows:

1   Inadequate review resources.
2   A growing workload.
3   Low-quality licence applications.

CVM reviewers cannot keep up with the growing workload, although more reviews are being completed because drug applications are increasing at the rate of 6% per year. The agency estimates that there is an upward trend of incoming NADAs and abbreviated NADAs. These applications are increasing at about 25% per year while application completions average only 8% per year.

Because of the heavy application workload the CVM can no longer keep up with updating guidance documents and some of these documents are 15 years out of date.

Another burden added to the growing problem is that the number of submissions needed to obtain approval for an NADA rose from an average of 8.2 in 1988 to 26 in 1993, due to the fact that the CVM reviewers are requiring additional information from the sponsors. The industry claims that the out-of-date CVM guidance documents are partially to blame for this situation.

With or without user fees, in order to improve the reviewing system the CVM has proposed four main goals, although it admits that any improvements will take time to implement and may still be incomplete, especially if additional resources are not available. These goals are as follows:

1   To achieve a 'submit once–review once' procedure. With this procedure drug sponsors will no longer need to resubmit applications for review. The onus of this goal is on the animal health industry. The drug sponsor will be required to improve the quality of applications. Validation of the quality control carried out on the submission before CVM review is being introduced. Also phase review of submissions is being encouraged, whereby a review will begin when one complete component of the application is submitted.
2   To 'improve current CVM policies and the dissemination of information to drug sponsors the CVM will solicit public comment on new standards applied to new animal drug applications' (CVM, 1995).
3   To increase the efficiency of the review through better training and increased productivity. With the implementation of computerized systems, coordination between the GMP inspections and the review process will be facilitated.
4   To improve procedures through the use of information technology.

The CVM realizes that the implementation of user fees is limited due to the fact that profit margins on most animal drugs are low. However, user fees would decrease R&D costs by 3–10% which translates into $10–35 million annually for the industry (CVM, 1995).

The animal health industry – the state of affairs in Japan

Japan – a difficult market to penetrate

In 1992 the animal health market in Japan represented the second largest in the world with sales of about $535 million. The Japanese market has been somewhat difficult to penetrate and few European companies have had success in developing this market. European market share at that time was approximately 5–10% which included licensed-out products.

Japan has imposed certain registration and import impediments on European animal health companies. For example, the Ministry of Agriculture, Fisheries and Food (MAFF) will not accept residue studies which are conducted outside Japan. Residue studies must be repeated twice within Japan at two different locations. Also the method of calculating residues presents another problem. Consequently, Japan will not register products which are well-accepted in other parts of the world. This is a costly proposition.

The zero-residue policy

Another point of contention has been Japan's strict adherence to its zero-residue policy, which is in direct conflict with the international acceptable daily intake (ADI). When there is sufficient evidence that residues are safe to humans the zero-residue concept is superfluous and only widens the gap between Japan and the rest of the world. Consequently, this policy deliberately keeps barriers up to outside trade.

The European business community is confident that if the Japanese authorities will accept the concept of ADI as well as maximum residue limit (MRL), sales will have the potential to increase 30–300% (from our Japan correspondent, 1992).

Further to this scenario and in order to be in accord with its commitment to GATT harmonization agreements, in 1995 Japan has made some policy changes and eventually plans to introduce some MRLs and ADIs for animal drugs. A number of animal drugs have already been evaluated and MRLs established under this new policy (Japan changes zero residue policy, 1995).

Regulatory authorities in Japan are also considering shortening the registration time for animal products. Approval times could potentially be shortened from 18 to 12 months.

MAFF has proposed that some clinical trials as well as some residue trials conducted outside Japan would be accepted. Also import quotas will be relaxed, especially in the vaccine products. These proposals may be approved by 1996 (Shorter Japanese approval time ahead? 1995).

Drug availability in Japan

As in the EU and USA, Japan's MAFF approved fewer animal drugs in 1994. Only 34 new animals drugs were approved, as opposed to 37 in 1993 and 54 in 1992. The Japanese Pharmaceutical Affairs Law defines new drugs as different in active ingredient, concentration, usage and dosage efficacy from drugs already approved (Fewer Japanese approvals in 1994, 1995).

Japan seeks harmonization

Despite communication difficulties and scientific and regulatory differences, Japan is slowly moving into the international scene. The USA and EU should take concerted action to include Japan in the harmonization process in order to achieve a truly international agreement (International harmonisation gaining ground, 1994).

The NAFTA treaty

Mexico: The effects of NAFTA on its animal health industry

Since the ratification of NAFTA with the USA and Canada, Mexico's animal health industry has had mixed feelings about how the treaty will affect the nation's economy. Since the agreement more animal health drug dossiers are being submitted; however, these dossiers are mainly for licences to import products from the USA and Canada. But many cheaper products are brought in from the USA illegally by local farmers.

The Mexican market has about 5000 licensed products. The registration time required varies between 1 month and 1 year, depending on the drug type. Registration fees are nominal. Some products cost more to register if they involve more detailed field trial evaluation.

Mexico falls behind the USA and Canada in the areas of patent protection and pharmacovigilance. In the area of pharmacovigilance a company whose product is found to cause an injury must compensate the farmer. Mexico's procedures for reported suspected adverse drug reactions are performed primarily on an *ad hoc* basis and it is open to interpretation as to how adequate these procedures are.

Another obstacle to increased trade links is in the area of improving its disease status. Diseases ear-marked for eradication over the next few years include swine fever, brucellosis and bovine tuberculosis. Veterinary drug residues are another important animal health-related topic of interest to its NAFTA counterparts. Mexico has 129 TIF (Tipo inspección Federal) plants, 35 of which comply with international export requirements. CENAPA, the national center of animal health validation, certifies that all meats shipped out of Mexcio are free of toxic residues.

At this point the Mexican regulatory authorities have not dealt with the harmonization of animal health procedures with the other NAFTA members but the International Office of Epizootics and the Codex Alimentarius guidelines provide guidance in the animal health area (Doyle, 1994). Legislation of veterinary products is slated for future discussions.

Under the NAFTA treaty Mexico has a unique opportunity to be competitive at the international level. They need to improve product quality while lowering production costs. It will take time for Mexican companies to upgrade their standards to be on equal ground with their US and Canadian veterinary drug producers, especially since Mexican companies lack the necessary technology and have produced little innovative R&D. A number of US and Canadian companies do not have production capabilities in Mexico; however, Mexican companies could become contract manufacturing facilities for these companies. But the NAFTA treaty is not the panacea it is touted to be in the animal health sector, since 80% of the multinationals are already in Mexico. While imports from the USA and Canada will increase, cheaper imports will probably not flood the market. Therefore, major gains from the NAFTA treaty in this area will not be apparent until the next decade.

What is happening in Mexico somewhat parallels the situation in the EU on the eve of the single market. The European Community believes that the implementation of the regulations would lead to a better regulated and more professional market in which to operate, even though it has proved time-consuming and costly in its initial stages. Mexico is heading in the same direction.

NAFTA has opened up the world's biggest animal health market. If the Mexican producers are up to the challenge they can take advantage of the newer technologies developed by their neighbours and improve quality control and distribution channels, which will translate into greater drug availability (Doyle, 1994).

Canada: the other side of the NAFTA coin

Recent political upheaval in Canada has forced the Canadian animal health industry to reassert itself. Prior to the switch from a Progressive Conservative to a Liberal government in Canada, the Canadian Animal Health Institute (CAHI) had been lobbying politicians on several issues. The importation of illegal veterinary products was high on this agenda since the Institute believed that illegal residues would result and target animal safety was at risk. The major problem facing the CAHI is that the animal health industry is relatively small and veterinary medicines are a low priority to politicians. But this prevailing attitude could have serious implications for food safety. Unfortunately, consumer advocate lobby groups are not strong in Canada, so the CAHI needs to convince the government that this is a serious matter.

In 1993 the CAHI had approached the Health Protection Branch (HPB) about illegal imports during the ministry's review of all regulations. It also proposed that illegal importers be fined up to $50 000 plus imprisonment, similar to fines imposed in the USA. But the association was disappointed when its recommendations were not accepted in the HPB's regulatory review document.

The CAHI has also recommended that distinct veterinary drug relations be proposed as opposed to being 'lumped in with human regulations'. Since the Canadian Bureau of Veterinary Drugs (BVD) has recently been moved to the Foods Directorate, this recommendation may be viable since the Foods Directorate is much more in step with food-oriented legislation.

Another issue facing the industry is the HPB's proposed cost recovery system with the introduction of fees similar to those in the USA for animal drug approvals. In the area of food animals these fees raise some ethical issues. It has been argued that food animal drug fees should be less than for pets.

Harmonization efforts between Canada and the USA

The BVD is very encouraged by the progress being made between Canada and the USA in the harmonization of veterinary drug regulations. The BVD realizes that there are opportunities available in reducing redundant review time, especially in the areas of drug withdrawal times and labelling (Rosato, 1994).

The FDA's CVM and the BVD have reached a number of agreements in the area of animal drugs as follows:

1 Adoption of the same tolerances for many veterinary drugs, the same tolerance-setting standards, and identical data requirements for new animal drug approval.
2 CVM's methods validation guidelines have been adopted by the Canadians through a memorandum of understanding (MOU).
3 Labelling standards are falling in line, with both nations using the Canadian PR symbol and the US prescription legend on Rx veterinary drugs. Human warning statements and instructions such as 'information for physicians' are being harmonized.

Current GMPs for medicated fees are being developed which are very similar between the two countries and a draft MOU on sharing feed inspection information has been prepared (Federal Preemption, 1990).

Harmonization of the Latin American countries

Latin America represents a land mass seven times greater than western Europe, yet its sales of veterinary products accounted for only 10% of the global market in 1992, while western Europe captured nearly 30% of the world market. Due to its growing population and constant need for more and better-quality food, the potential for the veterinary industry in Latin America is clearly evident.

FILASA, Federación de la Industria Latino Americana para la Salud Animal, the Latin American animal health industry association, recognizes that uniting the various industry associations in South America is one of its most pressing problems. A consolidated trading bloc must be established in order for Latin America to compete on a global basis (FILASA, 1993).

One of these trading blocs, the MERCOSUR federation, consisting of Argentina, Brazil, Paraguay and Uruguay, already has its own infrastructure, establishing guidelines for the registration of veterinary products for its member nations in June 1992. The MERCOSUR recognizes a number of international organizations as points of references – the FDA, the Federal Code of Regulations; the US Pharmacopaea; the Guidelines of the European Community; the British and European Pharmacopoeia; the Office International des Epizooties (OIE), and the World Health Organization (WHO) (Asunción Proceedings, 1992).

MERCOSUR members have accomplished a number of significant achievements towards harmonization, as follows:

- The definition of a registration procedure for veterinary products.
- The creation of a system of mutual recognition.
- The drafting of three application documents for the registration of pharmaceuticals, biologicals and medicated feedstuffs.
- A list of criteria for the naming of reference centres.
- A compendium of quality-controlled veterinary medicines (FILASA, 1993).

Another Latin American trading bloc, JUNAC, consisting of Bolivia, Columbia, Equador, Peru and Venezuela, which is a newly formed organization established in 1992 for the regulation of animal health products, is closely following MERCOSUR's lead. Major goals for this alliance are the following:

1 To implement a database of veterinary products.
2 To compile a list of pharmaceuticals and biologicals for harmonization.
3 To establish reference laboratories (International harmonisation, 1994).

Other FILASA members have not fully participated in Latin American harmonization programmes. For example, Chile does not appear to be sufficiently convinced of the benefits of belonging to FILASA. Mexico is another glaring exception. Mexico accounts for 21% of the Latin American market, which is the largest market after Brazil. However, Mexico tends to align itself with the NAFTA trading bloc of North America (FILASA, 1993).

Harmonization in the Americas will only move forward quickly if all the trading blocs, including NAFTA, can overcome their internal and external political issues and concentrate on their shared scientific and regulatory expertise.

The animal health industry – struggling to go global

The GATT treaty and the ICH

In 1994 the US Congress enacted legislation which marked the conclusion of 7 years of negotiation. At that time GATT was implemented. ICH had already succeeded in developing a centralized human drug regulatory policy in Europe as well as establishing common policy for developing and testing new drugs. The pharmaceutical industry has been particularly enthusiastic about these recent international developments due to the fact that GATT will effectively reduce the tariffs that interfere with free trade and also extend protection for intellectual property rights. GATT, over a 5-year period, will provide a reduction of over $1 billion in tariffs to both the pharmaceutical and medical equipment manufacturers. Also, GATT provides for increased patent protection, switching from a 17-year patent from time of award to a 20-year patent from time of filing. Most manufacturers will benefit from this lengthened patent coverage. Although the USA has agreed to these terms there are some companies – especially biotechnology firms, since they have the most difficulty obtaining patents – that fear that the new policy will in fact reduce patent coverage. The US Congress states that its policy will be flexible and will enact new legislation that will offer an inventor a choice between the old 17-year term from patent grant or the new 20-year term from date of filing (Wechsler, 1995).

Impact of GATT on veterinary drug regulations

Under the GATT treaty, veterinary drug tolerances and regulations promulgated by individual member nations must be based on health standards determined by risk assessment. Also international technical agreements are considered reference standards. Countries may differ from these standards if the standards are applied both domestically and internationally and if they are in the best interest of protecting human, animal or plant life. Scientific risk assessment is the key measure and the risk assessment process requires 'transparency'. Each nation can determine the appropriate level of risk as long as it is consistent with its other risk assessment policies.

Any changes to regulations and procedures must be made known as a notice of public record to other GATT countries.

The three major players in the harmonization process are Europe, Japan and the USA. International harmonization will require that each government must assess and revise its national procedures to accommodate its international obligations, and also be prepared for greater public scrutiny by fellow nations (CVM, 1994).

The FDA is also much more supportive of the considerable progress that the ICH is making. The ICH has made notable strides in the worldwide human pharmaceutical arena and the FDA has indicated that international harmonization is one of the top four priorities for the FDA's drug and biologics centre (Wechsler, 1995).

GHOST (Global Harmonization of Standards for Testing)

Europe (the EU), the USA and Japan's differences in registration requirements are particularly highlighted in the areas of product quality and safety testing, efficacy, manufacturing practices, residue studies and analytical methods. FEDESA's views on the process of harmonization are outlined in the document called GHOST (Global Harmonization of Standards for Testing) (Verschueren, 1992). Within the context of GHOST veterinary drug licensing should be guided by four basic principles:

1 Harmonization should specify requirements for testing and not procedures for registration.
2 Each issue should be revisited for scientific evaluation rather than the addition of requirements.
3 The initiative should be tripartite – What are the implications for other countries? How will it affect drug availability?
4 All new requirements should be considered within the framework of GHOST to eliminate further divergence.

How the GHOST document and the ICH guidelines will interface should be guided by the progress already made by ICH's lead (Verschueren, 1992).

Past efforts to standardize drug development and regulatory requirements have been convoluted and generally unsuccessful. Through several meetings with the industry and government groups, the ICH has hammered out a number of significant guidelines on the detection of toxicity to reproduction for medicinal products, studies in support of geniatric populations, dose–response studies and stability testing. In October 1994 'it approved a new standard for population exposure to assess clinical safety data, established definitions and standards for expedited reporting of clinical safety data, and agreed on what essential documents are needed to verify clinical trial data (Wechsler, 1995). Additional guidelines were developed for assessing systemic exposure in toxicology studies, dose selection for carcinogenicity studies and for repeated dose tissue distribution studies. With the rising cost of R&D expenditures these guidelines will reduce the need for redundant animal studies around the world.

On the animal health industry front the FDA's CVM is participating in this harmonization initiative with the OIE to harmonize veterinary drugs. The USA, Japan and the EU are the lead participants but all 140 members of the OIE will have access to the ICH veterinary guidelines (Wechsler, 1995).

The CVM sees any agreements made in the human pharmaceutical area as starting points for harmonization in the veterinary drug arena. However, the specific requirements of veterinary drugs, which are significantly different from human drugs, are not addressed in ICH.

In order to facilitate similarity between European and US requirements the CVM has also offered its assistance to the EU in developing terminology for veterinary products. Joint review of new animal drug applications between the CVM and EU has also been an area of general agreement; however, harmonization of registration requirements must be hammered out first, especially in those areas where there are significant differences. Food-producing animals, it was suggested, would be a good starting point for joint reviews (CVM, 1994).

The ICH guidelines will become mandatory in Europe and Japan, but they are not legally binding on the FDA or US companies and their effectiveness will depend on how closely the FDA will adhere to them. The results of the guidelines will depend on their implementation by the regulators and if they can convince the industry of their value and ability to cut costs (Wechsler, 1995).

Other issues given top priority in the harmonization process are human food safety, pharmacovigilance and manufacturing chemistry. These are the areas that have the most international impact and where there are no political constraints (International harmonisation gaining ground, 1994). With regard to the human food safety issue the Codex Alimentarius Commission (Codex), an international organization established by the United Nations Food and Agriculture Organization (FAO) and WHO to protect the health and economic interests of consumers and to encourage fair trade in food and food standards on the international level (International Standard, 1995), submitted four principles relating to the role of science on its decision-making process at its July 1995 session. The four principles are as follows:

1 The food standards, guidelines and other recommendations of Codex Alimentarius shall be based on the principle of sound scientific analysis and evidence, involving a thorough review of all relevant information, in order that the standards assure the quality and safety of the food supply.
2 When elaborating and deciding upon food standards Codex Alimentarius will have regard, where appropriate to other legitimate factors relevant for the health protection of consumers and for the promotion of fair practices in food trade.
3 In this regard, it is noted that food labelling plays an important role in furthering both these objectives.
4 When the situation arises that members of Codex agree on the necessary level of protection of public health but hold differing views about other considerations, members may abstain from acceptance of the relevant standard without necessarily preventing the decision by Codex.

These guidelines are especially relevant to the heated debates surrounding the use of growth-promoting hormones (International harmonisation gaining ground, 1994).

In the human health-related areas like food safety, consumer groups are highly suspicious of harmonization activities. They often believe that setting international standards means seeking the lowest common denominator among nations, when in reality this is not the goal of promoting harmonized standards.

Summary

National governments do not regard animal medicines and animal drug development with high priority; therefore, harmonization activities in the animal health area must be channelled through those organizations which will champion their cause, such as the OIE and the Codex Alimentarius. Although some countries are not yet ready to participate fully, the harmonization process needs to be put in motion as soon as possible. Short- and long-term goals need to be determined and agreed upon. Positive economic repercussions as well as good science must prevail if harmonization in the animal health industry is to meet with success (No time to lose, 1992).

References

Animal Health Institute (1994) *Understanding the Animal Drug Availability Crisis – Facts to Remember*, pp. 1–10.

Asunción Proceedings of the III Meeting of the Veterinary Sector of MERCOSUR, June 4–5, 1992, Asunción, Paraguay, pp. 5–6.

CVM striving for harmonization of animal drug standards (1994) *Food Chemical News* 35: 14 Feb.

CVM proposes $11 million user fee collection (1995) *ANIMAL PHARM* 316: 12.

Doyle, C. (1994) Mexico in the NAFTA era: new colonialism or land of opportunity? *ANIMAL PHARM* 314: 13–15.

EMEA approvals will be science-based, pledges new director (1994). *ANIMAL PHARM* 299: 1.

Federal Preemption still on table of GATT talks (1990) *Food Chemical News* 32: 2 July.

FEDESA's plea for time on good laboratory practice compliance (1993) *ANIMAL PHARM* 285: 3.

FEDESA assembly seeks solutions to animal health's 'imposed recession'. (1994) *ANIMAL PHARM* 302: p. 3.

FEDESA looks to EMEA to promote innovation (1995a) *ANIMAL PHARM* 319: 3.

FEDESA responds to need for clinical trials info (1995b). *ANIMAL PHARM* 322: 2.

Fewer Japanese approvals in 1994 (1995) *ANIMAL PHARM* 331: 22.

FILASA points the way to harmonization in Latin America (1993) *ANIMAL PHARM* 287: 16–17.

From our Japan Correspondent EBC-AHC (1992) *ANIMAL PHARM* 246: 14.

Good Clinical Practice for the Conduct of Clinical Trials for Veterinary Medicinal Products. GCPV: the EU note for Guidance (1995) Brussels, Belgium: FEDESA, pp. 2–17.

International harmonisation gaining ground (1994) *ANIMAL PHARM* 311: 8–9.

International Standard – setting activities (1995) *Federal Register* 60: 23 May.

Japan changes zero residue policy (1995) *ANIMAL PHARM* 329: 12.

Medicines availability at risk? The animal health industry's perception. (1994) *ANIMAL PHARM* 304: 12–13.

NADA/INAD and user fees head FDLI conference agenda (1994) *ANIMAL PHARM* 292: 8.

No time to lose in the run-up to harmonisation (1992) *ANIMAL PHARM* 256: 10.

Rosato, C. (1994) Canadian industry adapts to political upheavals. *ANIMAL PHARM* **296:** 12–13.

Shorter Japanese approval time ahead? (1995) *ANIMAL PHARM* **329:** 12.

Verschueren, C. (1992) Comparative aspects of registration requirements in the EC, USA, Japan – manufacture, quality and safety of residues. Brussels: FEDESA/COMISA, pp. 280–281.

Wechsler, J. (1995) Going global. *Pharmaceutical Executive* 15:18.

PART SIX

Biotechnology

17   The progressive implementation of good manufacturing practice in a biotechnology process, from research through development to routine production

V G Edy and P M Squibb

The development of a pharmaceutical produced by a biotechnology process involves the repeated successful resolution of an apparent contradiction. On the one hand, it is necessary to retain as much scientific freedom and flexibility during the programme as possible, to encourage the development scientists to create imaginative solutions to the problems that will undoubtedly occur during development, and thus to allow the programme to progress as rapidly as is possible. On the other hand, materials manufactured during development will be administered to humans, hence concerns about the quality and safety of the clinical trial materials are therefore paramount. For this reason alone the assurance of adequate product quality and safety through compliance with good manufacturing practice (GMP) must form an integral part of the development programme. Additionally, the goal of the whole development effort is to produce a submission (marketing authorization application, MAA, in Europe, establishment licence application, ELA, and product licence application, PLA, in the USA; equivalent systems exist elsewhere) that is acceptable to the regulatory authorities. Regulatory acceptability of the manufacturing process can only be gained if it is in compliance with GMP codes. The amount of work necessary to assure GMP compliance is large; it cannot simply be done at the final full-scale process stage but must build on foundations laid at various stages earlier in development.

Compliance with GMP is often seen as reducing, if not eliminating, scientific creativity, slowing progress and increasing costs. Even if this is not true (a matter of opinion), this perception means that the extent of application of GMP in development can be a subject of contention. The regulatory authorities have made it clear that GMP must be applied during manufacture of materials for clinical trials (Food and Drug Administration,

1991; Committee for Proprietary Medicinal Products, 1992) as far as possible, but do not give detailed guidance in the application of these requirements. In this present chapter, we describe one way of progressively implementing GMP throughout the lifetime of a development programme. The implementation programme, which we call the GMP gradient, is illustrated by references to a biotechnology development process, but there is nothing in the model that restricts its use to biotechnology products; with appropriate modifications we have also applied it to new chemical entities.

In developing the GMP gradient we have largely built upon our own experiences in development of biotechnology products, but have also been aided by a recent series of articles in *Pharmaceutical Technology Europe* by members of the Fast Trak validation team and others: Adner and Sofer, 1994; Akers *et al.* 1994a,b; Barry and Chojnacki, 1995; Bozzo, 1995; McEntire, 1994; Seely *et al.* 1994; Sofer, 1994. These articles are especially strong on validation issues surrounding purification and analytical procedures.

The GMP gradient is applied to the development process continuously, although in the current description we divide the whole programme into discrete steps. Although these steps do represent significant milestones in the development project, this division is purely for convenience and clarity of description. In real life some parts of development will be brought forward, others pushed back, others merged or run in parallel; the application of the GMPs must be correspondingly adjusted. However, in the 'typical' biotechnology process used as the basis for the description of the GMP gradient, we are going to describe progress in a simple linear fashion, from the research laboratory right through to regulatory submission. On the way between these two points we shall pass through initial process development, manufacture for toxicology studies, manufacture for phase I administration, process scale-up and improvement, manufacture for phase II trials, establishment of a manufacturing facility, and phase III trial production. In addition, the essential background tasks, such as development of analytical methods, which go on during this progress from laboratory to factory will also be covered.

The GMP gradient programme outlined here may seem quite heavily 'front-end loaded', with many GMP tasks being carried out relatively early in the development programme, before they are clearly essential. This is quite deliberate; even at the earliest stages of development the material manufactured, and the results obtained during processing, are being used to generate key information that may be referenced in future regulatory submissions. This information also forms the foundation for many of the critical decisions that are made as the project continues, and provides a baseline against which future process changes are compared. By setting up and applying many of the GMP requirements at an early stage of development the quality of the material and data derived from it can be assured. Additionally, the level of financial investment required rises very steeply, especially once a programme has entered the clinic. Therefore, the financial consequences of mistakes requiring work to be done again also rise very steeply; everything possible to reduce the risk of unnecessary delay and costs should be done. It is helpful therefore to have implemented GMP earlier rather than later, to avoid halting or slowing a programme whilst the quality systems are brought up to standard. The alternative, to push ahead and hope that the necessary GMP compliance will somehow 'catch up', is highly undesirable; the catching up is unlikely to occur until the last minute, when it is (almost) too late and will almost certainly cause the maximum delay and disruption to the whole programme.

The whole GMP gradient concept, like development itself, is built on an assumption that the target development programme will be successful. This is a higher-risk strategy in the sense that investments, both of money and of time, must be made under conditions of considerable uncertainty about the outcome of the project. However, the alternative is to take a much slower path towards a licensed product, with the consequence of delayed revenues, shorter exclusivity as the patent term expires, and the possibility that a competitor's product will seize a significant part of the market first. The GMP gradient concept is compatible with the rapid progress we believe to be essential in the successful development of a biotechnology product.

In describing the gradient we list activities as being carried out at certain arbitrary stages of the development programme. It is important to note that these are the stages at which we believe these activities should commence; they then continue for the duration of the entire programme. Each stage builds on the GMP-compliance activities set in place during the previous stages. Additionally, in the interests of completeness, we assume that the facility in which the development will be done is not already validated, and that all the processes are new. Where this is not so, then obviously much existing work does not need to be repeated, but should simply be critically reviewed to assure yourself of its continuing adequacy.

Exploratory research

In the research laboratory not only is the molecule that is to be subject of the development programme first produced and found to be of interest, but also the foundations for all development activities are laid. The requirements that must be applied at this stage for a subsequently successful and as far as possible trouble-free development process are few and simple, predominantly related to equipment, records and an awareness of likely subsequent development.

All equipment used in research must be adequately maintained and in an appropriate state of calibration; this is essential to give confidence in the reproducibility of the work that was done and the reliability of any measurements made. Second, all work must be adequately recorded. This can be quite a difficult task to instil into research scientists, but it is vital. Because it is mostly impossible at this stage to know what is important in the embryonic process, everything must be fully described. The review of lab notebooks by supervisors or managers must be thorough, asking the question: Is this experiment described well enough that in 5 years (for example) other scientists will be able unequivocally to reconstruct what was done? Third, it is very important that research scientists, whether they will be the people to carry the programme through from research into development or not, have an awareness of the needs and potential problems of development. It is not unknown for research scientists to use processes that cannot be scaled, or that are for some other reason impossible to use as the basis for development. An awareness of what is necessary to turn an idea into a product should help reduce the amount of re-invention that has to go on in development.

Initial process development and manufacturing for toxicology

It is in this phase that perhaps the most potential for conflict concerning the extent of GMP application arises. If too strict a line is taken, it is inevitable that creativity will be restricted (or felt to be restricted, which is just as destructive). However, too relaxed a line can mean that major headaches are created for subsequent steps in the development. Therefore, during these initial phases, we impose certain minimum requirements in the areas of raw materials, validation, documentation including specifications, training and auditing.

Raw materials control

A very loose degree of control of raw materials is enforced at this stage – little more than setting up specifications for each raw material as a need for it is identified. At this stage, the specification needs to be little more than a code number, a supplier, and the supplier's catalogue number for the item, storage conditions and a (usually arbitrarily decided) shelf-life. On receipt each raw material shipment is checked to determine that it is an item for which an approved specification is in existence, that it is from the specified supplier, that all the containers are clearly labelled with a unique lot number (in our case allocated by a computerized system), and that the packaging is not unacceptably damaged. It could be argued that such a minimal lack of control is of little value, but we would contend that setting simple systems in place early, then tightening them up as development proceeds, is much easier and faster than trying to impose complete control in a single step at a later stage. It also provides an opportunity to encourage scientists to use existing approved materials and suppliers wherever possible. This simplifies stock control and gives advantages when supplier audits are required at later stages in the development programme. Additionally, during the early development stage information on critical raw material parameters may be gained; this is obviously built into the raw material specifications more easily if the basics of the system are in operation.

Validation master plan

The development of a validation master plan (VMP) is not a specific requirement of any GMP code, as far as we are aware. In our experience, however, a simple VMP, tabulating the areas, utilities and equipment (including analytical equipment) likely to be used in the process, and setting out policy on the validation programmes, is an extremely valuable document. The VMP should describe, perhaps by reference to other documents such as standard operating procedures (SOPs), what is meant by the various phases of validation, how far each item described in the VMP will be taken through this validation cycle, and at what stage in the development programme. The VMP will undoubtedly be changed several times as development progresses, but to have a single master plan to refer to will help ensure that the validation approach is consistent, neither too much nor too little, and appropriately and consistently timed. Finally and perhaps most usefully, a VMP is essential for defining the resources that will be needed for validation during the programme. Without such a clear definition, these resources almost certainly will not be available when needed.

Facility and utility qualification

The facility in which development is undertaken needs basic qualification (if the development takes place in a new facility; if not, we would expect all the systems to be in place already) and monitoring. The major utility systems (heating, ventilation and air conditioning (HVAC), water, clean steam, etc.) appropriate to the process under development must be identified from the VMP, then put through installation qualification (IQ), commissioning and operational qualification (OQ) as early as possible. With the utilities validated, it is then necessary to set in place routine facility monitoring, both of air and water quality, although at this stage the actual quality of the environment and utilities is not likely to be very important. However, by starting to collect data early, it is possible to build a picture of typical operating conditions, so than when this monitoring is essential (during manufacture for administration to humans) there is a degree of assurance that the systems do perform as expected. Additionally, there will be sufficient background data to allow identification of unusual conditions and some experience of their consequences. Furthermore, if monitoring is not done early, there is a risk that sloppy working habits will be allowed to develop, as there is no feedback generated on the consequences of particular working practices. These inappropriate practices can then be hugely difficult to erase, as is absolutely necessary during production for administration to humans. We have found that it is very beneficial to administer the monitoring programmes, both of environment and utilities, via a laboratory information management system (LIMS) package. Not only does this make it very easy to tailor quite complex monitoring programmes with minimum administrative burden, but it also makes trending of the results (a GMP requirement) quite simple.

Equipment qualification and documentation

Again, based on the VMP drawn up earlier, development equipment, including that used for key assays and for product characterization, must be put through IQ and OQ, and calibration and maintenance programmes instituted. SOPs for each piece of equipment, covering (as appropriate) equipment start-up, operation, shutdown, cleaning, maintenance and calibration, must also be prepared. This is also the time when equipment logbooks should be started. Again, this is based on the assumption that the process uses new equipment; if not, now is the time to check that all the requirements given above are still met. In addition to the requirement for completion of IQ and OQ for the equipment used in the process, performance qualification (PQ) must be completed for all critical autoclave and sterilizing oven loads. Critical loads are those containing materials and components that may be used in aseptic processing of the product after it has been sterilized by filtration.

Training

The initiation of GMP training is critical at this phase of the programme. All the scientists involved in the development of the process and in manufacture of material for toxicology must have an understanding of the requirements of GMP and how it relates to their role. This training would normally take the form of presentations by quality assurance (QA) staff, supplemented by seminars by external consultants and possibly external training courses.

Process documentation

During the initial development phase, it is very difficult to produce final SOPs, but it is our opinion that the effort must be made, accepting in turn that revisions will be required due both to changes in the process, and experience being gained. Coupled to this programme of preparation of SOPs, most of the work should be recorded in lab notebooks, although there are instances when formal record forms are more valuable. However, as the manufacturing process is established, batch manufacturing records (BMR) should be drafted; again it is accepted that these will need considerable revision as development proceeds, but the value of a formal BMR, at least for manufacturing for toxicology, is inestimable. Without it, it becomes exceptionally difficult to find out how materials for toxicology really were made. Additionally, the use of BMRs in toxicology manufacture serves as a 'dry run' to ensure that these documents will be workable later, when used to record manufacture for administration to humans.

Assay development

During this initial development phase, much assay and analytical development work is ongoing. This will include the development of assays for batch release, and in particular the development of stability-indicating assays for stability studies. It is important for later work that effort is also put into the development of assays to support cleaning, including cleaning-in-place, which may not be seen as scientifically rewarding. However, without work on assays that will help in the assessment of equipment cleaning, it will obviously be impossible to test how effective cleaning procedures are, and there is a risk that development may have to be held up while an effective cleaning protocol is developed.

Specifications

Where batches of material are manufactured during development, there is a tendency to submit only those samples to QC that explore parameters of current interest; alternatively there is a tendency to apply all conceivable assays to all possible samples to gather information. Both of these approaches have their value. However, at the time of toxicology manufacture it is vital that a basic specification has been set for the product. This will be little more than a list of tests to be applied to samples; in only a few cases can and should acceptance criteria be set. Where this is done, great thought should be given to defining the acceptance limits; they must neither be so wide as to be meaningless, nor unnecessarily restrictive. Because at this stage it is probable that relatively little is known about the product, and because many of the assays used will not have been validated, it is probably very helpful to include a wide range of additional tests in the specification at this stage. These are tests that must be performed prior to batch disposition, but which are intended to help gather knowledge about the process and product rather than as release tests. The results of these additional tests should be reviewed periodically; if they are found to give useful information about the product then they should be moved to full formal specification tests; if they do not contribute useful information they can be dropped.

It is important to assure that the quality of material used in toxicology studies is as well-understood as possible, to allow comparison with the product of improved and up-scaled processes, to avoid making the toxicology programme already carried out irrelevant. (Although it must be accepted that as processes, both manufacturing and analytical, are improved during the development programme, some repeated or extended toxicology is almost inevitable.) Part of the process of assessment of the quality of materials used for toxicology is a full review by independent quality assurance (QA) staff of the production process actually used, and of the analytical methods employed as well as a review of the assay results generated. Without awareness of the methods used, the analytical results alone are of limited value in assessing the quality of materials.

Audit programme

Although the quality system specifications during this early stage of development are rather vague, we feel it is valuable to start an internal audit programme. This has two purposes: the obvious one of assessing compliance with the quality system such as it is, ensuring that staff understand that even in early development non-compliance is to be taken seriously; and a subsidiary purpose of familiarization, ensuring both that QA staff are aware of the development process, and that development staff are aware of, and if possible comfortable with, the audit process. At this stage, we feel that reports on audits should be informal, concentrate on corrective action, and be primarily addressed to the scientists responsible for the areas or functions audited, rather than the company management. On the other hand, few external audits (i.e. audits of suppliers or contractors) are appropriate at this stage. The main area needing attention is inspection of organizations supplying critical pieces of equipment, including software, to assess the adequacy of the supplier's internal quality systems. Those items judged as critical should have been so identified in the VMP developed earlier.

From toxicology to first administration to humans

Although many of the foundations of GMP compliance have already been laid in the preceding phase of development, it is in the period leading up to manufacturing of clinical trial product for phase I trials that the major building blocks of the GMP programme must be put in place. In addition to the programme started earlier in development, at this stage we introduce formal change control, additional requirements for validation, raw materials and documentation and introduce more specific training, formal QA review and batch disposition, a formal procedure for review of deviations and failures, a rudimentary stability programme and process flow charts. To monitor compliance with these extra requirements it is also necessary to tighten the audit programme.

Change control

Perhaps the most important procedure that ought to be set up at this stage is a formal change control system. The scope of the system needs to be carefully thought out, but it is better to review changes that need not have been formally reviewed than to lose sight, and thus control, of a part of the manufacturing process, facility in which it is run, etc. Always, changes must be clearly described and a detailed reason for the change given. Like laboratory notebooks and all GMP documentation, the level of detail and clarity in completing change control forms must be stressed; people must realize that they are writing not for the present, when everyone is familiar with the change and the background to it, but rather for a disinterested regulatory authority investigator, with no familiarity with the process, at some indeterminate time in the future. In reviewing requests for changes, the baseline that must always be used as the reference level is the process, equipment and facility as used to manufacture the material for toxicology. Obviously, we do not mean to imply that the process cannot be changed, merely that changes must be thoroughly documented, reviewed by all relevant functions (always including QA), and the implications fully assessed before implementation.

Assay validation

Key assays, for potency, purity and safety, must be formally validated (perhaps excluding the assessment of robustness where appropriate) before first administration to humans. The guidance produced by regulatory authorities on investigational products specifies that tests associated with product sterility (and most biotechnology products will be in the form of a sterile injectable) must be validated. Identification of which other assays are key depends on the product, and the specification should be formally reviewed to identify which they are. The other, non-key assays required by the process or product need not be validated at this stage; indeed, given that assay methods, and potentially the matrix will change during further development, fully validating these assays too early risks wasting effort.

Aseptic processing validation

Most products of biotechnology must be sterilized by filtration before aseptic filling into their final containers; occasionally additional processing is necessary after filtration and before final filling. Aseptic processing is probably the area in which it is easiest to compromise the safety of the product, and therefore it is obviously an area requiring considerable assurance that it has been adequately performed.

The statistics of the pharmacopoeial sterility test are such that there is a reasonable chance that quite considerable rates of contamination will not result in a failed sterility test. Therefore before preparation of materials for administration to humans it is essential that successful broth simulations of the aseptic process have been carried out, involving all the staff likely to take part in the aseptic processing. A very useful source of information on the execution and interpretation of media fills as an aid in aseptic processing validation is the *Parenteral Society Technical Monograph No. 4* (1993). Aseptic processing must be revalidated periodically even if the process is not changed; indeed, if the process is not run fairly frequently so that staff are continually practising aseptic techniques, it is probably best to repeat the media fills prior to each manufacturing run. If the aseptic process itself is changed, even if only in scale, then complete validation is again essential.

Cleaning validation

The cleaning process of equipment is perhaps all to easily overlooked; although there is undoubtedly a general recognition that cleanliness of equipment is important, it may not be seen as a scientifically challenging part of the programme. However, the main problem with cleaning and its validation is one of establishing reasonable limits, in the absence of any data on likely therapeutic doses and no-effect levels in humans. One is reduced to the selection of almost arbitrary limits, essentially using assays of the highest practical sensitivity on both final rinse fluids and surface swabs. It is essential that the assays used test not only for the specific product, but also for other potential contaminants such as other proteins (including denatured product) as well as for the cleaning agents themselves. As a non-specific assay of quite high sensitivity, we have found determination of total organic carbon (TOC) to be of value in assessing cleanliness levels. Although the approach to setting acceptance criteria for cleanliness is arbitrary, it is difficult to argue that the effluent from a cleaned pipe, vessel or piece of equipment can be accepted if it does not match the quality of the rinse liquid.

Raw materials

For those raw materials that are actually involved in the manufacturing process, the specifications need to be tightened. Besides testing for any parameters identified in earlier stages as important for successful production, it is now necessary to add, as a *minimum*, a requirement for identity testing and a certificate of analysis (*not* a certificate of conformance) for each batch of raw material. Identity testing should be performed on every container of starting material, unless the sampling process could damage the material itself (e.g. in sampling a sterile buffer there is a risk that sterility might be compromised; under these circumstances we have chosen to sample $\sqrt{n}+1$ containers), and to discard them once sampled. On certificates of analysis, our practical experience is that these cannot simply be taken for granted. They must be checked to ensure that all the expected tests have in fact been done, and that the results all 'pass' against the same limits applied to earlier batches of the material. Even with materials claimed to be of pharmacopoeial grade, it is sometimes found that the manufacture does not record all the tests specified in the pharmacopoeia on the certificate. Besides specifications for the raw materials used in the process, detailed specifications must be developed for the primary packaging materials.

Process documentation

After manufacturing for toxicology and before preparation of clinical trial materials, the SOPs for the process equipment and the BMR should be critically reviewed and if necessary revised and reissued. The BMRs used for clinical trial manufacture must be formally issued for a specific batch by QA. At this stage it should also be appropriate to introduce formal approved specifications, for the intended finished dosage form (including any placebo required by the trial protocol), for the bulk drug, and for various intermediate stages in the process. At this stage, limits on the tests can be established based either on known pharmacopoeial requirements or on the data generated from the earlier development batches. As this information is likely to be very limited, it is normal to set quite wide specifications at this stage, but to evaluate the data carefully before batch release. The limits will be reviewed and in many cases narrowed as experience is gained.

Training

In addition to the general training in GMP specified earlier, it is now essential to ensure that the key processing and analytical steps are identified, and staff trained in them. In the common situation that the staff who will operate the process are the same as those who developed it and wrote the SOPs, then formal training is rather pointless. However, a formal record must be made of the decision that training was inappropriate, and why. It may be useful to have all appropriate staff review the SOP and sign a record to indicate that they have read, had the opportunity to discuss, and understood it – a suggestion for which we are grateful to Mike Anisfeld of Interpharm Consulting. This is a useful approach for experienced staff, but is certainly insufficient for a novice operator, who should have the process explained and be closely supervised, with an assessment of competence before being left to run a process alone.

Deviations and failures

Despite all the intensive development work that has been done, and the care that has gone into preparation of documentation, it is probable that the specified process cannot be followed exactly as described, and that there will be test failures. Both must, from this stage of development onwards, be formally recorded, reviewed by scientific staff as well as QA, and be taken into account in deciding the disposition of the product. Any test failures must be investigated and the results recorded. The general principles established in the Barr case (see 'The Gold Sheet' for February 1993, and Madsen (1994) for a good exposition of the critical points in the Barr judgement and an assessment of their implications for pharmaceutical manufacturing and testing) should be followed, although the exact system for review and actions will probably be somewhat less rigorous.

Batch disposition

At present there is no legal requirement for batch disposition to be carried out by a qualified person (QP) when a product is in development. However, the type of review normally carried out by a QP of the batch records for a licensed product is equally as appropriate (or possibly even more appropriate) for investigational products. Although the toxicology batches were reviewed and released by QA, the level of rigour in the review was less than that required when the material is to be used in humans, and the tolerance of GMP deviations greater. When reviewing all records for a batch for clinical trial, QA must cast a critical eye over the whole batch records, including the environmental monitoring, and ensure that any omissions, errors and other discrepancies are reviewed and necessary corrective actions undertaken. Similarly, a thorough review of the complete QC records for the batch (including in-process and intermediate samples) is essential; it is not sufficient just to look at the summarized analytical results alone.

Stability

During this phase of the development programme, and before manufacturing for humans, materials should be set aside for preliminary or pathfinder stability work. This does not mean full formal studies for submission in support of the shelf-life claims as part of the licence application, but instead studies to establish one or more assays as stability-indicating. The more stability work that can be done now the better, as it will aid in ascribing realistic shelf-lives to clinical trial materials and reduce the always necessary extension to expiry dates on clinical trial supplies.

Audit programme

During this phase of development, the rudimentary internal audit programme must be built upon, to form a fully functioning internal self-inspection programme. Because of the fairly informal audits conducted earlier, the development staff will be familiar with the purpose and procedure of audits, and will be less likely to react defensively. Additionally, the auditors should be fairly familiar with the process being evaluated. Each audit must be formally written up in an audit report, giving the audit subject the chance to correct any efforts of fact, and submitted to the scientist responsible for the area or function, and to the senior management responsible for the development programme. The prime purpose of giving reports to management is to ensure that they can make any necessary resources available for corrective action; it may be necessary to stress this to audit subjects. The responsible scientist must be required to draw up a formal audit response, dealing with all the points in the initial report, detailing corrective actions, and giving (realistic) time frames for the implementation of these corrective actions. The QA group must review the audit response and decide whether and when a follow-up is appropriate; alternatively the achievement of corrective actions should be assessed in the next audit.

Prior to this stage, informal audits were not logged, but now it is essential both to have a formal internal audit programme, described in an SOP or equivalent document. Part of this SOP should require a log of audits, recording the area or function covered, the date and reference number of the audit report, the date and reference of the response, and any follow-up activities.

It is important that QA staff carrying out audits are well-trained and have an up-to-date knowledge of current regulatory expectations. It is also important that they are able to maintain an objective view of the process under development, the working practices and the development facilities despite their close working relationship with the development groups. For both reasons, it may be extremely useful to bring in an experienced contract auditor as a consultant at this stage, to look at the process with a fresh pair of eyes as well as making sure that the internal QA staff are aware of current inspection concerns and practices.

Finally, on the subject of audit, it is at this stage that formal audits of suppliers and contractors must be implemented. There must be written criteria for assessing suppliers and contractors, for deciding who shall be audited, against what standards, and how often; the audits must be written up and logged in a similar fashion to internal audits.

Process flow charts

Flow charts to illustrate parts of the manufacturing process are required by the Food and Drug Administration (FDA; *Biotechnology Inspection Guide*, 1991). In addition to being a regulatory requirement necessary to satisfy an investigator at, for example, a preapproval inspection, flow charts can usefully be introduced fairly early in development. Although the *Inspection Guide* suggests that flow charts are only required for extraction, isolation and purification, a basic flow chart of the manufacturing process (from raw materials right through to finished dosage forms) should be drawn up at this stage. It is accepted that it will have to be revised repeatedly during the remainder of the development programme; even so, the effort required to create the chart is well worthwhile. The purpose of the flow chart at this stage is not to aid an investigator in understanding the process, but as a framework around which a logical system of batch manufacturing and packaging records can be designed. Given the length and complexity of most biotechnology processes, it is convenient to split the process documentation into manageable parts; a flow chart aids in the assessment of what are appropriate 'break points'. Additionally it provides an excellent template to check on equipment needs, to ensure that equipment used in the process is clearly identified, triggering a review of SOPs, equipment logs, qualification status, etc.

First administration to humans (phase I) to phase II

In this stage of development, the major imperative is the manufacture of materials for further clinical trials to show evidence of efficiency, but simultaneously to up-scale the production process so as to be ready for phase II. In the background, much work must also go on to help select the final dosage form, formulation, etc. All this work is to a greater or lesser extent covered by the existing parts of the GMP gradient programme, and involves specification reviews, the initiation of batch analysis reports, and preparation work for the regulatory inspection that will follow shortly on submission of a PLA to the US authorities.

Specifications

As more batches of product are made, and more batches of raw materials consumed, the specifications should be periodically reviewed and refined. In this process, as in all changes, great attention must be given to ensuring that the rationale for the change is adequately recorded, and that all identifiable implications are fully assessed.

Batch analysis report

Again, once more than one or two batches have been made, it is very useful to implement what we refer to as a batch analysis report, but which is in reality little more than a huge table, with one column per batch, listing in the rows all the analytical results for intermediates and for finished products. Although preparing this table can be a huge amount of work, and its design can be very taxing if it is to deal with changed processes, we find it an invaluable tool in QA review of batch quality control (QC) results, and in the review of specifications as well as in the preparation of regulatory submissions.

Initial preparation for preapproval inspection

At this stage, and working on the (essential) assumption that the programme will be successful, it is very useful to review operations in the light of regulatory expectations, perhaps most notably in the knowledge that, if the programme is successful, an FDA preapproval or pre-licence inspection is inevitable. This inspection will follow shortly on the submission of the product and establishment licence applications (or new drug application for a chemical entity). Although much help can be obtained from consultants familiar with current regulatory authority thinking, a very large amount of information about the regulatory requirements and expectations can be gleaned quite easily from FDA publications. Although these will doubtless have been consulted at various stages throughout the project's history to date, a critical review, looking at them as audit checklists, at this stage can help ensure that when the investigators do visit, the inspection goes smoothly.

Phase II to phase III

It is during this phase that the final process and final formulation should be established. Although changes are still possible, the additional work these generate is very large, and should be avoided it at all possible by careful planning and sheer hard work at the current stage.

Specifications

Although the periodic specification reviews suggested earlier should continue, we believe that from this present stage the assumption should be that specifications are frozen. No changes should be introduced without pressing need, and care should be taken to avoid unnecessary fine-tuning.

However, where a product is made in one country and will be tested, and eventually marketed, in others, the question of national pharmacopoeias must be addressed. Whilst it may be acceptable to test raw materials, bulk drug and finished dosage forms using the methods specified in a single pharmacopoeia during early development, it is probably essential that materials and products are tested according to the local pharmacopoeial requirements for each country for phase III clinical trials and beyond. Therefore, it is necessary to establish and test out these assays now, to ensure that they will work acceptably and are adequately documented in time for their use when actually needed.

Stability studies

Although pilot studies have been set up earlier, it is essential to set up full formal studies on bulk drug, and on dosage forms in their packaging as early as possible, in order to have the maximum data to support shelf-life claims at time of registration. The advantages of establishing good stability data early must, however, be set against the risk of necessary significant changes in manufacturing process or dosage form design that would render all the work that had gone into earlier stability studies without value. This is a factor that must be considered in assessing proposed changes.

Assay validation

Some initial analytical method validation was specified before first administration to humans, but now the remainder of the analytical programme must be reviewed and priorities set for validation. All assays must be validated prior to production of materials for phase III; this includes both the assays on the final bulk drug and on the dosage form, as well as assays on intermediates and in-process stages. Additionally, assays used in the formal stability studies discussed briefly above must be validated (including being shown to be stability-indicating) before these studies are initiated. Although the validation of a biological assay can be a complex undertaking, the International Conference for Harmonization (ICH) *Harmonised Tripartite Guideline Validation of Analytical Procedures* makes a good starting point for designing plans for validation. The article by McEntire (1994) is also directly relevant to determining how and when to perform validation of analytical methods.

Phase III to licence application

In this, the final phase of time development (it must be borne in mind that some development support will be necessary throughout much of the life of the product) it is essential to move a complete GMP compliance. Most topics are already appropriately addressed, however, and it is now a matter of dealing with a few, albeit major, items.

Validation

By the time of phase III trials it is essential that the final process is established, and if possible being run in the facility, although possibly not at the final scale, that will be used for manufacturing the licensed product. This means that process operators must be trained (including production QC if this is distinct from research and development QC), and the actual manufacturing process must be validated. All this work, so easy to specify and so hard to do, must be accomplished, including writing and review of the reports, before the grant of the licence, if the claim that manufacturing is to follow GMP is to be true.

Conclusion

In this chapter, we have presented, in an excessively simplified way, the GMP gradient concept, starting with a fairly easy climb but rapidly steepening, as appropriate for materials being put into humans. Of course, for simplicity we have presented development as a single strand; in fact it is probably never like this. For example, we have discussed the manufacture of material for toxicology studies and the level of GMP compliance necessary for this as if such manufacture only occurred once. The key idea here is that a single standard should be applied at any one point in time; the manufacture of material for toxicology at a time later than mentioned in this article must be done to the (higher) standard applicable at the time of production. To tighten the level of GMP compliance continuously is difficult to manage; to shift back and forth between higher and lower standards would be almost impossible.

This then is the GMP gradient as applied to a biotechnology development programme. As will be obvious, all of it is simply common sense; we believe that adoption of this common-sense approach will both smooth and speed any development programme.

References

Adner, N. and Sofer, G. (1994) Biotechnology product validation, part 3: chromatography cleaning validation. *Pharm. Tech. Europe* **6**: 22–28.

Akers, J., McEntire, J. and Sofer, G. (1994a) Biotechnology product validation, part 1: identifying the pitfalls. *Pharm. Tech. Europe* **6**: 32–34.

Akers, J., McEntire, J. and Sofer, G. (1994b) Biotechnology product validation, part 2: a logical plan. *Pharm. Tech. Europe* **6**: 38–41.

Barry, A. R. and Chojnacki, R. (1995) Biotechnology product validation, part 8: chromatography media and column qualification. *Pharm. Tech. Europe* **7**: 34–38.

Biotechnology Inspection Guide (1991) Washington DC: US Department of Health and Human Services, Food and Drug Administration.

Bozzo, T. (1995) Biotechnology product validation, part 9: a former FDAer's view. *Pharm. Tech. Europe* **7**: 40–44.

Committee for Proprietary Medicinal Products (1992) *Good Manufacturing Practice for Investigational Medicinal Products: Annex 13 to the EC Guide to Good Manufacturing Practice for Medicinal Products* Brussels: European Commission.

Guideline on the Preparation of Investigational New Drug Products (1991) Washington DC: US Department of Health and Human Services, Food and Drug Administration, Center for Drug Evaluation and Research.

ICH Harmonised Tripartite Guideline Validation of Analytical Procedures (1994) Commission of the European Communities III/5626/94 Final.

McEntire, J. (1994) Biotechnology product validation, part 5: selection and validation of analytical techniques. *Pharm. Tech. Europe* **6**: 48–55.

Madsen, R. E. Jr. (1994) US vs Barr Laboratories: a technical perspective. *PDA J. Pharm. Sc. and Tech.* **48**: 176–79.

Parenteral Society Technical Monograph No. 4: The Use of Process Simulation Tests in the Evaluation of Processes for the Manufacture of Sterile Products (1993).

Seely, R. J., Wight, H. D., Fry, H. H., and Flack, G. F. (1994) Biotechnology product validation, part 7: validation of chromatography resin useful life. *Pharm. Tech. Europe* **6**: 32–38.

Sofer, G. (1994) Biotechnology product validation, part 4: clearance of impurities from protein and peptide biotherapeutics. *Pharm. Tech. Europe* **6**: 29–32.

'The Gold Sheet' (1993) *Quality Control Reports* **27**: 1–12.

18   GLPs in a biotechnology setting

R Kaplan

When I first joined the biotechnology industry in late 1988, I immediately experienced some unexpected and some new good laboratory practice (GLP) concerns. The unexpected concerns arose as a result of questions of applicability. Some basic researchers who worked with cell lines or with gene splicing were unsure as to whether GLPs applied to their work. GLPs after all is the acronym for good laboratory practice. These questions were those of scientists who were new to the pharmaceutical industry. Since GLPs are about good practice, they reasoned, why should they not apply to them? Training programmes were established to review the history and development of GLPs and to explain the scope of coverage of these regulations, especially in the USA. None the less, the scope of coverage as I had known it was to expand.

The questions of applicability concerns were the result of my background. Testing of the cell lines that produce the therapeutic products for microbiological contamination is probably just as important, or more so, as classical toxicity testing. I had spent the previous years working for drug companies in which GLPs applied to toxicity testing and some pharmacokinetics and metabolism testing, but not to testing of production processes. The latter were the stuff of good manufacturing practice (GMP) regulations. But biotech is an industry regulated in the USA by the Food and Drug Administration's (FDA's) Center for Biological Evaluation and Research (CBER), not the Center for Drug Evaluation and Research (CDER) which regulates drugs in the USA. And CBER has its *Points to Consider* documents (1994), which recommend various kinds of testing on cell lines used to produce the active ingredient. CBER expects such testing to be done under GLPs (Marous-Sekura and Kozak, 1994).

Added to these GLP considerations is the assessment of the recipient's antibody response to exogenous proteins. I came to learn about HAMA (human antimurine antibodies) and HACA (human antichimeric antibodies) in my company. The potential generation of such responses during clinical trials raises concerns about both efficacy and safety. Thus HAMA and HACA testing of clinical trial serum samples also became a GLP issue. In the discussion that follows, I shall give an overview of GLP implementation in a biotechnology environment.

Toxicity testing

The company for which I had worked during the last 6 years develops monoclonal antibodies as therapeutic agents. Toxicity testing was generally contracted out, as I suspect it is for most biotechnology companies. This use of contractors is based on several reasons. Toxicity testing is often nowhere as extensive as that for a chemical drug, because the results from animal testing of human (or humanized) proteins do not give meaningful information for predicting human safety concerns. Second, some of the testing requires simians because they are biologically closer to humans than rodents and dogs. These are expensive to acquire and maintain. Third, developing companies with limited capital need not (and may not be able to afford to) invest in an animal colony and testing facilities to support limited testing. Therefore, it is much cheaper to contract the needed studies. Lastly, some testing requires specialized services. One type of testing that has been routinely performed for antibodies under development is cross-reactivity with human tissue. It is hoped, of course, that an antibody is specific for one receptor on one cell type in one tissue. Although this is a restatement of the pharmacologist's dream of a *magic bullet* it has been found that antibodies do act on other tissues. Therefore, these studies require the use of samples drawn from human tissue banks. These contracted safety studies were routinely performed under the GLPs.

The implementations of GLPs for routine and specialized toxicity testing in my former company consisted of typical contract toxicity testing work. The Regulatory Compliance department which was responsible for audit worked closely with Pharmacology/Toxicology. The latter prepared overall toxicology strategies, developed and reviewed protocols, selected contractors, monitored studies and data on an ongoing basis, reviewed all amendments and issues arising, reviewed and approved reports, and worked with the company's regulatory affairs staff to report to and respond to regulatory authorities. These activities were all proceduralized – standard operating procedures (SOPs) were prepared to describe the various functions and responsibilities. Thus, Pharmacology/Toxicology's SOPs included preparation and review of protocols, protocol amendment review, contractor site visit and selection, study monitoring and report review.

Compliance supported these efforts by performing several types of audits and making recommendations. A pre-award audit of a potential contractor occurred during the development of a schedule of studies to be done. Often done jointly with Pharmacology/Toxicology, this audit is a typical GLP facility and quality inspection with an emphasis on the quality control and assurance practices of the facility. Quality assurance unit (QAU) SOPs for facility, procedure, data and report audits are reviewed to determine their acceptability. The facility is questioned about sharing study audit findings with the sponsor as well as reporting all pertinent study activities to the company study monitor. The audit would typically take 2 days and would inquire about FDA inspectional history. Visual inspection of all major areas would occur. Since the company's protein products are temperature-sensitive, the contractor's facilities, equipment and operations involved in receipt, logging, storage, taking inventory and issue of test article are closely assessed to ensure that no loss of quality could happen. Dose preparation would also receive scrutiny. The contractor's animal facilities, laboratory areas such as histopathology and clinical pathology and archives would be inspected. Any computer-supported activities would be assessed for validation and documentation.

At the conclusion of such an audit, a close-out meeting is held with the contractor to review major findings, if any. Upon return to the company the compliance group prepares an audit report that describes the audit, findings and contractor responses, and makes recommendations concerning the acceptability of the contractor. Any unresolved issues are communicated in writing by Pharmacology/Toxicology to the contractor. Written responses are reviewed jointly for acceptability.

Once a contractor has been selected, the Compliance Department performs several other audits. Audits of ongoing studies have been done to ensure that the protocols and contractor's SOPs are being followed, any protocol amendments agreed to by the sponsor have been appropriately implemented, and that data are appropriate and acceptable. Maintenance of the test article, the antibodies, under required conditions, such as refrigerated storage, is scrutinized.

Although the in-life audit has been infrequent, the third type of audit – audit of a completed study report – has been frequent. Compliance has attempted to audit, at the contractor, each significant GLP toxicity testing report. The audit consists of comparing the report to the protocol and amendments and the drug log as well as assessing the quality of the report by determining its internal consistency (the latter can be done at the sponsoring company prior to the site visit). Data audit is also performed. Major summary data tables are compared to individual data tables and raw data to ensure that the report accurately, completely and verifiably reflects the raw data.

Results of this audit are communicated to the Pharmacology/Toxicology study monitor who contacts the contractor. Responses and any report changes sent to the study monitor are presented to Compliance for an assessment and final acceptability of the report. Compliance has submitted a statement of audit with product licence application (PLA) submissions to CBER that describe the audits. The statement includes dates of audit, type of audit and contractor. These are in addition to the contractor's QAU statement.

For contractors with whom the company has developed a history, pre-award and procedural audits do not occur. However, Compliance's goal is to visit each contractor used routinely once every 18–24 months.

Contract cell line testing

As noted above, biotechnology products derived from cell lines are under the aegis of an FDA *Points to Consider* document (Center for Biological Evaluation and Research, 1994), which requires testing of the cell lines for *Mycoplasma* and viruses, depending on the origins of the cell line. If an antibody-producing hybridoma cell line was derived from human and mouse cells, then testing of the cell line for human and mouse viruses is required for lot release. These tests are quite specialized and are usually done at several contract laboratories. A PLA must identify these laboratories. Most biotechnology companies, to the author's knowledge, use these contractors. The contractors specify GLPs in their performance of these studies. This means, operationally, that a study director is appointed, the testing is kept on a master schedule, each study follows a protocol, there are SOPs for all study activities, and that personnel are trained in GLPs.

The test systems for many of these studies are cell lines – the indication of viral presence is destruction of cells. Thus, the cell lines must have inventories, documentation of origin and traceability, specifications for growth characteristics and suitable media, and other performance criteria to support positive and negative controls in the cell line testing. They must be maintained under suitable storage conditions and be free of contaminants. The preparation, maintenance and use of media require SOPs and documentation. As a facility issue, the control of media brings GMP-like considerations under a GLP programme. These considerations include the sterilization of media containers and transfer lines, validation of the sterilization cycles, etc.

Since the results of these tests are used in release, including release of product, the control of the communication process between contractor and sponsor is quite important. Specifications must be set, against which each study's results are compared by the sponsor. The results, then, must be submitted directly or indirectly to a quality control/quality assurance group which determines whether a lot of product can be released. Since these studies are done under GLPs the sponsor must receive the results in a study report, signed by the study director and audited by the contractor's QAU, accompanied by a QAU statement. Only upon receiving a final study report with verified results should release proceed. The specifications must be set by the sponsor because the sponsor is responsible for the product, its release and regulatory agency specifications. Instructions must also be given to the contractor for handling residual sample and for retesting. The sponsor and contractor must agree as to the basis for performing a retest, must develop procedures that describe the circumstances under which retesting is allowed, and must establish that the sponsor is contacted any time that a result is considered invalid by the contractor. The contractor must understand that it must report all results, including any invalidated data and the basis for invalidation, to the sponsor.

The FDA has requested copies of the sponsor's contract with the contractor that delineates the testing and responsibilities. This request was seen as part of the licensing requirements for a biologic in the USA. Such contractors are routinely inspected by CBER, often looking at the testing for specific clients.

The company's Compliance Department audits these cell-testing contractors just as it does the toxicity-testing contractors. Audits of the facility to determine acceptability have been done in conjunction with the sponsor's Quality Control Department and the development groups responsible for cell lines. The audit assessed the contractor's facilities and equipment for storage of cell lines and sponsor samples. The contractor's provision for segregation and quality control of these cell lines and the provisions for prevention of biological contamination were also assessed. The functions of the QAU, its audit procedures and training were reviewed as well as documentation practices and testing procedures. Included in the facility aspects were media preparation and storage, glass wash and sterilization and sterilizer validation.

Periodic audits of these contractors include report audits, which are essentially comparisons of the reported data to the raw data. The sponsor's documentation of the samples was compared to that of the contractor. Documentation of sample processing, culture media preparation and preparation of the cell lines for the specific tests were also reviewed. Since the test data are usually straightforward and not voluminous, these audits could compare all the data in a short amount of time.

HAMAS, HACAs, Hetc.

Injection of exogenous proteins into humans can elicit an antibody response. If the administered protein is of murine origin, the resulting antibody is known as HAMA. If the administered protein is chimerized then the resulting antibody is known as HACA. There are more potential antibody responses (human antihuman antibody or HAHA (*sic!*), etc.).

Typically, in human clinical trials, blood samples are taken from the patients to analyse for the generation of HAMAs or HACAs, depending on the administered material. The generation of such a response may limit efficacy, especially for chronic administration, and/or it may impact upon safety. Because the effect needs to be characterized, the blood samples are returned to the sponsor for these tests. Because these are human blood samples, the GLPs do not apply. None the less, the company for which I was working established a GLP laboratory to handle the testing. GLP principles were followed except that neither master schedules nor protocols were used. Audit as well as the remainder of the GLPs were part of the programme which included extensive documentation of the activities.

The quality programme for this testing started with method qualification. Since the test methods were immunochemistry-based and since there were neither reference standards (human antibodies) nor standard methods, the development of a method was no easy task. The method that was to be developed had to be specific, accurate, linear over the expected range of concentrations, and quantifiable, as well as having reasonable precision. The assay had to demonstrate these characteristics when used to test in human blood, a complex mixture that varies from patient to patient.

Once the method was qualified, suitable documentation of samples as well as physical lay-out to handle samples needed to be created. Depending on the materials, the blood samples were shipped at 2–8°C. Therefore the documentation of the samples included a statement of their condition upon receipt as well as evidence of maintenance of the appropriate temperature during shipment. A log was created that captured the sample number (or site, patient, and sampling date, depending on whether the samples were blinded or not), the date of receipt, condition upon receipt, initials of the person receiving the samples, and any comments.

The laboratory was set up to receive, log and store the samples under suitable controls. Thus, a designated freezer or refrigerator with a limited (locked) access, calibrated temperature monitoring and recording devices and alarm was employed. Samples would be stored in an organized fashion, to prevent mix-ups.

Strict documentation practices were employed in the processing. Notebooks were used. All reagent and chemical entries included manufacturer, lot number and expiration date. Calculations for preparation of solutions and for dilutions were included. Data from printouts were clipped to the notebooks, unless they were so voluminous as to be kept separately. Date, initials, assay, sample identification and similar information were written on the printout. Any computer-generated standard curves were also kept. All documentation and data were archived.

To have adequate control necessitated writing SOPs for these assays, handling samples and reporting of results. All the equipment in the laboratory was under maintenance and calibration programmes. Records were kept of any cleaning of the equipment.

Upon completion of the testing of all the samples from a clinical protocol, a report of the results or a separate section of a clinical report would be prepared.

As for any well-managed facility, training records were maintained. These included job descriptions, curriculum vitae and training for all staff. Training would include review of appropriate procedures, technical review of specific assays and/or techniques, demonstration of successful conduct of assays (as appropriate) and regulatory/legal training. This last training became a routine part of training and covered the Investigational New Drug (IND) process, GLPs, good clinical practices (GCPs), basics of the Food, Drug, and Cosmetic Act and Public Health Services Act as well as 18 United States' Code 1001 (fraud statute). These sessions were well-attended and elicited much discussion.

As noted, audit was an integral part of this programme. Since HAMA/HACA data were potentially significant safety data, the audit programme focused significant resources on the data and the laboratories. For pivotal trials, the laboratory facilities, equipment and materials were audited. The calibration and maintenance status of the equipment were inspected, as were use logs, the security and orderliness of the storage freezers and refrigerators, as well as the handling and tracking of samples.

Audit also handled data quality. Reports were audited just as a GLP or GCP report would be. This audit would assess the report's internal consistency: agreement of statements and data, correct table of contents, pagination and tabulation. Data quality was audited comparing a sampling of data (using Military Standard 105E) against the raw data as well as reviewing selected calculations.

An audit report is issued after meeting with the supervisory laboratory staff to discuss findings and issues and correct any errors. The audit report would describe any systematic problems, make recommendations for improvement and describe any corrective actions that resulted from the supervisory meeting.

Conclusion and recommendations

Implementation of a GLP programme for a biotechnology company demands an understanding of the types of studies and their included objectives. Because the companies are often small, it is easy to communicate the quality/regulatory message to those who make managerial decisions. The implementation of such quality programme depends on instilling a strong sense of the need for such programmes. Such necessities not only include regulatory compliance with FDA expectations but also validity and quality of the data. Assessments of safety are, after all, only as good as the quality of the data on which they are based.

Another set of issues for a new developing company consists of limited resources and the need to move forward rapidly. The ability to move forward is often supported by strong quality practices in preventing mistakes and in well-managed programmes. Much of the GLP principles and practices go far in supporting the success of innovative technologies. The alternative can be false starts, meaningless studies and the wasting of scarce resources.

During my tenure at my previous company, I had long, philosophical discussions about implementing GLP throughout Research and Development (R&D) with R&D and regulatory management. The practical implications are substantial. The issues we discussed included the interaction of control and basic research – how much control is necessary. Generally, basic concerns for the quality of data were not issues in developing quality systems. All agreed that measuring equipment must have good procedures for operation, calibration, maintenance, and cleaning and concomitant documentation of performance of these to assure the quality of data, and thereby the validity of studies.

Data found unanimity as to control under GLP standards. Thus, the basic considerations for recording, in controlled notebooks, the materials, equipment, test systems and experimental conditions were agreed upon. The details of experimental set-up were looked upon as useful in analysing an experiment's success or failure. Data too needed to be controlled. Thus, printouts, chromatograms and the like needed to have identification, date, equipment and cross-reference to the notebook. Records of calculations and dilutions all were to be recorded in the notebooks.

For the implementation of other GLPs in early R&D we found that some were appropriate, some not. Those activities described above needed SOPs, but many activities do not, particularly for a new experiment that may not work and/or may never be used again. Protocols in early research were seen as only an obstacle with nothing to recommend their use as a means of controlling quality. Master schedules were viewed in a similar way.

Audit was not dismissed. It was thought by all parties that a periodic audit of basic research would be useful, particularly as a management tool to assess the state of compliance with policies, practices and procedures. Thus, an audit could be conducted annually throughout R&D to review the maintenance of equipment, material and facility quality as well as data audits of selected key study reports against the raw data.

As I was leaving the company, these policies were being developed. Clearly, the understanding of the principles of study and data quality grew considerably during my tenure. These understandings were reinforced by product approvals in which many studies received considerable scrutiny. The ability of these studies to stand up to this intense scrutiny attests to the implementation of quality practices that support the science.

References

Center for Biological Evaluation and Research (1994). *Points to Consider in the Manufacture and Testing of Monoclonal Antibody Products for Human Use*. Rockville, MD: Food and Drug Administration.

Marous-Sekura, C. S. and Kozak, R. W. (1994) Continuous cell lines and contaminant testing. In: Lubiniecki, A. S. and Vargo, S. A., eds. *Regulatory Practice for Biopharmaceutical Production*. New York: Wiley–Liss, p. 72.

PART SEVEN

Laboratories –
implementation of GxPs

19   Good laboratory practice vs ISO 9000 for laboratories not directly involved in non-clinical projects

H D Plettenberg

Introduction

What kind of work are we concerned with?

Since the first publication of good laboratory practice (GLP) regulations, science has proceeded remarkably, and especially astounding is the progress in analytical work performed in laboratories. Some of this work could be called routine, but major improvements have been achieved in reproducibility and in cost reduction using advanced equipment. Other work deserves a description as being on the cutting edge of technology, where sensitivity and specificity have been pushed to limits previously beyond reach.

In both cases, dedicated analytical laboratories seem to have advantages over small divisions, which cannot afford modern techniques or expensive equipment. Many measuring units become economically feasible only with a throughput way above the number of specimens generated in a small non-clinical laboratory. Thus, specialized analytical laboratories have evolved which investigate specimens from clinical trials as well as from non-clinical laboratory studies. These laboratories contribute to the projects; however, they are not directly involved in study or trial performance.

The existence of these laboratories is well-known to the authorities, and reference to laboratories with expertise in analytical and clinical chemistry testing forms a specific section in the annual overviews of the national GLP monitoring programmes to the Organization for Economic Cooperation and Development (OECD, 1992).

GLP compliance is explicitly requested by many sponsors of analytical work, but producing evidence for GLP compliance may become difficult: analysis of specimens generated in clinical trials is not governed by GLP. Where contribution to non-clinical studies is not intended, GLP inspection and, hence, GLP certification, may be impossible to obtain.

On the other hand, contributing to at least some non-clinical studies may be very attractive for a laboratory, as a trickle of specimens collected from rats or dogs may be the beginning of a flood of specimens generated in clinical trials. Where at least a certain aspect of non-clinical work, as governed by GLP, is planned or being performed, the title question 'GLP vs ISO 9000' must by no means be interpreted as the alternative 'GLP *or* ISO 9000'. A quality system according to ISO 9000 includes, under any circumstances, the fulfilment of *all* requirements of society, i.e. of 'obligations resulting from laws, regulations, rules, codes, statutes, and other considerations'. The only alternative to laboratory management therefore is GLP alone or integration of ISO 9000 and GLP.

Regulations and standards addressed

For the present comparison, the only GLP document referred to will be the OECD's *Good Laboratory Practice in the Testing of Chemicals* (1982). Studies performed to these principles are acceptable throughout the world and, moreover, they are immediately legally binding in the states of the European Union (EU; after request by Council Directive 87/18/EEC). All other GLP source documents represent variations on this theme, without major additions or omissions. References to specific sections in the OECD *Principles of GLP* are included in this chapter; a reference to for example, the section on 'study plan' will read '[*GLP* II.8.1]'.

ISO 9000 is a short name for an approach to quality systems. It is described in a group of standards, the ISO 9000 family (see clause 3.6 in ISO 9000–1: 1994), which at present comprises 'a) all the International Standards numbered ISO 9000 through to ISO 9004, including all parts of ISO 9000 and IS 9004; b) all the International Standards numbered ISO 10 001 through to 10 020, including all parts; and c) ISO 8402'.

Special emphasis is given to ISO 9004–1 (1994) and ISO 9001 (1994). Both standards often address the same topic from their respective different points of view of either utilizing quality management for the internal benefit of an organization (ISO 9004–1) or of providing confidence to a customer (ISO 9001). References to specific clauses of either or both standards are included in the text; a reference to the respective clauses addressing, for example, control of inspection, measuring and test equipment will read [9001: 4.12/9004–1: 13]. Other standards will be mentioned and referred to as well.

Terminology

A comparison of GLP and ISO 9000, two systems for quality management, must recognize that different concepts and goals are reflected in the different use of quality-related terms (Plettenberg, 1994).

The most difficult term in this context is quality assurance (QA).

'Quality Assurance Programme means an internal control system designed to ascertain that the study is in compliance with these principles of GLP' [*GLP* I.1.2(3)]. Incorporation of this GLP objective into ISO 9000 is certainly possible, but some careful adjustment in wording is required.

In order to avoid misunderstandings, the various aspects of quality assurance will be addressed specifically either as activities to provide confidence about quality (to reassure) or to ascertain quality (to ensure). The GLP approach is described consistently with 'QA programme' or activities of the QA unit (QAU).

Within ISO 9000, a wide-ranging program to ensure and ascertain quality would be named quality system or quality management system. (In the good manufacturing practice (GMP) regulations of the EU, quality assurance and quality management are used synonymously.)

In almost all GLP facilities the responsibility for the quality of the study is assigned to the study director; quality surveillance is assigned to line management. The task performed by the QAU can be described as 'systematic and independent examination to determine whether quality activities and related results comply with planned arrangements and whether these arrangements are implemented effectively and are suitable to achieve objectives' – and this is exactly the definition of ISO 8402 for the term 'quality audit' (clause 4.9 in ISO 8402: 1994). There is an explanatory note in the standard, which is absolutely in line with the current approach to GLP: 'An audit should not be confused with "surveillance" or "inspection" activities performed for the purpose of process control or product acceptance'.

Thus, there is no contradiction between GLP and ISO 9000, if independent QA auditors are explicitly requested not to let themselves be pushed into a position of *de facto* assuming responsibility for the quality of the study.

The term quality control is avoided in this chapter, in favour of more specific aspects like quality surveillance and quality improvement.

A written plan for analytical investigations is called analytical protocol to differentiate it from study plan or, where a differentiation is irrelevant, simply protocol. The one person responsible for the project is called the responsible analyst.

Problems and options for either system

Problems with GLP

Most activities performed in analytical laboratories are not preconceived in GLP regulations. The principles barely mention, under 'reporting of study results', that cooperating scientists may be involved [*GLP* II.9.1(4)]. On the other hand, if a laboratory is asked to perform a subset of a GLP study, for example, specimen analysis, many of the core elements of GLP do *not* apply.

Above all, a project like analysis of drug residue in tissues does not represent a study in the definition of GLP. GLP defines a study as the complete work from its plan, proceeding to selection and exposure of test systems, observations of the test systems, including specimen collection, specimen analysis and evaluation of all findings in a comprehensive report [*GLP* I.3(1)–(2)]. Laboratories which are not directly involved in GLP work thus by definition are excluded from the privilege of having a study director, of writing study plans etc.[1]

The author knows of at least one example where a local GLP monitoring authority claimed that study director and study plan are indispensable core elements for GLP compliance, and explicitly requested that an analytical laboratory had to write study plans and nominate study directors for its contribution to GLP studies. This caused a lot of trouble for the sponsor's laboratory, where the animals had been treated, as the study director there had to reconcile two mutually exclusive interpretations of GLP regulations in order to finalize the study report.

In a non-clinical laboratory, the QAU is expected to ensure adherence to protocol and standard operating procedures (SOPs) 'by periodic inspections of the test facility and/or by auditing the study in progress' [*GLP* II.2.2(b)]. If a test facility is sufficiently diversified to perform all aspects of a complex non-clinical study, including specimen analysis, it would be unlikely that the analytical laboratory will be visited by the QAU in each study – or at least, not more than once. However if the analytical work is contracted out to an external laboratory, multiple activities of the QAU have been requested by contract managers, who redefined a segment of a study as a study in its own right. As a result, the inherent tendency of GLP to abuse the QAU as a surveillance instrument may become even more pronounced.

Options with GLP

Without compliance to the formal framework of GLP an analytical laboratory could contribute to a GLP study only if the sponsor's QAU would perform the necessary monitoring of the project. Compliance to (applicable aspects!) of GLP, including an internal QA programme, allows the

---

[1]There is however one exception to this statement: analytical method validation projects, where sample generation is an integral part of the analytical work, may stand for themselves as complete studies, as defined by GLP.

laboratory to participate in GLP studies without triggering (or requesting) activities of an external QAU.

With perfect understanding (and observation) of GLP techniques, the laboratory's contribution will blend easily into the major part of the study. This again increases the value of the service provided: not only can the results be substantiated, but also incorporation without effort into the study report is achieved.

Problems with ISO 9000

GLP is so widely acknowledged that adherence to GLP is specifically requested by many sponsors of analytical work even for projects where application of GLP is excluded by definition in the regulations (clinical laboratory work, bioanalytical investigations in the context of clinical trials investigating absorption, distribution, metabolism and excretion of drugs, etc.). Obviously such sponsors consider a GLP certificate as the instrument to provide confidence in a laboratory, irrespective of the applicability of GLP. The certificate indicates proficiency in a type of work reasonably similar to the one requested.

ISO 9000 on the other hand is applied so generally that certification to ISO 9001 does not imply any proficiency of an organization to perform laboratory work. Moreover, no health authority has so far indicated its willingness to accept an ISO 9001 certificate as sufficient for quality assurance. For regulatory purposes, confidence cannot be provided outside the tools of GLP, by an independent QAU working according to GLP and by a GLP monitoring programme.

Options with ISO 9000

ISO 9000 describes an extremely generalized approach to a quality system; thus it is applicable to any product, including the analytical services of a laboratory not directly involved in GLP projects. People accustomed to the tight guidance provided by GLP will at first feel disoriented when they start consulting the ISO 9000 standards. A series of documents equally applicable to organizations providing car rentals, manufacturing video screens, offering training courses or constructing railway bridges can by no means address any type of business as detailed as how the *Principles of GLP* cover the performance of non-clinical studies.

On the other hand, the very same generalized approach of ISO 9000 allows application of the standard to any aspect or segment of GLP-governed studies, including those not addressed specifically in the GLP regulations, such as performance of analytical work in the laboratory.

An increasing number of chemical and pharmaceutical manufacturers for their own interest are addressing ISO 9000 within their organizations, and with increasing knowledge of the strengths of this standard they will start looking for suppliers applying the same standard.

Upgrading of GLP by ISO 9000

Management involvement [9001: 4.1/9004–1: 4]

GLP always requires laboratory management to ensure compliance to its principles, but especially in larger laboratories there is a strong trend to shift much of this responsibility to the QAU. For a quality system according to ISO 9000, top management involvement is requested explicitly. 'The responsibility for and commitment to a quality policy belongs to the highest level of management' [9004–1: 4.1], and no independent group assigned with quality surveillance is suggested. Only top management can define the quality policy; it has to determine quality objectives and request that lower levels of management follow suit.

An evasive approach of management to its own responsibilities may be defensible in a quality system according to GLP; it becomes impossible when accepting the challenge of ISO 9000.

Quality system: advanced guidance [9001: 4.2/9004–1: 5]

GLP has been widely accepted as a quality system. Unfortunately, GLP concentrates completely on quality surveillance. Important as quality surveillance is in order to prevent an unexpected deterioration in established procedures or quality system elements, surveillance alone never can and never will create improvement.

The thorough explanations in ISO 9000, especially in ISO 9004–1, provide a much advanced guidance to develop a quality system geared for improvement. Additionally a collateral ISO 9004–4 exists which 'describes fundamental concepts and principles, management guidelines and methodology (tools and techniques) for quality improvements' (clause 7.12 in ISO 9000–1: 1994).

This standard, ISO 9004–4, gives a perfectly well-suited summary of the reason why GLP alone cannot be the future quality system of a laboratory:

> Correcting process outputs reduces or eliminates a problem which has occurred. Preventive and corrective actions eliminate or reduce the causes of a problem, and hence any future occurrence. Thus, preventive and corrective actions improve the processes of an organization and are critical to quality improvement (clause 3.1.5 in ISO/DIS 9004–4: 1992).

Several aspects of the quality system described in ISO 9000 extend beyond the scope of GLP. The concept of planning for quality, as expressed in quality plans [9004–1: 5.2.3], goes well beyond a study plan or protocol for analytical investigations.

The documentation of the quality system is much more comprehensive if organized according to ISO 9000 as compared to GLP. (People afraid of excessive paperwork may relax, as the standards on several occasions strongly recommend documentation to be limited to the extent required in a specific situation.)

Another strength compared to GLP is the assignment of another, additional purpose to quality records: they not only serve to provide evidence for fulfilment of requirements, they are also considered as a valuable tool for improvement [9001: 4.16/9004–1: 17].

Link between economic success and quality

Financial considerations [9004–1: 6]

GLP, like all good practice regulations, does not address the interrelation of quality and the economic success of a laboratory. Whether an organization is economically successful or not, compliance is indispensable. In the past, the three needs of a laboratory's clients (quality of data and report, timeliness and low price) or laboratory management (sponsor satisfaction, deadline and turnover) have often been dealt with as a conflict of interest ('pick any two'). People seriously asked: 'Do you want it on time, or do you want to have it done right?'

Most laboratories are exposed to the forces of a highly competitive market, where prices for routine as well as sophisticated analyses tend to stagnate or even drop against inflation's trend. In a laboratory requiring several review cycles to ascertain data integrity, timeliness and reliability are inversely correlated. When a laboratory responds to complaints about deviations from data integrity or GLP requirements with an increase in efforts at error detection, it is creating restrictive costs for quality. Departments lose their ability to create the revenues needed for measuring equipment with higher sensitivity, more powerful computers, more user-friendly and reliable software. Confronted with increasing costs locked up in the requirement to maintain quality, not a small number of department heads ended up as perceiving quality as a counter-productive concept, opposed to scientific relevance.

ISO 9000, especially the standard ISO 9004–1, provides the tools to avoid such a deadlock. In the introduction, economic production and competitive prices are listed at the same level of goals as customer satisfaction and compliance. Clause 6 of ISO 9004–1 (financial considerations of quality systems) offers a variety of approaches to investigate quality-related costs and implicitly suggests that quality improvement (e.g. by elimination of error sources) should be utilized for economic success.

Whenever a quality-related problem is detected, corrective and preventive action is to be installed. Local correction may be sufficient for GLP compliance, but a prospective approach to quality includes all steps from 'investigation of possible causes' through 'analysis of problem' to 'elimination of causes' – not forgetting appropriate 'process controls' to avoid recurrence of the problem [9004–1: 15.4–15.7].

Customer orientation

Whether the needs of the sponsor of a project have been explicitly stated or only implied, they must be satisfied in order to make the project a full success. Thus it is of utmost importance to investigate the needs of the sponsor [9004–1: 7.2, 'Defining product specification'] to explore whether there are any specific requirements as yet unstated (the ominous tacit assumptions), and to develop a product brief, for which both sides are confident that it contains all requirements which, when fulfilled, will satisfy the client's needs.

Most sponsors react rather anxiously to perceived changes in the regulatory environment, especially if the final submission of data is still years ahead. A laboratory is well-advised to establish a documented system to analyse information about future trends [9004–1: 7.1, 'Marketing requirements'] in order to adjust its internal procedures. A timely contact with the authorities (workshops, seminars) allows internal procedures to be developed proactively in line with future requirements. A pertinent example was the discussion on analytical method validation in 1990, where active participants could check their procedures and perform any necessary updates before today's standard requirements became published.

The focus of the sponsors of analytical work is shifting continuously. Next to repetition of relevant questions raised by regulatory authorities (computer validation being the hottest topic), they concentrate increasingly on the format of reporting and on communication during the project (e.g. on-line data transfer).

Without a system in place to ask for feedback [9004–1: 16.6], the response from the sponsors after delivery of results and report is unpredictable. Some perform an in-depth review for acceptance, others prefer to include the report directly into their submission, and the earliest comments – if any – come years later from a health authority. Whenever a sponsor or a regulatory agency complains about an aspect of a laboratory's work, an established procedure should ensure that it is not only dealt with on a case-by-case basis, but that it is analysed for general applicability [9004–1: 16.5), and corrective action installed.

In addition, sponsors of analytical work today expect that a laboratory is capable and willing to amend the report if additional requests are brought forward. Such servicing activities [9001: 4.19] may not create income, but they do offer an excellent opportunity for close contact with health authorities. Still, even a successful defence of analytical work by submission of additional data (e.g. from the validation process) is costly, and any procedure to prevent recurrence is worth the effort.

Contract review [9001: 4.3]
A formal system of contract review [9001: 4.3] should be established in a laboratory, and review performed before accepting a contract or submitting a tender. Readers unfamiliar with ISO 9000 may think that this describes a lawyer's activity, but the review has other aims: to make sure that the laboratory has the capability to meet contract requirements [9001: 4.3.2.c)], and even more, to make sure that these requirements are adequately defined and documented [9001: 4.3.2.a)]. To illustrate these two approaches, a laboratory first has to make sure that it can analyse, for example, a drug from plasma, with a sensitivity of down to 2.5 ng/ml with a method validated to accepted standards. However, if the request for this service does not contain requirements for the time-frame, there is a risk that an analyst gives a 'go-ahead' to management (because analyses can be performed to specifications), although it may be impossible to meet an implied (and as yet uncommunicated) deadline, or meeting this deadline may need major rearrangements of workload. A request for analytical services without specifications on deadline, on reporting format, on paper as well as by electronic data transmission, on frequency and intensity of communication and interim reporting is not yet adequately defined, and contract review will reveal that there is ample space for horrible misunderstandings.

Project planning: quality in specification and design [9001: 4.4/9004–1: 8]

ISO 9000, especially the complete section 8 in 9004–1, provides an in-depth description of how quality of a specific study starts with its specification and design. This section certainly does not contain any secrets, but it gives a highly organized description of a successful planning process: it should be regarded as essential reading for all study directors who want to improve.

There is a long list of specifications which need attention. On the one hand there is sensitivity, selectivity, precision, accuracy, specimen stability and robustness of the analytical method, including the evidence required to demonstrate these parameters, while on the other hand there are requirements for project performance, such as records for specimen handling providing evidence for specimen integrity, calibration range, acceptance/rejection criteria for analytical runs and single determinations, sequence of measurements, documentation, review procedure, communication of results, including requirements for record authentication, record keeping and archiving.

If these requirements do not completely reflect the needs of the sponsor of the study, unpleasant shortcomings are programmed into the work, and outright failure cannot be excluded.

Measuring equipment: ISO 10 012 [9001: 4.11/9004–1: 13]

The standard ISO 10 012–1 (1992), an acknowledged member of the ISO 9000 family, provides in-depth guidance for the most critical equipment in an analytical laboratory – measuring equipment. Even a short review of the standard goes beyond the scope of this chapter; it is highly recommended that it should be read and applied.

The more general GLP requirement for maintenance of all equipment, including that which does not perform any measurements, can easily be treated under the requirements for documented procedures under process control [9001: 4.9] or, more specifically, under 'equipment control and maintenance' [9004–1: 11.3].

Project control

The core product of an analytical laboratory, the performance of analytical services, may gain by considerations all over the ISO 9000 standards: from purchasing [9001: 4.6/9004–1: 9] and handling of incoming, customer-supplied products [9001: 4.7] to handling, storage and preservation [9001: 4.15] – the whole range of logistics is covered with more detail than in GLP.

During the analyses, an organized system of inspection, testing, verification (of chromatograms or similar records) and documented test status [9001: 4.10, 4.12/9004–1: 12] will improve control of the project.

Whenever an analysis fails, it must be clear that its results are prevented from entering the report or, if the flaw is detected retrospectively, that all its traces are removed. A well-established 'Control of nonconforming product' [9001: 4.13/9004–1: 14] will prevent inadvertent inclusion of erroneous data, and at the same time trigger corrective action [9001: 4.14/9004–1: 15].

Staff involvement [9001: 4.18 9004–1: 18]

The OECD *Principles of GLP* limit the responsibilities of personnel working under the study director to safe working practice and health precautions [II.1.3], and there is very limited further reference to personnel: management has to 'ensure that sufficient personnel is available' [II.1.1(2)(k)], and summaries of qualifications, training, experience and job descriptions have to be retained in the archives [GLP II.10.2(1)(c)], which implies that personnel should be qualified and well-trained.

It is correct that responsibility cannot and must not be delegated. With assignment of a responsible analyst for each project, there is actually no room left where further staff members can assume responsibility *in* or *for* an analytical project.

In GLP only two functions are mentioned, which go beyond responsibility for projects: those of the archivist and independent QA staff. However, an ISO 9000 quality system provides ample opportunities to increase staff involvement: staff members can not only be *authorized* to perform tasks critical for quality within the projects, they may also be in an excellent position to assume responsibility for defined activities in the quality system. The implementation of a responsibility matrix organization in a laboratory will encourage staff participation without generating ambiguity; when, for example, columns stand for quality system elements, and lines for projects, staff members can be assigned with reference standard administration, generation and administration of standardized report formats and continuous update of records on personnel qualification.

Thus, the experience and dedication of staff members are acknowledged, and contributions to quality improvement are encouraged.

Quality audits: ISO 10 011 [9001: 4.17/9004–1: 5.4]

With regard to quality audits, extremely valuable guidance is given in the standards ISO 10 011–1 to 10 011–3, recognized members of the ISO 9000 family. The volume and depth of these texts exceed any guidance available under GLP.

'GLP light' in a laboratory organized to ISO 9000

Reducing the burden of surveillance

A quality system limited to GLP does not plan for improvement; it is stuck in its emphasis on surveillance, which, necessary as it is under all circumstances, by definition does not include improvement. The term 'GLP light' has been coined for a quality system with reduction of quality surveillance in favour of planned efforts for quality improvement. It is a truism well-known to GLP experts that removal of error sources is much more effective than surveillance of error-prone processes. ISO 9000 provides the organizational framework for exactly this shift in emphasis.

In the transformation of the quality system from 'GLP alone' to 'GLP and ISO 9000', efforts should be made to define a set of internal procedures which allow bioanalytical work to be done to the same SOPs irrespective of the origin of specimens to be investigated – whether from a non-clinical study governed by GLP or from a clinical trial performed under good clinical practice (GCP). Where regulations differ, the laboratory has to decide which approach to different requirements is more cost-effective: close surveillance of alternative rules, or the development of procedures allowing the more stringent requirement to be fulfilled in any case.

Formal relation between GLP studies and derived analytical projects

Protocol

In a very strict approach to GLP, the indirect contribution of a laboratory to a GLP study should be planned either by explicit description in the study plan or by writing an amendment to the study plan, which defines the specific aspects of the analyses. It is obvious, however, that this document (or section of the study plan) contains only a fraction of the topics required for the overall study plan.

When laboratory work is not explicitly tied to a non-clinical study or clinical trial, a written protocol is still necessary in order to agree with the sponsor on the specifications to be reached.

Responsible analyst

Similar to the definition of the study director in *GLP*, ISO 9000 requests very clear assignments of responsibility and authority to contribute [9001: 4.1.2.1/9004–1: 5.2.2.]. Although specimens from a GLP study are not analysed under supervision of the study director, there must be a single responsible person for the laboratory's contribution.

Dilution of responsibility cannot provide confidence: there is no way to create reliable data in a laboratory, where responsibility for the work is distributed over an anonymous conveyor belt, i.e. several technicians perform their portions of work without central supervision.[2] Thus, a responsible analyst[3] has to be named, who accepts full responsibility in

[2]It is *not* sufficient if the head of the laboratory makes a review of the somehow generated final results in order to discuss findings and sign a report.
[3]A laboratory contributing to clinical as well as to non-clinical projects cannot use the GLP-derived term 'principal scientist' [*GLP* II.9.1(4)], because it is in strong disagreement with the meaning of the term 'principal investigator' used in GCP.

writing, including provisions for adequacy of the analytical method applied, sample integrity, performance and documentation of analyses, and reporting. There is no 'light' with regard to responsibility!

The only difference between a GLP study director and a responsible analyst is the scope of work for which he or she is responsible.

'*QA light*', *in line with GLP requirements*

Master schedule
Every reasonable laboratory must have something like a master schedule in order to plan its resources, and a quality auditor of the laboratory must have access to this information.

In some GLP facilities the task of maintaining this master schedule is assigned to QA.[4] Such an evasive attitude of laboratory management could not be upheld in an ISO 9000 environment: information on upcoming and active projects (as well as previous projects) is needed by management for process control, and thus it becomes available to the auditors by default. No auditor should be required to collect or administer this information! An auditor is better occupied with an examination of whether process control is effective or not.

Monitoring each project
Although the OECD *Principles of GLP* do *not* explicitly require monitoring *each* study, many laboratories feel that some extra assurance can be afforded to satisfy clients accustomed to the wording of the Food and Drug Administration's GLP.

The most critical phase in any project, from an ISO 9000 point of view, is specification and design (see section on project planning, above). A laboratory with adequate internal procedures for this project definition phase could ask the QA auditor to examine each project, whether a comprehensive listing of requirements for quality has been agreed upon. The form of this agreement (e.g. 'Protocol for analytical investigations' or 'Amendment to the study protocol' or another contractual agreement) is obviously secondary in importance as compared to its contents.

Without altering the policy that responsibility for the quality of the laboratory's services, including compliance to applicable GLP requirements, lies with the responsible analyst, the quality auditor may further be asked to examine each project, whether the laboratory's validated procedures have

---

[4]The reason is because of the lack of a specific requirement in the GLP regulations under management responsibilities to maintain a master schedule, while for QA a specific requirement is spelt out to 'maintain a *copy*'. Thus management in a GLP facility can, by simply doing nothing, push the QAU to perform this task.

been followed throughout and, most importantly, whether there is evidence for continuing and final review of records and data by the responsible analyst.

Any other repetitive QA activity in *each* project carries the risk of shifting responsibility. The limitation of mandatory QA involvement in laboratory projects to the two situations described above however does not mean that further audits would be neglected.

An internal audit programme

Shift in emphasis
In many laboratories practising GLP, the QA programme and related QA internal SOPs define involvement in projects or studies to such a degree that there is little time left to look at the laboratory's quality system or to think about error prevention or, more generally process improvement (see Table 19.1).

Table 19.1   *Options for distribution of quality assurance workload in a laboratory not directly involved in non-clinical projects*

GLP-driven	ISO 9000-driven, GLP-respected
Repetitive project monitoring (75%)	Basic project audit, including quality assurance internal administration (25%)
	In-depth audit of selected projects or project sections (25%)
	Process, system audits (25%)
GLP system audits (15%) Proactive work (10%)	Proactive work (25%)

By adoption of ISO 9000, emphasis will be shifted to examinations of process capability, away from error detection to error prevention. In the beginning laboratory personnel accustomed to reliable, repetitive QA monitoring may complain that they feel uneasy without a safety net. As long as the procedures in a laboratory are like tightrope walking, this can well be understood. But if processes lack robustness, they have to be changed. For someone walking on rock-solid ground, safety nets are not only superfluous, they even become an obstacle.

Capacity for process and system audits
Reduction of project-related audit activities is the best approach to creating the resources needed for process quality audits, and positive audit findings

in turn justify the reduction in project-related activities. On the other hand, findings of inadequate or ineffective procedures lacking the capability to build quality into the projects from the very beginning can be identified and corrected.

The process of performing laboratory projects has been compared to requirements for producing sterile products (Hutchison, 1994). Sterility has to be designed into the product by application of processes ensuring sterility; retrospective control cannot provide confidence, and retrospective correction is altogether impossible. Similarly, laboratories should strive for the development of error-free processes, and quality auditors are employed most effectively in examining process capability and cooperating in process improvement.

Targets for process audits can be anything from project specification and protocol writing to equipment maintenance, specimen handling, treatment of reference standards and solutions, reagents and chemicals, data management, and retention of records. One of the most important quality system elements is certainly its own documentation – in GLP terms the SOP system. Has the procedure for writing and updating the flexibility necessary to facilitate innovation and avoid retention of outdated procedures? Are distribution and training adequate? Moreoever, a comprehensive audit of the complete quality system can be planned and performed, providing further information to management and staff members, where improvement is possible and indicated.

Project-related audits: depth instead of repetition
Specific projects or sections of a project should be selected for a really thorough audit. Selection criteria would typically be for cause, specific management request, and a random choice from completely normal projects. It is highly preferable to reduce the number of projects or project sections examined in this way in favour of the depth applied to the audits.

For in-depth audits a number of clearly defined consecutive modules should be available. The number of projects hit at random by at least one module of in-depth audit is increased, preventing any misunderstandings that for normal projects a substandard performance might be acceptable.

The case for a merger

In the early 1980s, a small group of analytical laboratories determined the market by offering services not available before, and in some cases not available at any other site. At that time, technical expertise was so important that sponsors treated GLP compliance as a nice-to-have only, happy to find a place able to provide scientifically meaningful data. Within 10 years technology has advanced so far that sponsors now have a choice whether to ask for analytical services from internal laboratories or from one of a dozen or more contract laboratories capable of performing the required analyses. A laboratory which has difficulties in working to GLP standards will find it difficult to convince a sponsor who prefers a site with expertise as well as GLP compliance.

For all laboratories indirectly involved in non-clinical projects, maintaining or setting up a quality system in line with GLP is highly recommended, with careful interpretation to minimize administrative burden and to maximize effect (see above). A much more general quality system according to ISO 9000 should be wrapped around the narrow GLP approach, with benefit for all stakeholders.

Advantages to inspectors from either GLP or GCP monitoring programmes are the least obvious, as they are bound by their own regulator internal regulations. Certainly a carefully planned presentation of the interrelation between GLP and ISO 9000 is essential to avoid confusion of the inspectors. On the other hand, real improvements cannot but impress positively: every laboratory that has ever been submitted to the scrutiny involved with an in-depth inspection by health authorities shows that the inspectors are everything but inflexible box-checking clerks. With an increasing number of positive findings, more and more preliminary questions may be skipped in order to proceed faster to the most critical and relevant details. Thus both sides, inspector and laboratory, will find their burden reduced.

Sponsors of laboratory work will find better organized evidence of internal control mechanisms in the quality manual and at work, and may reduce their own surveillance activities based on positive audit findings.

Analysts, who carry responsibility for scientific value and regulatory appropriateness of the projects, gain from an improving environment for analytical work, including everyone and everything in staff, equipment and processes.

Staff members in line, i.e. those working under the scientists who assume responsibility for the projects, will appreciate the opportunities to contribute and receive acknowledgement. They may expect more acknowledgement for good work, reduction in frustrating defects and participation in economic success.

QA personnel will be released from surveillance activities: extensive and successful quality management activities provide laboratory management with the possibility to rely upon staff and processes working in line, just needing reassurance by independent audits. Quality auditors can be invited or encouraged to provide a diagnostic function as well, and they can be incorporated into improvement and training programmes – as long as management assumes directly the task of assessing the effectiveness of these activities.

Laboratory management may expect even in the short term some savings by reduction of quality-related costs, with further mid-term benefit from increased qualification of personnel and development of error-free (validated) processes (or steps in processes), in order to reduce surveillance costs. A culture of improvement is finally a prerequisite of the long-term economic success of the laboratory.

The research process on new drugs includes work controlled by various regulations, e.g. GLP, GCP, parts of GMP, legislation with regard to the clinical laboratory, etc. Unfortunately, there are remarkable discrepancies between these regulations, although it is obvious that all share the same purpose: to provide reliable data as the basis for decisions by physicians, scientists and regulators. ISO 9000 can be used to integrate the specific requirements of all these regulations into a consistent quality system of a research organization. Such an integration has not yet been performed in many organizations, but experience is increasing and will be communicated to the public soon.

Appendix 1:   Incorporation of applicable GLP requirements into the ISO 9000 framework for an analytical laboratory

There is very little similarity in the formal structure of GLP regulations and ISO 9000 standards. Although collations of both systems for quality management in a laboratory have been prepared for internal use in several companies or by industry associations, there is no fixed prescription available of where to place all the detailed GLP requirements in a quality manual or related procedures according to ISO 9000.

However, readers should be warned that in some cases cross-references were assigned based upon superficial similarities, and more detailed disassembling and reorganization may be needed.

To convince a more conservative GLP inspector of the fact that a laboratory's quality system described according to ISO 9000 does contain all details expected from a GLP point of view, the description of the quality system should contain an explicit road map of where to find each single requirement. This approach is highly recommended, as the cross-references suggested below are by no means the only convincing way, and the quality manuals of other laboratories with a different range of services may address GLP-related items in a more or less different arrangement.

Test facility organization and personnel [*GLP* II.1]

Management's responsibilities [GLP II.1.1]

The responsibilities assigned to test facility management are described in a rather specific way in *GLP*, and it is easy to incorporate these details into the broader approach of ISO 9000 [9001: 4.1/9004–1: 4].

Study director's responsibilities [GLP II.1.2]

In a GLP test facility, performance of the study is the key product, leading to information contained in data and report. Analogously, performance of a project is the key product of any other laboratory. With responsibility for the overall conduct of the study (or the project), the study director (or responsible analyst) will find his or her activities described in many sections of a quality system according to ISO 9000:

1   Agreement to protocol, protocol amendment procedure: see below, under protocol.
2   Ensuring protocol adherence [9001: 4.9 (process control), especially the statement 'Controlled conditions shall include the following ... c) compliance with reference standards/codes, quality plans and/or documented procedures;'/9004–1: 11 (Control of processes)].
3   Ensuring documentation and record-keeping [9001: 4.10.3 (In-process inspection)/9004–1: 12.2 (In-process verification)].
4   Signature of study report [9001: 4.10.4 (Final inspection)/9004–1: 12.3 (finished product verification)].
5   Transfer of study file to the archives: see the section on storage and retention of records and material, below.

The QA programme [*GLP* II.2]

Of all terms used in the OECD *Principles of GLP*, most can be incorporated into a quality system according to ISO 9000 without any change. However, the GLP concept of a documented QA programme has to be addressed twice in the description of an ISO 9000 quality system.

Generally, it will be described in the quality manual and, with regard to its details, in 'documented procedures' [9001: 4.2.1, 4.2.2/9004–1: 5.3]. In the current perception of GLP, it is the responsibility of the test facility management to ensure or ascertain study performance in compliance with GLP [*GLP* II.1.1.(1): Management should ensure that the *Principles of GLP* are complied with ...].[5]

More specifically, independent audits have to be described as 'audit programme' [9004–1: 5.4.2]. The independent QA personnel [*GLP* 2.1.(3)] are referred to as 'QA auditors' (same term as suggested in GCP), and they perform internal quality audits [9001: 4.17/9004–1: 5.4].

Facilities [*GLP* II.3]

GLP lists several requirements on facilities, which in ISO 9000 are to be incorporated into the general aspect of 'quality of processes' and 'process

---

[5]In the past, the *GLP* text was sometimes interpreted such that the independent QA function would be the single acceptable tool to fulfil this management responsibility. However, today it would be considered outrageous if facility management, study directors and any line management in between did not care for GLP compliance and requested that QA alone had to enforce these principles.

control' [9001: 4.9, e.g. 'Controlled conditions shall include ... b) ... a suitable working environment;'/9004–1: 10, especially 10.3 on environmental conditions].

As far as the description of facilities in the *Principles of GLP* implies requirements for certain activities (e.g. quarantine or separation requirements implied in the requirements on the facilities), these have to be located in the context of the activities themselves.

Apparatus, material and reagents [*GLP* II.4]

Requirements for measuring equipment are located at various sections of ISO 9000, primarily under 'equipment control and maintenance' [9004–1: 11.3], and 'control of inspection, measuring and test equipment' [9001: 4.11/9004–1: 13], including long-term storage requirements for project reconstruction when applicable. Requirements for records related to measuring equipment are dealt with in the context of quality records [9001: 4.16/9004–1: 17].

GLP requirements on reagents and material, like glassware or disposable pipette trips, should be described in the contexts of identification and traceability [9001: 4.8], inspection and testing [9001: 4.10.2 Receiving inspection and testing/9004–1: 9.7 Receiving inspection], process control [9001:/9004–1: 11.2 Material control, traceability and identification] and verification [9004–1: 12.1 Incoming material and parts].

Test systems [*GLP* II.5]

In a laboratory not directly involved in non-clinical projects, GLP requirements on test systems do not apply. Specimens investigated in the laboratory are not test systems in the terms of GLP: 'Specimen means any material derived from a test system for examination, analysis, or storage' [*GLP* I.1.3(5)].

Analytical laboratories receive specimens for investigation, and any requirements on identification and integrity to long-term storage, where applicable, have to be addressed in the context of 'control of customer-supplied product' [9001: 4.7], with proper care for handling [9004–1: 10.4]. In an organization with other divisions next to the laboratory, where specimens are collected, for example, in a clinical pharmacology unit, these obviously represent an intermediate product, and the description fits perfectly under 'handling, storage, packaging, preservation and delivery' [9001: 4.15/9004–1: 16.1–16.2] of products.

This is an example for the case that a certain activity can be linked to various aspects of the quality manual. In this situation care must be taken to avoid redundancies, because redundancies represent future discrepancies. A possible solution is a reference in both chapters of the quality manual to a set of 'documented procedures', i.e. SOPs, where specimen handling, from receipt over storage to shipment, is described in detail.

Test and reference substances [*GLP* II.6]

In the terms of GLP, test and reference substances are defined as the chemical substances under investigation. In a laboratory performing the core activity of GLP studies, i.e. administration of test and reference substances, requirements on handling of these substances would be summarized under 'control of customer-supplied product' [9001: 4.7].[6]

Requirements on reference standards (i.e. pure substances used for either calibration or standardization) are best described in the context of measuring equipment: they represent a close logical analogy to 'templates, patterns and gauges', which are routinely listed under equipment [9004–1: 11.3]; moreover, in the sections on 'control of inspection, measuring and test equipment' [9001: 4.11.1/9004–1: 13.1] explicit mention is made of the use of 'comparative references'. Any long-term storage requirements have to be addressed in the same context. Aspects of identification and traceability have to be considered as well [9001: 4.8/9004–1: 11.2)

Standard operating procedures [*GLP* II.7]

SOPs required from a GLP perspective have the same function as 'documented operational procedures' in ISO 9000 [9004–1: 5.2.5, 5.3.2.4].

The administration of the SOP system, including distribution and requirements on immediate availability in the work area [*GLP* II.7.1(2)], has to be considered under document control [9001: 4.5] and 'control of quality records' [9001: 4.16/9004–1: 17].

Any pertaining GLP requirement for specific SOPs should be emphasized under the description of the topic.

Performance of projects [compare to *GLP* II.8]

Protocol

The formal approval and distribution of the protocol may be covered under document control [9001: 4.5.2 and 4.5.3 (on document approval, issue and changes)].

[6]Requirements on storage in the context of test and reference substances are obviously addressing totally different questions compared to storage of products. Placement of all storage requirements in the context of postproduction activities [9004–1: 16] of 'Handling, storage, packaging, preservation and delivery' [9001: 4.15] would be quite unusual in the ISO 9000 framework.

The process of designing a project, as described in the protocol, is a topic beyond the objective of GLP, but can be located in the context of quality in specification and design [9001: 4.4/9004–1: 8].

The procedure for changes to the originally planned project will be described specifically [9001: 4.4.9 (design changes), 4.5.3 (on document changes)/9004–1: 8.8 (design change control)].

Identification of items related to the project

The GLP requirement on unique identification of each project should be addressed under product identification and traceability [9001: 4.8/9004–1: 11.2].

Requirements on recording of data, including those for changes

Records allowing reconstruction of the details of any laboratory project can best be dealt with under the aspect of product quality records [9001: 4.16/9004–1: 17.2], together with records on many other aspects, like quality of processes.

Reporting of results [compare to *GLP* II.9]

The report is the tangible end-product, containing the most relevant product of a laboratory – information derived from data. Standard requirements on product specifications should be included in the aspect of design control [9001: 4.4/9004–1: 8]; any review activity on the report will be covered under 'inspection and testing' [9001: 4.10/9004–1: 12.3].

Storage and retention of records and material [*GLP* II.10]

As the ISO 9000 standards are not specifically written for the product 'laboratory investigations', records of the type needed for and generated during and after such investigations are not explicitly mentioned.

The records routinely summarized as test facility-related records, like SOPs, equipment logbook, floor plans, audit reports, can easily be identified as quality records [9001: 4.16/9004–1: 17].

Requirements on archiving of project files are to be described as important subset of product quality records within the provisions for 'quality records' as well. This becomes evident in a note to terminology: 'A quality record provides objective evidence of the extent of the fulfilment of the requirements for quality (e.g. product quality record)' (Note 1 on clause 3.15 in ISO 8402: 1994).

Long-term storage of samples, specimens or even equipment needed for reconstruction of the project is best addressed in the context of these items themselves.

References

Hutchison, R. L. (1994) Is good laboratory practice compatible with total quality management? *Drug Information Journal* **28**: 1041–1045.

ISO 9000–1:1994. *Quality Management and Quality Assurance Standards – Part 1: Guidelines for Selection and Use.* Trilingual version EN ISO 9000–1:1994. Berlin: Beuth Verlag.

ISO 9001:1994. *Quality Systems – Model for Quality Assurance in Design, Development, Production, Installation and Servicing.* Trilingual version EN ISO 9001:1994. Berlin: Beuth Verlag.

ISO 9004–1:1994. *Quality Management and Quality System Elements – Part 1: Guidelines.* Trilingual version EN ISO 9004–1:1994. Berlin: Beuth Verlag.

ISO 10 011–1:1990. *Guidelines for Auditing Quality Systems; Part 1: Auditing.*

ISO 10 011–2:1991. *Guidelines for Auditing Quality Systems; Part 2: Qualification Criteria for Quality System Auditors.*

ISO 10 011–3:1991. *Guidelines for Auditing Quality Systems; Part 3: Management of Audit Programmes.* German–English–French edition, Berlin: Beuth Verlag.

ISO 10 012–1:1992. *Quality Assurance Requirements for Measuring Equipment; Part 1: Metrological Confirmation System for Measuring Equipment.* German–English–French edition. Berlin: Beuth Verlag.

ISO/DIS 8402:1994. *Quality Management and Quality Assurance; Vocabulary.* Trilingual version EN ISO 8402:1995. Berlin: Beuth Verlag.

ISO/DIS 9004–4:1992. *Quality Management and Quality System Elements; Guidelines for Quality Improvement.* Berlin, Beuth Verlag.

OECD (1982) *Good Laboratory Practice in the Testing of Chemicals.* Final report of the group of experts on good laboratory practice. Paris.

OECD (1992) *Draft Guidance for GLP Monitoring Authorities for the Preparation of Annual Overviews of Laboratories Inspected.* Document no. 1. OJ No L 15, 17 January 1987, pp. 29–30.

Plettenberg, H. D. (1994) Quality-related terminology in 'good practice' regulations and ISO standards. *Drug Information Journal* **28**: 921–929.

20 GMP and the pharmaceutical manufacturing environment

G Prout

Introduction and background

Over the past 25 years many standards have been used as determinants of air quality requirements for the manufacturing environment in which pharmaceutical products are prepared.

Until the current time the pharmaceutical industry has adopted and adapted standards, primarily intended for other industries, to its particular need.

The matching together of available air quality standards and good manufacturing practice (GMP) has proved an elusive goal. Perhaps this is not surprising since there are many widely divergent views on air quality requirements and few points where there is universal consensus.

The fact that air-borne particles of various kinds can and do contaminate products, as well as packaging components, people and processes, is well-known and has been the subject of many papers across a wide range of industries over many years. Indeed, one of the earliest applications of the use of filtered air to protect a product occurred in the early part of this century at a brewery in the north of England (Howorth, personal communication).

More recently, the use of air filtered through specially manufactured filters, high-efficiency particulate air (HEPA), revolutionized the ways in which aerospace components and assemblies were handled and the earliest published standards were very much directed towards the aerospace industries.

It is generally accepted that environmental control was pushed forwards in the early 1960s in the desire to increase product reliability in the field of defence products and later the manned space programme.

Willis J. Whitfield, working with a group from Sandia Laboratories, is credited with the invention of the unidirectional air flow cleanroom. The first, an 80 ft^2 (24 m^2) room, was built in 1961 and it was soon demonstrated that the application of the concept and principles would lead to an environment virtually free from contamination.

Very soon after this the description laminar flow was adopted for the system.

At the same time, in the pharmaceutical industry there was increasing recognition that end-product tests were often not reliable as a determinant of product quality and that a good way of reducing the probability of cont-amination either by microorganisms or by non-viable particles was to protect the exposed product and product containers using directed air flow. The main emphasis of the use of environmental protection has been in the manufacture of sterile products but it has been recognized that lower grades of protection can be very useful in reducing the potential for contamination in non-sterile products.

Much of the work that has been done and many of the papers that have been written have described activities that take place in cleanrooms or controlled areas. On the basis that all pharmaceutical manufacturing should be carried out in clean areas under controlled conditions, it is only the degree of application that varies and not the concept or principles.

Definitions

Absolute rated filter

A filter that theoretically and essentially retains all particles whose smallest dimension is equal to or greater than the absolute filter pore size.

Aesthetic (social) cleanliness

The condition of clothing when the fabric is cleansed of soiling and human residuals such as perspiration as well as being visually pleasing.

Agglomerate

A process of contact and adhesion whereby the particles of a dispersion form clusters of increased size.

Air lock

A small chamber located at an entry to a clean area, the doors of which are so interlocked that only one can be opened at a time. This acts as an air seal for the cleanroom to prevent flow of contaminated air from the outside into the cleanroom.

Air shower

When an air lock is equipped with a device for directing cleaned air on to the occupant of the lock while both doors are closed, this is called an air shower.

ASTM F 51/68 garment contamination standard

The only standard which specifies and classifies a permitted level of particulate contamination on clothing or textiles.

British cleanroom standard

BS 5295: 1989; *Environmental Cleanliness in Enclosed Spaces.*

Cleanroom

An area which incorporates high standards of control of humidity, temperature and air pressure and all forms of particulate matter and contamination.

Contaminant

Any material, substance or energy which is unwanted and adversely affects the product or environment.

First air

The air flow which issues directly from the HEPA filter before it passes over any work location.

HEPA filters

HEPA filter units characterized by having particle efficiencies better than 99.97% for 0.3 µm diameter particles.

Horizontal laminar flow room

The name given to unidirectional, non-turbulent air moving horizontally in a cleanroom or work station.

Laminar air flow room

A room having laminar (streamlined or non-turbulent) air flow characteristics throughout the entire work area.

Laminar air flow work station

A work station having laminar air flow characteristics in the entire work area where the air flows in unidirectional layers, and is non-turbulent.

Micron

A unit of length equal to 1/1000 of a millimetre or 0.000039 in (39 millionths of an inch).

NASA standard MSFC-STD-246

Design and Operational Criteria of Controlled Environment Areas, 29 July 1963.

Non-laminar (conventional) flow cleanroom

A cleanroom characterized by turbulent or non-uniform air patterns and velocity.

Operation levels

Dust or particulate counts taken in a facility during any activity period.

Particle size

Expressed as the apparent maximum linear dimension of diameter of the particle.

Particulate count

The term given to the action and results of measuring the volume of particles in the micron size range on a substance or in the atmosphere.

Particulate matter

A small portion of matter. A particle.

Sterilization

The act or process of destroying or removing all life forms in or on a substance. To make sterile.

Vertical laminar flow

The name given to unidirectional, non-turbulent air moving vertically from the ceiling or the roof in a cleanroom or work station.

Viable organism

An individual organism, such as a bacterium, capable of maintaining a separate existence and of reproduction and growth.

Visual cleanliness

The degree of freedom from contaminants that may be detected by the unaided human eye.

Origins of contamination

To maintain the specified level of cleanliness a manufacturing environment requires continuous and disciplined effort. However, any area will have a basic level of contamination based on several parameters.

Particulate contamination is generated from a wide range of sources from dust to dandruff, from bacteria to pollen, from ash and tobacco smoke through earth, sand, hair and textile fibres. However in the pharmaceutical industry contaminants are generally deemed to originate from three major sources in the following approximate proportions.

1   People – 80%.
2   Filtration inadequacies – 10%.
3   Process, materials and equipment – 10%.

It is well-known that personnel activity is by far the greatest danger to clean conditions. Contamination can be caused by layers of skin flaking or by the shedding of hair particles; it can be dislodged from the clothing or even produced by the very act of breathing out! The breath contains moisture retaining solid particles and is usually acidic in nature. Perspiration from the skin is a similar hazard and this is the reason why operatives are often required to wear gloves or fingerstalls when handling components. Tests carried out show that contaminants at the rate of 100 000 particles per minute at 0.3 μm can be emitted from a person at rest, increasing through 1 million particles per minute with average movement, to 20 million particles per minute with violent movement. It can therefore be seen that careful attention must be paid to operator movement and placement.

Estimates have been made that the quantity of particles that are carried on an operator's cleanroom apparel, outdoor clothes and skin surfaces adds up to a sum of 2×10^9 particles, all of which could be released within the room.

Air filtration systems are not 100% efficient and some particles will penetrate the system. Any moving part or workpiece can and will generate contamination.

The movement of equipment and workpieces involved in normal functioning is also a source of contamination. This movement may either dislodge contaminants not previously cleaned off, or create new contaminants by abrasion. Even cleaning fluids and material used to improve the situation may instead aggravate it because of the impurities they contain.

The usual sizes of air-borne contaminants are shown in Figure 20.1.

The size distribution of a typical atmospheric dust sample is shown in Table 20.1

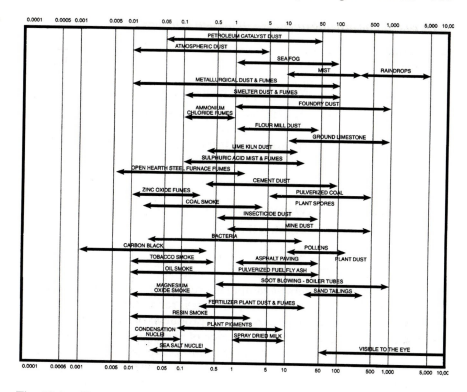

Fig. 20.1 *Sizes of air-borne contaminants: range, in micrometer size (0.0001–10 000 μm), of the commonest air-borne contaminants.*

Table 20.1 *Size distribution of a typical atmospheric dust sample*

Particle size range (μm)	Proportionate particle count	% by count	% by weight
10–30	1000	0.005	28
5–10	35 000	0.175	52
3–5	50 000	0.25	11
1–3	214 000	1.07	6
0.5–1	1 352 000	6.78	2
0–0.5	18 280 000	91.72	1

Ratio of viable to non-viable 1 : 500–1 : 20 000.

As an example of the extreme contribution made by human beings Table 20.2 shows the rate of shedding of particles whilst different activities are being carried out.

Table 20.2   *Contamination indices of human activities*

Particles 0.3 µm	Description of activity
100 000	Motionless in either sitting or standing position
500 000	Hands, arms, trunk, neck or head motions
1 000 000	Hands, arms, trunk, neck or head motions with some lower foot movements
2 500 000	Sitting to standing or standing to sitting position
5 000 000	Walking motion at 2.0 mph
7 500 000	Walking motion at 3.5 mph
>10 000 000	Walking motion at 5.0 mph

Probably the most extreme example of creating air-borne contamination in the processing of pharmaceutical products is represented by the spinning of overseals on to rubber stoppers for vial products. It has been found that this activity yields many tens of thousands of particles per minute.

A typical series of particle counts related to a cleanroom operation is shown in Figure 20.2.

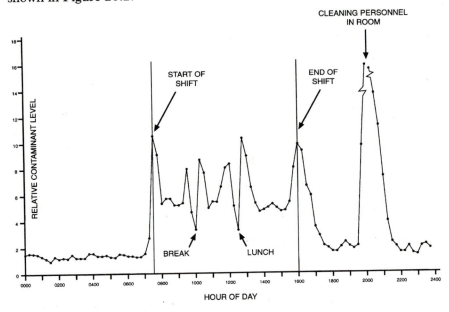

Fig. 20.2   *Typical series of cleanroom particle counts*

Non-viable particles are usually present in any pharmaceutical manufacturing environment at a higher level than viable particles. Again the major source of viable particles is the human being and various estimates have put the ratio between viable and non-viable particle levels at 1 : 100 or 1 : 1000. It seems that the ratio is relatively constant for any environment whilst actual numbers may vary fairly widely.

Typically the viable particles are bacteria, attached to other particles such as general dust, skin flakes or hair. Fungal spores and occasionally bacterial spores are found unattached to other particles. It is most unusual to find free-floating vegetative bacteria in an air sample and even more unusual to find anaerobic bacteria in a viable state in air samples.

The bacteria found are *Staphylococcus*, *Micrococcus*, *Corynebacterium*, *Streptococcus* and *Bacillus* species unless the air is moist air, when some Gram-negative bacteria may be present.

Requirements for non-sterile medicinal products

It is generally accepted that non-sterile medicinal products should be manufactured under clean, controlled conditions. What have failed to materialize over the years are definitive guidelines or requirements defining clean and controlled.

In the principles laid down in the original *Guide to Good Pharmaceutical Manufacturing Practice* (1971; the *Orange Guide*), it is stated that 'Appropriate precautions should be taken against product contamination risks of all kinds' and in the section on buildings and surrounding areas in the general subsection:

> The building should be effectively lit and ventilated, with air control facilities appropriate both to the operations undertaken within them and to the external environment... The operations carried out... should be such as to minimise contamination of one product by another.

By the 1977 edition little had changed and there was no other guideline available. It was considered acceptable for non-sterile products to be manufactured under 'socially' clean conditions, without any real definition of what that meant. At the same time, virtually none of the available standards specified acceptable (or even tolerable) levels of microbial contamination in the environment.

Much of the pharmaceutical industry covertly measured levels of microbial contamination in the non-sterile manufacturing environment and guarded the values obtained more closely than state secrets.

In most cases regulatory authorities did not ask for the data and so little use was made of the relationship that could have been developed between air-borne levels and product contamination levels. The available data were often only withdrawn from the file when there was a product complaint.

There have been a number of incidents where microbial contamination of non-sterile medicinal products has been shown to have originated from the manufacturing environment. These include yeast, mould, Gram positive and Gram negative bacterial contaminants in syrups, and bacterial contamination of creams and emulsions for topical use.

It is generally accepted that US Federal Standard 209E class M6.5 (1992) (Grade D in the EU *Good Manufacturing Practice for Medicinal Products*, 1992) is suitable for the manufacture of non-sterile products, with the caveat that the acceptability of such environmental conditions must be determined with due regard to the product or products being manufactured, and its susceptibility to microbial contamination.

However the regulatory guidance for the requirements remains scant. In *The Rules Governing Medicinal Products in the European Community* volume IV, *Good Manufacturing Practice for Medicinal Products* (1992: EU *GMP*) it is stated in section 3.12: 'Production areas should be effectively ventilated with air control facilities (including temperature and, where necessary, humidity and filtration) appropriate both to the products handled, and to the operations undertaken within them and to the external environment'.

Requirements for sterile medicinal products

For the environmental conditions required for the manufacture of sterile medicinal products, however, there is an enormous volume of literature, both in terms of official guidelines and literature references.

In Annex 1 to the EU *GMP*, it states in the principle and then in the general section:

The manufacture of sterile preparations has special requirements in order to minimise the risks of microbiological contamination, and of particulate and pyrogen contamination... Production of sterile preparations should be carried out in clean areas whose entry should be through airlocks for personnel or for goods. Clean areas should be maintained to an appropriate cleanliness standard and supplied with air which has passed through filters of an appropriate efficiency.

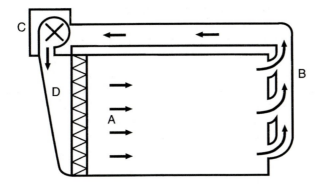

(a)

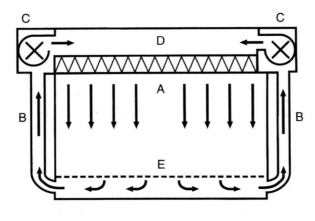

(b)

Fig. 20.3   *(a) Horizontal and (b) vertical unidirectional flow system. A = High-efficiency particulate air filter bank; B = return air ducts; C = fan; D = plenum chamber; E = perforated floor*

In the UK *Orange Guide* of 1983 (*Guide to Good Pharmaceutical Manufacturing Practice*) there is a table which defines the appropriate efficiency, although this definition is strangely absent from the EU document.

There are a number of different ways to achieve the required appropriate cleanliness standard for the air. These include a total unidirectional flow system, either vertical or horizontal (Figures 20.3 and 20.4) or the use of conventional turbulent flow rooms with horizontal or vertical laminar flow surrounding critical product or sterilized product container and closure areas (Figures 20.5 and 20.6).

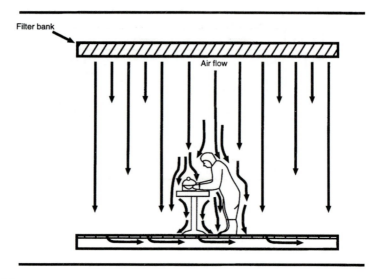

(a)

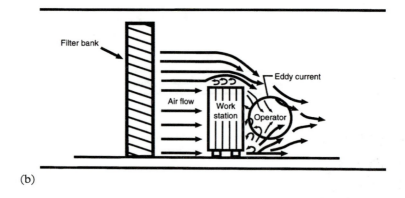

(b)

Fig. 20.4   *(a) Emission pattern in vertical laminar flow cleanroom; (b) air pattern in horizontal laminar flow cleanroom.*

Conventional
clean rooms
5-50 air changes
per hour (ch/h)

LAF rooms
500 ch/h

Hybrids
100 + 5-20 ch/h

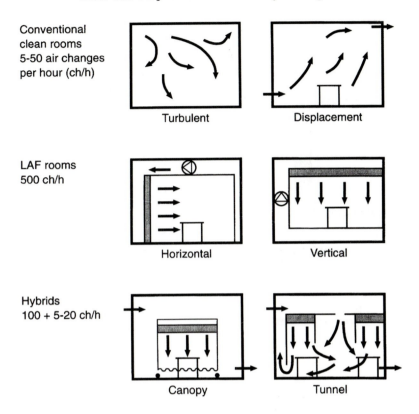

Fig. 20.5   *Air flow patterns in different operational conditions.*

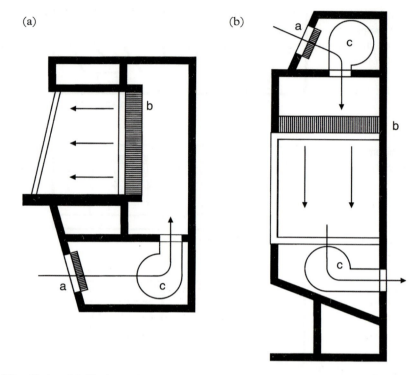

Fig. 20.6   *(a) Horizontal and (b) vertical laminar flow cabinets.* a, *Pre-filter*; b, *fan*; c, *high-efficiency particulate air filter.*

To ensure that conditions remain satisfactory for the manufacture of sterile preparations it is necessary to control many parameters. These include but are not limited to those listed in Table 20.3.

Table 20.3 *Conditions to be controlled in the manufacture of sterile preparations*

Particulate levels	See Table 20.9
Temperature	Usually 18–22°C is acceptable
Humidity	40–60% relative humidity (depending on the nature of the product)
Air flow patterns	To demonstrate that there is no risk of cross-contamination
Air changes	See Table 20.4
Integrity tests of HEPA filters	Using DOP test or similar Minimum frequency: annual
Overpressures	Minimum pressure differential between areas of different grade or class 12 Pa (0.05 in water gauge)
Pressure drop across HEPA filters	Minimum frequency of check quarterly
Microbiological conditions	Table 20.8

Cleanroom operators	Minimum number, carefully selected
	Responsible attitude
	Regular health checks
	Suitable clothing
	    Material
	    Design
	    Testing and monitoring
	Strict operating discipline
	Minimum movement
	Training/retraining, education (initial/continuing)

Air cleanliness quality standards and guidelines

As indicated earlier, there are a number of documents which describe air cleanliness requirements for various manufacturing operations (Tables 20.4–20.13)

Table 20.4 *UK Orange Guide (Guide to Good Pharmaceutical Manufacturing Practice, 1983): Basic environmental standards for the manufacture of sterile products*

Grade	Final filter efficiency (as determined by BS 3928)*	Recommended minimum air changes per hour	Maximum permitted number of particles per cubic metre equal to or above†		Maximum permitted number of viable organisms per cubic metre†‡	Nearest equivalent standard classification		
			0.5 µm	5 µm		BS 5295§	US Federal Standard 209B¶	VDI 2083, p.1**
1/A (unidirectional air flow workstation)	99.997%	Flow of 0.3 m/s (vertical) or 0.45 m/s (horizontal)	3000	0	Less than 1	1	100	—
1/B	99.995%	20	3000	0	5	1	100	3
2	99.95%	20	300 000	2000	100	2	10 000	5
3	95.0%	20	3 500 000	20 000	500	3	100 000	6

Air pressure should always be highest in the area of greatest risk to product. The air pressure differentials between rooms of successively higher to lower risk should be at least 1.5 mm (0.06 in) water gauge.

*BS 3928: *Method for Sodium Flame Test for Air Filters.* British Standards Institution, London, 1969.

†This condition should be achieved throughout the room when left unstaffed and recovered within a short 'clean-up' period after personnel have left. The condition should be maintained in the zone immediately surrounding the product whenever the product is exposed. (Note: It is accepted that it may not always be possible to demonstrate conformity with *particulate* standards at the point of fill, with filling in progress, due to generation of particles or droplets from the product itself.)

‡Mean values obtained by air sampling methods.

§BS 5295: *Environmental Cleanliness in Enclosed Spaces,* British Standards Institution, London, 1976.

¶US Federal Standard 209B, 1973.

**Verein Deutscher Ingenieure 2083, p.1.

Table 20.5 *Environmental classification: BS 5295 (1989)*

Class	Class limits, in particles per cubic metre, of sizes greater than or equal to sizes shown (µm)				
	0.3	0.5	5.0	10	25
C	100	35	0		
D	1000	350	0		
E	10 000	3500	0		
F		3500	0		
G	100 000	35 000	200	0	
H		35 000	200	0	
J		350 000	2000	450	0
K		3 500 000	20 000	4500	500
L			200 000	45 000	5000
M				450 000	50 000

Occupancy state: as built; unmanned; manned.

Table 20.6 *US Federal Standards 209E (1992): Air-borne particulate cleanliness classes in cleanrooms and clean zones*

Class name		0.1 μm Volume units		0.2 μm Volume units		Class limits 0.3 μm Volume units		0.5 μm Volume units		5 μm Volume units	
SI	English	(m³)	(ft³)	(m³)	(ft³)	(m³)	(ft³)	(m³)	(ft³)	(m³)	(ft³)
M 1	1	350	9.91	75.7	2.14	30.9	0.875	10.0	0.283		
M 1.5		1240	35.0	265	7.50	106	3.00	35.3	1.00		
M 2		3500	99.1	757	21.4	309	8.75	100	2.83		
M 2.5	10	12 400	350	2650	75.0	1060	30.0	353	10.0		
M 3		35 000	991	7570	214	3090	87.5	1000	28.3		
M 3.5	100			26 500	750	10 600	300	3530	100		
M 4				75 700	2140	30 900	875	10 000	283		
M 4.5	1000							35 300	1000	247	7.00
M 5								100 000	2830	618	17.5
M 5.5	10 000							353 000	10 000	2470	70.0
M 6								1 000 000	28 300	6180	175
M 6.5	100 000							3 530 000	100 000	24 700	700
M 7								10 000 000	283 000	61 800	1750

Class limits are given for each class name. The limits designate specific concentrations (particles per unit volume) of air-borne particles with sizes equal to and larger than the particle sizes shown.

Table 20.7 *The Rules Governing Medicinal Products in the European Community, Volume IV (1992): Air classification system for manufacture of sterile products*

Grade	Maximum permitted number of particles per m^3 equal to or above		Maximum permitted number of viable microorganisms per m^3
	0.5 µm	5 µm	
A Laminar air flow workstation	3500	None	Less than 1*
B	3500	None	5*
C	350 000	2000	100
D	3 500 000	20 000	500

Notes:
- Laminar air flow systems should provide a homogeneous air speed of 0.30 m/s for vertical flow and 0.45 m/s for horizontal flow.
- In order to reach the B, C and D air grades, the number of air changes should generally be higher than 20 per hour in a room with a good air flow pattern and appropriate high-efficiency particulate air filters.
- *Low values involved here are only reliable when a large number of air samples are taken.
- The guidance given for the maximum permitted number of particles corresponds approximately to the US Federal Standard 209C as follows: class 100 (grades A and B), class 10 000 (grade C) and class 100 000 (grade D).
- It is accepted that it may not always be possible to demonstrate conformity with particulate standards at the point of fill when filling is in progress, due to generation of particles or droplets from the product itself.

Table 20.8   *Environmental Contamination Control Practice: Technical Monograph no. 2 (1989): Environmental microbiological classes*

Class	Level (see note)				Summary of processing operations
	Settle plate	Air sample	Surface sample (contact plate)	Finger dabs	
V1	1 per 2 plates	1 (see note)	2	1	Manipulations associated with aseptic filling
V2	2	5	2	5	
V3	5	10	5		
V4	20	40	20		Manipulations associated with processing for terminal sterilization and preparation of components
V5	40	80	40		

Table 20.9 *Environmental Contamination Control Practice: Technical Monograph no. 2 (1989): Selection of classes for aseptic manipulations*

Activity	Operational microbial classification	Operational cleanroom (particle) classification (US Federal Standard 209)	Note (see below)
Point of fill or other location where product and components are exposed	V1	100	1
Transfer of partially stoppered containers	V2	1000	
Transfer and storage of sealed packages or containers, sterile components or of product for use in aseptic filling	V3	10 000	2
Location of isolator unit where all sterilization and transfers are carried out within the closed system		None specified	
Transfer and storage of sealed packages of sterile components for use in isolator unit	V3	10 000	3
White area of changing rooms where garments are stored and donned	V3	10 000	
Grey area of changing rooms where washing is carried out	V4	10 000	4
Black area of changing rooms where factory and personal garments are removed		None specified	

Note 1: It is recognized that some processes, e.g. powder filling, may prevent the operational particle level from being achieved.
Note 2: It should be noted that in order to achieve V3 in situations of high personnel occupancy, greater quantities of clean air may need to be provided. This may have the effect of enabling the operational particle classification to be reduced to e.g. 3000.
Note 3: The environmental class can be relaxed for deployment of isolators where transfer is in a closed system or double wrapping and isolator disinfection entry procedures are adopted.
Note 4: Depends on design of changing suite and company procedures.

Table 20.10   *Environmental Contamination Control Practice: Technical Monograph no. 2 (1989) Filling of products to be terminally sterilized*

Activity	Operational microbial classification	Operational cleanroom (particle) classification (US Federal Standard 209)	Note (see below)
Filling suite	V4	10 000	1
White area of changing rooms	V4	10 000	
Grey area of changing rooms	V5	100 000	
Black area of changing rooms		None specified	

Note 1: Many Users fill under conditions which meet classes V1 and 100. This is not essential for maintaining control of total and viable contamination, but may provide data which could be included in supporting a case for parametric release of terminally sterilized product.

Table 20.11   *Environmental Contamination Control Practice: Technical Monograph no. 2 (1989): Preparation of components*

Activity	Operational microbial classification	Operational cleanroom (particle) classification (US Federal Standard 209)	Note (see below)
Preparation of bulk solution prior to filtration	V4	10 000	1
Preparation of components for sterilization by moist heat	V4	10 000	2
Preparation of components for sterilization and depyrogenation by dry heat	V5	100 000	
White area of changing room	V4/V5	100 000	3
Grey/black area of changing room		None specified	

Note 1: It may be possible to relax the microbial and particle classifications to V5 and 100 000 if the process is totally enclosed. If, however, if the product is known to support microbial growth and cannot be manipulated in a closed system, classifications of V3 and 10 000 are appropriate.
Note 2: Components sterilized by moist heat do not undergo a depyrogenation step. Therefore a tighter environmental classification is proposed to facilitate control of pyrogenicity during preparation. The loading of an enclosed tunnel process may be carried out in area classified to proposed B.S. Standard 5295 Class M provided that the tunnel system is protected from inducing unfiltered room air.
Note 3: Relaxation may be appropriate.

Table 20.12 *Environmental Contamination Control Practice Technical Monograph, no. 2 (1989)*

Standard	Class					
US Federal Standard 209	100	1000	10 000	100 000		
BS 5295 (1976)	1	Not defined	2	3	4	

(A controlled area, for which no limits were specified, is also described in this standard. Class M, for which limits are specified, is described in the proposed version of this standard)

Standard	Class					
BS 5295 (proposed)	E/F	G/H	J	K	L	M
Guide to Good Pharmaceutical Manufacturing Practice, 1983 (*Orange Guide*)	1 A/B	Not defined	2	3	Not defined	
PIC 1989	A/B	Not defined	C	D	Not defined	
EEC *GMP* (1992)	A/B	Not defined	C	D	Not defined	

Table 20.13   *Proposed standards for the EC Guide to GMP (1992)*

Grade	Maximum permitted number of particles per m³ $\geq 0.5\ \mu m^*$	$\geq 5\ \mu m$	Maximum permitted number of viable microorganisms per m³	Settle plate counts per 100 cm²/h†	Air filter efficiency (%)‡
α	3500	20§	1§	0.2§	99.97
β	35 000	200	5§	1	99.97
γ	350 000	2000	50	10	95
δ	3 500 000	20 000	500	100	90–95

*The $\geq 0.5\ \mu m$ particle threshold should be used only to measure the performance level of the cleanroom. The standards to be achieved are those given for the $\geq 5\ \mu m$ particle threshold and the number of microrganisms per m³.
†Settle plate counts are given as cfu/100 cm² per h. Small plates usually have an internal area of ~60 cm², large plates ~150 cm². Plates can be left for as long as 6 h in a unidirectional flow airstream and, if necessary, for as long as 24 h in a conventionally ventilated room.
‡Air filter efficiency is based on Eurovent 4/4 for grades α, β, and γ and Eurovent 4/5 for grade δ.
§Reliable only when large samples are taken.

Notes
- Grade α can be achieved using a unidirectional airflow of 0.3 m/s for vertical flow and 0.45 m/s for horizontal flow.
- Monitoring of the levels of inanimate particles and microorganisms should be carried out during normal production.
- Grades β, γ and δ can be achieved using a conventional airflow system with an air supply volume determined by the air standard required and the number of personnel in the room.
- The suggested maximum permitted number of particles corresponds approximately to the US Federal Standard 209E as follows: class 100 (grade α), class 1000 (grade β), class 10 000 (grade γ) and class 100 000 (grade δ).
- When filling is in progress, it may not be possible to demonstrate conformity with particulate standards at the point of fill due to generation of particles or droplets from the product itself.
- The level of contamination of a product is directly proportional to the area of the neck of the container, the period of exposure and the concentration of bacteria-carrying particles in the room, and so can be calculated.

Control and monitoring of the pharmaceutical manufacturing environment

Air-borne particulate contamination is minimized, in cleanroom operations, by the use of HEPA filters. Whether the room is a conventional turbulent flow room with critical zones protected by unidirectional air or is a horizontal or vertical flow room, such filters play a major role in the protection of the product. A typical filter structure is shown in Figure 20.7.

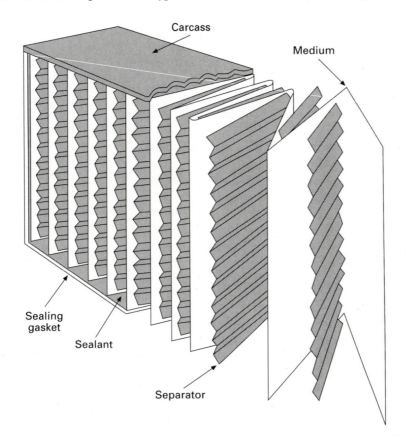

Fig. 20.7   *High-efficiency particulate air (HEPA) filter. Efficiency: 99.9997% removal of particles >0.3 μm.*

Primary control of cleanroom areas is required by GMP and can be effected by a number of tests, described in the literature (British Standard 5295, 1989; *Environmental Contamination Control Practice: Technical Monograph no. 2*, 1989; US Federal Standard 209E, 1992).

For clean areas these tests include:

1   Particle counts.
2   Overpressure (pressure differentials).
3   Temperature.
4   Relative humidity.
5   Rate of air change.
6   Integrity tests of HEPA filters.
7   Pressure drop across HEPA filters.
8   Microbiological counts in air and on surfaces.

For laminar flow units the tests include:

1   Integrity test of HEPA filters.
2   Pressure drop across HEPA filters.
3   Air velocity.
4   Air flow patterns under working conditions.
5   Particle counts.
6   Microbiological counts in air and on surfaces.

In both cleanrooms and when using laminar air flow devices, personnel activities are critical and essential adherence to gowning practices and thorough training is required by GMP.

Details of typical methods for the physical tests in the cleanroom environment can be found in the literature (British Standard 5295, 1989; US Federal Standard 209E, 1992). For microbiological tests monitoring can be qualitative or quantitive.

The qualitative test is the use of settle plates. Details of this and the quantitative tests involving slit to agar samplers, centrifugal samplers, liquid impingers, membrane filtration and cascade impactors are found in the Parenteral Society Monograph Number 2 (1989).

Surface microbial monitoring can be effected using swabs, contact plates (Rodac) or agar overlay methods. Descriptions of these tests are found in the literature (*Environmental Contamination Control Practice Technical Monograph no. 2*, 1989).

The same reference also gives some guidance on permissible levels of microbiological contamination for various activities. However, it is recommended that the proposed limits for alert and action are discussed with the appropriate regulatory authority before being cast in stone.

All such control and monitoring activities will, of course, be in vain if the design of the facility is not suitable for its intended use and this is a prerequisite for successful operation and the manufacture of a product which complies with its specification and is suitable for its intended use.

The future

Work is well under way on a number of International Standards for clean-rooms and associated controlled environments under the auspices of the International Standards Organization ISO/TC 290.

In 1993 the US Institute of Environmental Sciences (IES) was appointed as the ISO Secretariat for this activity by the American National Standards Institute (ANSI). It is believed that when the standards are completed they will define how to design, build, operate and control a cleanroom environment.

Working Group 1 (WG01) has reviewed a document on *Classifications of Air Cleanliness* and this is now with industry for its comments. The modified document will be presented at the next ISO/TC 209 technical committee meeting and, if accepted, the draft standard will be circulated to all participating nations for comment and then a final acceptance vote. It is expected that the full process will be completed in 1996.

Working Group 3 (WG03), *Metrology and Test Methods*, is reviewing a list of tests and methods to assist with the maintenance of the integrity of the clean environment. These tests include how to test a HEPA filter *in situ* and in a test rig, how to measure air flow, distribution patterns and so on. The next meeting of WG03 is scheduled for March 1996. Working Group 5 (WG05) on *Cleanroom Operations* will meet at the same time. Working Group 2 (WG02) is dealing with *Biocontamination Standards*, WG04 is working on *Cleanroom Design and Construction*, WG06 on *Terms, Definitions and Units* and WG07 on *Clean Air Devices*.

The whole area of biodecontamination will, of course, be observed by a considerable number of government agencies in a number of countries. Some regulatory issues may go beyond the scope of TC 209.

The new standards will have immediate impact in Europe since ISO standards can be adopted as CEN standards. In principle the standards will be voluntary in the USA but the Food and Drug Administration has already been closely involved with the US technical support activity groups (TAGs) and has delegates on many IES working groups.

October 1996 is the target date for publication of the first parts of the standard.

At the same time as these standards are being developed, newer technologies are being introduced and improved. In the past few years isolation technology has emerged as a promising solution to some of the difficulties involved in aseptic filling. The integrity of the isolator is a crucial factor and other aspects such as sterilization of the internal surfaces of the isolator and passthroughs are under continuous development. In the absence of human intervention during the process it is considered that there is a significant reduction in the probability of microbial contamination.

However, thorough training in the correct use of the entire system is still a principal requirement.

Further advances in isolator design and auxiliary equipment inside the isolator will take place to increase the assurance, required by GMP world-wide, that the products manufactured in such systems will be suitable for their intended purpose.

References

Guide to Good Pharmaceutical Manufacturing Practice (1971) London: HMSO.

US Federal Standard 209E (1992) *Airborne Particulate Cleanliness Classes in Cleanrooms and Clean Zones* Fort Worth TX: G.S.A.

The Rules Governing Medicinal Products in the European Community, volume IV. Good Manufacturing Practice for Medicinal Products (1992). Luxembourg: Office for Official Publications of the European Community.

Guide to Good Pharmaceutical Manufacturing Practice (1983) London: HMSO.

British Standard 5295 (1989) *Environmental Cleanliness in Enclosed Spaces.* London: BSI.

Environmental Contamination Control Practice Technical Monograph No. 2 (1989) Swindon: The Parenteral Society.

Whyte W. *et al.* (1992) Suggested modification to the clean room air standards of the EC *Guide to GMP. Pharmaceutical Technology* Jan/Feb.

Further reading

Agalloco, J. P. and Gordon, B. M. (1987). Current practices in the use of medil fills for validation of aseptic processing. *Journal of Parenteral Science and Technology* **41:** 128–141.

Avallone, H. (1989). Control aspects of aseptically produced products. *Journal of Parenteral Science and Technology* **43:** 3–7.

Beer, C. L. (1991) Gowning training: the use of video recording together with microbial assessment. *Journal of Parenteral Science and Technology* **45:** 128–131.

Commission of the European Community (1989). *Guide to Good Manufacturing Practice for Medicinal Products* Luxembourg: Office for Official Publications of the European Community.

Farquharson, G. J. (1987). Picking a route to cleanliness. *Manufacturing Chemist*, September: 39–41.

Farquharson, G. J. (1989). Developments in clean room regulations and standards. *Manufacturing and Chemicals* July 19–23.

Farquharson, G. J. (1990). Using current environmental standards and guidelines in pharmaceutical clean room application. INTERPHEX Conference, November.

Favero, M. S. *et al.* (1968). Microbiological sampling of surfaces. *Journal of Applied Bacteriology* **31:** 336–343.

Favero, M. S. *et al.* (1996) Comparative levels and types of microbial contamination detected in industrial clean rooms. *Applied Microbiology* **14:** 539–551.

Federal Standard 209D (1988). *Clean Room and Work Station Requirements, Controlled Environment* Fort Worth TX: G.S.A.

Food and Drug Administration (1987) *Guidelines on Sterile Drug Products Produced by Aseptic Processing* Rockville MD.

Frieben, W. R. (1983) Control of the aseptic processing environment. *American Journal of Hospital Pharmacy* **40:** 1928–1935.

Galson, E. L. (1988). Controlling microbial contamination standards, techniques and case study. *Medical Development and Diagnostic Intervention,* Febr, 34–39.

Kaye, S. (1988) Efficiency of Biotest RCS as sampler of airborne bacteria. *Journal of Parenteral Science and Technology* **42:** 147–152.

Kraidman, G. (1975) The microbiology of of airborne contamination and air sampling. *Drug and Cosmetic Industry* **116:** 40–43, 108–111.

Lee, J. Y. (1988) Environmental requirements for clean rooms. *Biopharmacy* **2:** 42–45.

Lingnar, J. *et al.* (1990) EEC Guide to Good Manufacturing Practice for Medicinal Products. Supplementary Guidelines: Manufacture of Sterile Medicinal Products: Air Classification System: Discussion of the Cleanliness Class Requirements. *Drugs Made in Germany,* **33:** 20–24.

Ljunqvisst, B. and Reinmuller, B. (1991). Some aspects on the use of the Biotest RCS air sampler in unidirectional air flow testing. *Journal of Parenteral Science and Technology* **45:** 177–180.

Lu, A. *et al.* Reliability of the settling plate method in monitoring laminar airflow benches. *American Journal of Hospital Pharmacy* **40:** 271–273.

Luna, C. T. (1988). Training the clean room employee. *Pharmaceutical Engineering* **8:** 34–36.

McCollough, K. Z. (1987). Environmental factors influencing aseptic areas. *Pharmaceutical Engineering* **7:** 17–20.

Mistalski, T. S. (1987). Microbiological contamination troubleshooting. *Pharmaceutical Engineering* **7:** 13–16.

Niskanen, A. and Pohja, M. S. (1977). Comparative studies on the sampling and investigation of microbial contamination of surfaces by the contact plate and swab methods. *Journal of Applied Bacteriology* **42:** 53–63.

Pascual, P. (1987). Cualificacion y validacion de sistemas y procesos en areas esteriles. Doctoral thesis. Facultad e Farmacia, Madrid.

Pascual, P. (1990). Validacion de areas limpias. Madrid.

PDA (1980). Validation of aseptic filling for solutions of drug products. Technical monograph no. 2 Philadelphia PA.

PDA Environmental Task Force (1990). *Fundamentals of a Microbiological Environmental Monitoring Program*. Technical Report no. 13.

PDA Gowning Task Force (1990). Report on survey of current industry gowning practices. *Journal of Parenteral and Science Technology* **44:** 223–227.

Rech, M., Panaggio, A. and Bontempo, J. A. (1991). Current trends in facilities and equipment for aseptic processing. *Pharmaceutical Technology International*, March, 48–52.

Richard, J. (1980). Observations on the value of a swab technique for determining the bacteriological state of milking equipment surface. *Journal of Applied Bacteriology* **49:** 19–27.

Sharp, J. (1989). Manufacture and control of sterile products. *Manufacturing Chemist*, March, 57–61.

The Pharmaceutical Inspection Convention (1989). *Guide to Good Manufacturing Practice for Pharmaceutical Products*. Document PH 5/89.

Thornton, R. M. (1990). Pharmaceutically sterile clean rooms. *Pharmaceutical Technology* **14:** 44–48.

Waldheim, B. J. (1988). Microbiological control of clean rooms. *Pharmaceutical Engineering* **8:** 21–23.

Wrightson, M. and Jardine, N. (1991). Cost control in clean room design. *Manufacturing Chemist*, August, 19–21.

21 The quality control situation under review in Poland as a role model for hospital laboratories

D Bobilewicz and A Brzeziński

Laboratory diagnostics in Poland

Over 25 years ago the term laboratory diagnostics replaced another word that had been in use – analytics – and ever since, the constant process of changing its range has been noticed. Traditionally laboratory diagnostics included all activities performed *in vitro* and related to medical diagnosis and monitoring of treatment. Gradually, especially in district and other hospitals of equivalent size, bacteriology and blood transfusion became independent under separate professional supervision. Clinical chemistry, including haematology, haemostasis and some other routine tests (urine, stool etc.) created the core of the laboratory discipline named laboratory diagnostics. Obviously a sharp division can never be achieved and several tests are grouped and performed not according to their origin (bacteriology, clinical chemistry), but according to the technology (enzyme-linked immunoassay, polymerase chain reaction applied to different parameters), and setting them up depends mainly on the local conditions and facilities. Generally, the principal clinical or medical laboratories do not perform morphological tests, apart from urine sediment, peripheral blood and bone marrow smears, and they try to avoid radioimmunoassays.

As the process of separation of bacteriology and blood transfusion is quite new, for organizational reasons emergencies at nights and weekends were often covered by staff working on duty in the main laboratories.

Parallel to separation tendencies, which are very strong and seem to be one of the tools providing better quality, on the other hand Poland has been influenced by European trends to coordinate efforts in the promotion of ideas and philosophy of laboratory medicine with its cooperating subdivisions.

In 1993 the College of Laboratory Medicine was founded and started its activities, with the participation of pathology, haematology, genetics, clinical chemistry, nuclear medicine, toxicology and pharmacology. It is mainly intended to enable contacts between the above-mentioned disciplines to develop guidelines for the implementation of the total quality management concept.

Structure of Polish clinical laboratories

Clinical laboratories include laboratories performing clinical chemistry, haematology, coagulation and urinalysis. There are about 2000 state laboratories, half of which perform only basic tests and do not have fully qualified staff. The number of hospital laboratories slightly exceeds the number of hospitals, which is about 700; some of them, because of the different location of the wards, run more than one laboratory. About 100 laboratories, including 12 university hospitals, 10 health research institutes and 49 county hospitals, can be considered the leading laboratories offering a broad spectrum of tests. Since 1992 there has been a list of 12 laboratories entitled by the Ministry of Health to perform the medical evaluation of new instruments and reagents coming on to the Polish market.

The central laboratory, as understood in western Europe, does not really exist. It might function as a group of hospitals or outpatients departments working within the same management committee, at a distance of not more than a few miles. The central laboratory does not refer to the diagnostic centre created for particular purposes, such as clinical trials. However several tests are centralized, mainly viral infection, such as human immunodeficiency virus (HIV) confirmation test, sexually transmitted diseases and rare tests.

Until now there has been no fully documented legislative base for the functioning of laboratories and even if there were, in many cases it is very difficult to fulfil the official requirements regarding equipment, personnel qualifications and safety without totally reconstructing everything. State laboratories exist as part of the hospital or different sizes of outpatient health centres and are fully financed either from local or central budget. Unfortunately they have very little influence on how much money they can get so they cannot make any detailed financial plans in advance.

The situation of private laboratories from the legislative point of view is much less clear and more complicated. Often they function as part of a private doctor's office and so are neither registered by the local health authority nor have any certificates to recognize their capacity to perform the tests they offer. Physicians' qualifications do not ensure proper professional laboratory supervision.

There are also small so-called research clinical laboratories situated in teaching hospitals, attached to clinics with clearly defined profiles, performing specific non-routine tests, mainly for research purposes.

Staffing

One of the criteria for laboratory classification into small, medium and large is the number of professional staff employed. Less than 10 persons is considered as small, 11–25 medium and above 25 large. It is not exceptional to have 1–3 persons working in very small laboratories, mainly in rural areas or in the suburbs of larger towns.

There are two categories or professional staff in clinical laboratories: technicians with qualifications below university degree and those with a degree. Some have graduated from medical school – whether faculty of medicine, pharmacy, general or diagnostic division, and the special newly created branch of so-called clinical analytics – while others represent different disciplines, such as chemists, biologists, veterinarians. Since 1986 all, both medical and non-medical, can carry on postgraduate education in different forms. After 5 years' experience, several courses and a successful two-step final test, they become specialists in the field of laboratory diagnostics if medical graduates, and clinical analytics (the others). At present, of 5000 degree-employees, only about 10% have completed full postgraduate education; among these about 30% are graduates from the faculties of medicine.

It is true that the vast majority of experienced laboratory staff with no postgraduate certificates represent a high level of technical skill and awareness of the quality of work. Nevertheless, the shortage of well-qualified personnel with a good general medical background is to some extent a drawback for the development of laboratories of all kinds.

Assessment of quality of results

Quality assessment, closely related to quality of laboratory performance, has a long-standing tradition in Poland. Apart from intralaboratory control samples produced by local manufacturers mainly for precision evaluation, there is a strong recommendation, published by the Ministry of Health as laboratory guidelines in 1978, for daily accuracy control in large laboratories and at least once a month in smaller ones.

Accuracy is assessed on the basis of good quality and generally accepted international control materials, preferably with target values, but for economical reasons those with assigned values estimated by standardized routine methods are also accepted. Interlaboratory surveys have been carried out for over 20 years. The external quality assurance (EQA) scheme was introduced in 1974 first at the regional level, followed by a national programme supported by the Ministry of Health and the Polish Society of Laboratory Diagnostics. At present regional EQA functions in some districts, on the basis of the enthusiasm of local people traditionally being involved in the problem.

The national programme has a clear organization. The scheme is fully computerized and since 1975 it has operated regularly (Bobilewicz and Brzeziński, 1994). It consists of:

1   A central clinical chemistry survey for over 100 laboratories, including 49 county hospitals – 2 samples, 12 parameters, every month since 1975.
2   A general clinical chemistry survey for over 1500 laboratories – 5 samples, 22 parameters, twice a year since 1981.
3   Blood gases survey for 700 laboratories – 3 samples once a year since 1982.
4   Basic haematology survey for about 1000 laboratories automated only – 3 samples twice a year since 1992.

The results reported directly after the survey and annually are expressed against the general mean (truncated) of all participant values and assigned values according to the manufacturers. The final report contains the ranking of precision.

EQA is free and to some extent mandatory. However there is no clause for those laboratories which choose not to participate. Neither is there any formal need to apply for EQA as the laboratories are already on the updated list.

Recently a bacteriology survey operating in a similar manner has been introduced.

The question arises as to what information can be gained from EQA results. First, there is the quality of analytical performance but also general trends in methodology can be observed, as well as the evolution of enzyme estimation and enzymatic substrate tests (Tables 21.1 and 21.2).

As, for example, now almost all laboratories use the most popular version for creatine kinase activator for aminotransferases, only a few years ago most laboratories were using the colorimetric Reitmann–Frankel's method and even now some still use it (Table 21.1). The most common analytical procedure is the International Federation of Clinical Chemistry (IFCC) method and it shows the highest percentage of accepted results according to reference method values.

Evident progress can be observed in enzymatic methods (Table 21.2) for glucose and cholesterol estimation; however, only 31% of Polish labs apply that technology to the urea ultraviolet test. Parallel to the increased number of labs using substrate enzymatic methods, the percentage of accepted values according to assigned values can be clearly noticed (Table 21.3). The situation is even better in the group of 100 laboratories included in the central clinical chemistry survey. Among them the percentage of accepted results (mean participant values) is around 87%, and for assigned values 84%.

Table 21.1 *Aspartate aminotransferase and alanine aminotransferase estimation over the last 3 years.*

Method	Percentage of labs			Percentage of accepted results	
	1992	1993	1994	1992	1994
DGKC[1] Phosphate buffer	18.2%	25.4%	21.8%	74%	76%
IFCC Tris buffer	13.6%	33.2%	44.2%	70%	83.5%
IFCC Tris, PLP[2]	1.8%	2.4%	4.4%	55%	78%
Colorimetric	66.4%	39%	29.8%	24%	21%

Percentage of accepted results = reference method values ± 10%. IFCC, International Federation of Clinical Chemistry. Data from the general clinical chemistry survey; results from about 1000 laboratories.
1. DGKC = Deutsche Gesellschaft für Klinische Chemie.
2. PLP = Pirydoxal phosphate.

Table 21.2 *Percentage of laboratories using enzymatic methods for cholesterol, glucose (oxidase) and urea (urease ultraviolet)*

Analyte	1982	1988	1990	1994
Cholesterol	0.8%	2.8%	14.8%	90.5%
Glucose	3.4%	10.1%	59.7%	90.9%
Urea	1.0%	1.0%	5.0%	31.4%

Table 21.3 *Accepted results for glucose, cholesterol and urea calculated against A – all participants mean ± 10% B – assigned values obtained by enzymatic method ± 10%*

Analyte	1986		1990		1994	
	A	B	A	B	A	B
Cholesterol	73%	49%	64%	36%	82%	79%
Glucose	73%	58%	71%	63%	74%	76%
Urea	70%	57%	74%	71%	79%	78%

Data from the general clinical chemistry survey: about 1500 laboratories.

The haematological survey is limited to 1000 laboratories equipped with automated and semiautomated electronic cell counters. Accuracy criteria according to the manufacturer's values (Streck Laboratories USA) were fulfilled for haemoglobin by 78%, for haematocrit by 64% and for erythrocytes by 70% of laboratories.

The final protocol and its evaluation are sent back to the person in charge of the laboratory as well as to county consultants; otherwise the results are confidential.

The annual general summary of the surveys is published in the *National Journal* 'Laboratory Diagnostics' (in Polish) and the results are discussed on different occasions, such as society meetings and at symposia.

The existing system of nationwide quality assessment covers all hospital laboratories and most others. Until now it has mainly had an educational goal, with no impact on further laboratory functioning. In contrast, for 20 years regular contacts with the quality control centre has become a tradition and is now treated by participants as a voluntary must. The additional advantage of that system is the possibility of obtaining up-to-date information about laboratory status and the position regarding personnel, equipment and methods.

Apart from national programmes there are several laboratories, also private, taking part in different international EQA schemes, such as Instand, Murex, Randox and recently Labquality, which offers a broad spectrum of parameters, including the evaluation of morphological features (a peripheral blood smear). There is a great need for immunoassay control, mainly endocrinology.

Attempts to improve the quality of results

Quality assurance – the final goal of laboratory results as well as the other medical activities – has three components: structures, process and outcome. Structure mainly concerns personnel qualification and equipment, while process includes the analytical procedure, quality control, reporting and interpretation of the results. Outcome is represented by the results obtained in proficiency testing schemes. The attitude towards those components will vary depending on the degree of expected fulfilment of standards (Burnett, 1993). In the USA under Clinical Laboratory Improvement Amendment (CLIA'88) and in Germany the outcome is emphasized; the Danish philosophy of quality goals concentrates more on the educational role of quality assessment.

At present Poland, like a number of countries throughout the world, makes an effort to ensure the expected reliability of laboratory results. Developing the full accreditation scheme for clinical laboratories, including proficiency testing, is going to be a lengthy process and a very difficult

Accreditation – first phase

To accredit: to certify or guarantee that someone or something meets the required standards

Certification if the laboratory is capable of providing reliable test results

Licensing – a continuous process
Whether the laboratory is actually
providing reliable test results –
negative selection

Good laboratory practice
Organizational structure and process
of laboratory work

Recommendations
Positive selection of the best laboratories
based on their structure, analytical process
and reliability of test results

Figure 21.1   *Ideas of accreditation, licensing, good laboratory practice and recommendation.*

one until basic changes in the organization of the health service and the insurance system are introduced and fully established. The most realistic way of starting the procedure seems to be focusing on structure and processes, ignoring the outcomes for the time being. This form of accreditation, viewed in terms of its application to different aspects of organization (structure) and performances (processes) has much in common with good laboratory practice and might be considered as an initial phase (Figure 21.1). Licensing, closely related to proficiency testing, is a continuous process that has to be related to the economical situation and the financial regulations of the health care system. Poland's health services, funded by the central or local budget, are free to all citizens, and the insurance and reimbursement systems are still under discussion. Lack of financial regulations concerning method of payment, whether annual contract or fee-for-service, for laboratory tests makes it difficult to introduce any official mandatory requirements regarding proficiency testing, even if its idea would be acceptable. Nevertheless, professionals, including members of scientific societies, are trying to implement step by step the following procedures that are expected to improve the quality and reliability of results:

1   To interest laboratory staff in what they are doing. As they have little financial motivation, some other motivators such as desire to work better and to be ahead of the competition are emphasized.
2   To introduce good laboratory practice (GLP) requirements, according to the Coordinating Committee for the Promotion of Quality Control in the Health Care Sector (CCKL). For many laboratories it is only a matter of changing the documentation and responsibility system according to GLP; this can easily be done with the help of experts.
3   To follow the existing regulations concerning personnel qualifications.
4   To make internal and external quality assurance a routine procedure and an obvious part of laboratory activities.

As the implementation of GLP will take some time, so it is believed that the temporary certification of the potential ability of laboratories to meet the required standards of quality will be advantageous. At present it will be issued by the College of Laboratory Medicine and the Polish Society of Laboratory Diagnostics and it will only concern personnel qualification and participation in EQA. It will apply to both state and private sectors, hospitals and outpatients clinics and it will eliminate at least some of the small laboratories of doubtful quality. As a process of reorganization in health care proceeds, the proper accreditation system will develop. In the Polish situation, the accreditation of the hospital laboratory should occur first and be one of the conditions for accreditation of the whole hospital.

References

Total quality management. *Clinical Laboratory Management* October 1994, 4–7.
Bobilewicz, D. and Brzeziński, A. (1994). Clinical laboratory accreditation in Poland. *Drug Information Journal* **28**: 1197–1199.
Burnett, D. (1993). Laboratory accreditation. *J. IFCC* **5**: 146–151.
CLIA '88. Federal Register. 28 February 1992 and 19 January 1993.
Guidelines for Laboratory Diagnostics and Microbiology (in Polish) (1978) Warsaw: Ministry of Health.
Quality System–Practical Guidelines for Implementation in laboratories in the Health Care Sector. (1991) CCKL. The Netherlands: Bilthoven.

Regulatory agencies and GxPs

22 The World Health Organization: its normative activities, in particular in the pharmaceutical area

M ten Ham

History

International health cooperation has gone, and is still going, through a period of stormy development. The first International Sanitary Conference held in Paris in 1853 can be seen as the starting point. Its objectives were mainly to harmonize the existing requirements of quarantine, in place in different countries in Europe, and directed mainly against the importation of plague from Eastern Mediterranean countries. At a later stage yellow fever outbreaks and epidemics of cholera were inducements for subsequent sanitary conferences to include the three diseases in the International Sanitary Conventions.

After several of these International Sanitary Conferences had been held without achieving an effective, internationally accepted public health policy, it was decided at the 1903 conference that a permanent international health bureau should be established, and in 1907 the Office International d'Hygiène Publique (OIHP), with a permanent secretariat, was established in Paris.

After the First World War there was a universal desire to construct a machinery to build a better world: the League of Nations. One of its tasks was 'to endeavour to take steps in matters of international concern for the prevention and control of disease', and to this end the Health Organization of the League of Nations was created.

On the other side of the Atlantic the Pan American Health Organization constituted a third international health organization.

Many new practices, procedures and activities were established within and between these three organizations that are still being applied in the current activities of the present World Health Organization.

After the Second World War all international activities had to be re-established almost from scratch. This turned out to be a blessing since the newly formed United Nations (UN) could now accept a proposal from Brazil and China to start an international health organization without having to count with existing structures. The result was the Constitution of the World Health Organization (WHO) in July 1946, which came into force on 7 April 1948, now marked as World Health Day each year.

Structure and organization

WHO is part of the UN family. This means that it forms part of the so-called UN system, sharing the administrative procedures, pension fund and personnel policies. However, it is in no way subordinate to the UN, but it is a specialized agency, carrying out specific tasks that are not in the terms of reference of the UN itself. It collaborates closely together in numerous projects with other specialized agencies of the UN, such as the Food and Agricultural Organization (FAO), the International Labour Organization (ILO) and the UN Children's Fund (UNICEF).

The organization is truly international and intergovernmental. It owes responsibility exclusively to its governing bodies, the member states. The organization consists of three organs: the World Health Assembly, the Executive Board and the Secretariat. The member states are represented in the Assembly, which meets once a year, and decides on matters of general policy. Each member of the Assembly has one vote, irrespective of the contribution his or her country pays into WHO's budget. The Board is the main executive body of the Assembly. The Secretariat is the staff of the WHO. In fact, one may say WHO is its staff; its technical advisory and advocacy role relies entirely on staff competence and staff activities.

From its position as an international, or, better, intergovernmental body it follows that WHO does not have the possibility, nor the intention to impose any regulation upon its member states. It tries to influence long-term health policy decisions through convincing advice, not by issuing binding regulations. Even resolutions adopted by the World Health Assembly may be ignored by the member states, although normally such resolutions will be implemented at national level.

An important characteristic feature of the WHO is its decentralization of power. WHO headquarters are located in Geneva, Switzerland, but there are six regional offices, each with a considerable degree of autonomy. As a matter of fact, WHO is the most decentralized of all UN agencies. This allows for flexible and, if necessary, fast action at the regional and national level. Activities at country level in many member states are coordinated by a resident WHO representative, who supports the government in the planning and management of national health programmes.

Objectives and activities

The constitution of the WHO was adopted by the International Health Conference held in New York from 19 to 22 June 1946. Its first article formulates the objectives of the organization as: 'the attainment by all peoples of the highest possible level of health'. In this statement health is defined as: 'a state of complete physical, mental and social well-being, and not merely the absence of disease or infirmity'. WHO considers such standards of health as one of the fundamental rights of every human being.

In 1978 the objective was extended by a joint WHO/UNICEF International Conference in Alma-Ata, (former) USSR, which adopted a Declaration on Primary Health Care, stating the target of governments and WHO to be 'the attainment of all the people of the world by the year 2000 of a level of health that will permit them to lead a socially and economically productive life'. This does not mean that disease and disability will no longer exist, but that resources for health will be evenly distributed, and that essential health care will be accessible to everyone.

Disease-oriented approach

WHO's activities in the early years were almost exclusively disease-oriented, and several efforts to control widespread diseases turned out to be successful. A few examples are given here.

For centuries people living in hot countries have been confronted with *yaws* (framboesia), a crippling and disfiguring disease. A large-scale WHO programme organized treatment with antibiotics, and millions of patients have now been successfully treated.

In 1974 the WHO launched a programme, together with three other UN agencies, to combat *onchocerciasis* (river blindness). The framework of this programme ranged from spraying the rivers to eradicate the disease-carrying blackflies, to providing (in collaboration with the manufacturer) a new, effective drug (ivermectin) to infected patients.

The parade-horse of WHO's activities is doubtless the eradication of *smallpox*, a disease that every year killed some 2 million people and left several millions of survivors disfigured or blinded. Thanks to a global vaccination programme, the disease simply no longer exists: the last known case was detected in Somalia in 1977, and as there is no animal reservoir of infectious organisms, re-emergence of the disease is not possible.

However, a lot is left to be done. Many infectious diseases, including measles, diphtheria, tuberculosis and poliomyelitis, are preventable by timely vaccination. WHO aims at total eradication of polio by the year 2000, and tries to bring other illnesses under control through extensive immunization programmes. Tropical diseases, malaria, diarrhoeal diseases and sexually transmissible diseases, in particular acquired immuno-deficiency syndrome (AIDS), receive focused attention in WHO through specialized programmes.

Since the Alma-Ata conference WHO has taken on the task of not only providing technical advice and assistance on medical matters, but also advocating changes in health policy. This activity is reflected in programmes on safe motherhood, chemical safety, environment, health protection and promotion, health of the elderly (becoming more important as ever more people reach advanced age, also in developing countries), and many others.

Normative functions

Classically WHO has three functions: to provide advice, to help developing health policy, and to set normative standards. Through the years of WHO's existence the last function has been the mainstay of its activities, on which its reputation for scientific excellence is based. Standards, definitions and limits have been set in numerous fields of public health. To name but a few: the Programme for the Promotion of Chemical Safety produces values for the acceptable daily intake (ADI) of chemicals and for maximum acceptable concentrations (MAC) of chemicals. Guidelines are published on such various subjects as management of cancer pain, the clinical management of AIDS, development of on-site sanitation, female sterilization, legislation on tobacco use, and many other areas of public health. Normative activities in the pharmaceutical area will be described below.

WHO's tools

As indicated above, WHO's work is done by its scientific secretariat. However, many issues require very specialist competence and experience that cannot be expected to be available within the organization. Moreover, WHO does not have research facilities or laboratories. In order for the staff to be able to carry out its duties WHO relies heavily on external expertise.

Competence from outside WHO can be obtained in several ways. Once an issue has been identified, a background paper is prepared by a competent staff member or by an external consultant. To provide for expert discussion and advice to WHO, resulting in concrete recommendations, usually an *ad hoc* consultation is organized, bringing together well-known experts in the field.

Such technical meetings often produce valuable advice, but, on the other hand, it is difficult for a small group of highly specialized experts to cover all the various branches of knowledge of relevance to the subject, and to represent the sometimes widely different experience and views prevailing in different parts of the world.

To utilize available scientific resources effectively WHO has established expert advisory panels, from which individual members of expert committees may be drawn as circumstances require. Such experts may contribute either by correspondence or in person during special expert committee meetings. In order to maintain actuality and geographical representation the composition of the panels is flexible and membership normally does not exceed 4 years. Reports of expert committee meetings are the organization's most authoritative documents, usually published in the Technical Report Series.

A large number of programmes within WHO have a need for research at laboratory level. At an early stage of WHO's existence scientific institutions offered help to WHO. The National Institute for Biological Standards and Control in the UK, and the State Serum Institute in Denmark acted during the years of the League of Nations on behalf of the Health Organization as worldwide centres for the storage and maintenance, preparation and distribution of standard preparations of biological materials, and established potency units for many of these substances by biological assays. This collaboration was continued at the establishment of WHO and signified the starting point for the nomination of a large number (currently some thousand) of institutions as collaborating centres. They serve the organization in all the various facets of its work, including dissemination of information, development of appropriate technology, training and standardization of terminology and nomenclature, often collaborating in a global network.

In carrying out its function as the directing and coordinating authority on international health matters WHO may make suitable arrangements for consultation and cooperation with non-governmental organizations (NGO). NGOs admitted to official relations with WHO are usually international in scope and structure. Their area of competence lies within the purview of WHO and in conformity with its spirit. In return for the support an NGO provides to WHO it has access to relevant meetings and documentation, and may correspond directly with the Director-General of the Organization.

Normative activities in the pharmaceutical area

Introduction

Article 2 of the Constitution of WHO, which describes its functions, states, among others, that one of WHO's tasks is 'to develop, establish and promote international standards with respect to food, biological, pharmaceutical and similar products'. According to article 23 of the Constitution the Health Assembly has authority to adopt regulations concerning 'standards with respect to the safety, purity and potency of biological, pharmaceutical and similar products moving in international commerce'; and on 'advertising, labelling of all biological, pharmaceutical and similar products moving in international commerce'.

On the basis of this article the Division of Drug Management and Policies within WHO headquarters is responsible for technical matters relating to safety, efficacy and quality of pharmaceutical products. Its natural counterparts are the Drug Regulatory Authorities in the national Ministries of Health. The division also maintains close working relationships with various non-governmental organizations, in particular the International Federation of Pharmaceutical Manufacturers Associations (IFPMA) and the World Federation of Proprietary Medicines Manufacturers (WFPMM), organizations which represent the pharmaceutical industry.

Quality assurance of pharmaceutical products

Certification scheme

The quality of pharmaceutical products, in particular in developing countries, has been of concern to the Health Assembly for many years, and several resolutions have requested WHO to develop means to assist these countries in their battle against substandard drugs. Discussions in the Assembly initially invited member states to subject drugs for export to the same regulations and control as for drugs for domestic use. Soon it became clear that this did not work as expected and the need for international guidance became apparent.

The lack of adequate drug regulatory systems in some countries entails concrete risks of drugs being offered for sale that do not comply with quality standards. The WHO has sought to develop a certification system, based, at least partially, on systems already operated by health authorities of exporting countries who issue a certificate on request to foreign importers with respect to drugs subjected to statutory control in the exporting country.

The first version of the WHO Certification Scheme on the Quality of Pharmaceutical Products Moving in International Commerce was issued in 1975. In order to promote and facilitate its use, guidelines for the use of the scheme were issued in 1992 (WHO, 1992b, 1995a). They identify the scheme as an administrative instrument that requires each participating member state, upon application by a commercially interested party, to attest to the competent authority of another participating member state, whether:

1   A specific product is authorized to be placed on the market within its jurisdiction or, if it is not thus authorized, the reason why the authorization has not been accorded.
2   The plant in which it is produced is subject to inspections at suitable intervals to establish that the manufacturer conforms to good manufacturing practice (GMP) as recommended by WHO.
3   All submitted product information, included labelling, is currently authorized in the certifying country.

Currently more than 130 countries participate in the scheme; practically all major exporting countries adhere.

The scheme was initially intended for finished dosage forms of pharmaceutical products, but has been extended to include certification of veterinary products administered to food-producing animals, starting materials, and information on safety and efficacy.

When the Health Assembly recommended the first version of the scheme it accepted at the same time the GMP text as an integral part of the scheme.

Good manufacturing practices

In 1968 the first WHO text on *Good Manufacturing Practice in the Manufacture and Quality Control of Drugs and Pharmaceutical Specialities (GMP)* was published, focusing on the concept that quality control has to be built into the product, and that the primary responsibility for good quality is with the manufacturer.

The current version of the guidelines outlines the general concepts of quality assurance as well as principal issues such as hygiene, validation, self-inspection, personnel, premises, etc. (WHO, 1992a)

The provisions in the guide are fully consonant with those published by the Commission of the European Community and with those operative within countries participating in the Convention for the Mutual Recognition of Inspection in Respect of Pharmaceutical Products, and other major industrialized countries. It is intended to be used as a standard to justify GMP status and as a basis for the inspection of manufacturing facilities. It may also be used as training material for government drug inspectors.

As with all WHO guidelines, the GMP guidelines should be considered general guides, and they may be adapted to meet individual needs.

In the course of the last decade several supplementary guidelines have been developed, addressing specific issues, including investigational products, herbal medicinal products, excipients and for training.

Analytical testing

An absolute prerequisite for effective pharmacotherapy is the availability of drugs of good quality. Many countries have elaborate systems in place to control their drug market in this respect, but a much larger number unfortunately do not have sufficiently qualified staff or sufficiently sophisticated equipment to carry out comprehensive control.

But analytical quality control does not need to be highly sophisticated in all cases: adequate assurance of pharmaceutical quality can often be obtained by relatively simple methods. WHO put together a collection of such tests in two volumes, *Basic Tests for Pharmaceutical Substances*, and *Basic Tests for Pharmaceutical Dosage Forms* (WHO, 1986, 1991). Both volumes provide easily applicable methods for verifying the identity of a drug substance, in particular when a fully equipped laboratory is not available. They may also be used to indicate if gross degradation has occurred, for instance during storage or transport under adverse conditions.

For condition of quantitative specifications and of purity and potency of pharmaceutical products the *Basic Tests* are inadequate. The *WHO International Pharmaceopeia* provides specification on these characteristics for essential drugs, widely used excipients and dosage forms. While having no legal status at national level, the *International Pharmacopoeia* can be helpful to national authorities to establish national standards of quality.

Reference standards

Through one of its collaborating centres WHO issues reference standards to be used in conjunction with the *International Pharmacopoeia*. Since standards for sera and vaccines were omitted from the *Pharmacopoeia* at an early stage, WHO now produces standards for these compounds in the form of Expert Committee Reports.

Drug nomenclature

Drugs are an essential element of health care. But an identification is required: drugs need a name. Health professionals usually take it for granted that pharmaceutical compounds do have a unique name, but do not realize that this international nonproprietary name (INN) (*International Nonproprietory Names*, 1992) or generic name has been given by a WHO programme that has been in existence since 1953. WHO encourages the use of these names in order to avoid confusion and to ensure unequivocal reference to the product.

Drug safety and efficacy

Introduction

The thalidomide tragedy in the late fifties and early sixties, resulting in thousands of severely malformed children born to mothers who had been treated with the drug during pregnancy, was the impulse for many countries to establish drug regulatory agencies or to strengthen existing ones. At almost the same time the World Health Assembly requested the WHO to set up a programme securing exchange of information between these regulatory agencies on the safety and efficacy of pharmaceutical preparations, and, in particular, information on serious side-effects.

Several initiatives resulted from these resolutions.

Information exchange

It occasionally happens that regulatory authorities are confronted with an aspect of drug safety that is of immediate relevance to their colleagues. In such instances WHO may send out an alert to all authorities. More often though, regulators, in particular in developing countries, need evaluated information on regulatory issues. To this end WHO produces a monthly *Pharmaceuticals Newsletter*, sent to all drug regulators in member countries. The periodical *WHO Drug Information* is issued three-monthly and contains articles on current controversial issues, regulatory issues, new developments, and prescribing information on essential drugs.

The information WHO provides may help countries to define their position in drug regulatory questions and to take adequate action in case of safety issues.

International Drug Safety Monitoring

Some years after the thalidomide disaster the WHO set up a pilot project to investigate the feasibility of an international programme of monitoring adverse reactions. This has finally, some 30 years later, resulted in a programme joined by some 45 countries, who share the reports of adverse reactions to drug treatment, received from health professionals. These reports are collected in a database – currently containing some 1 300 000 reports – maintained by a WHO collaborating centre in Uppsala, Sweden.

During its existence the programme has exerted considerable influence in harmonizing the management of spontaneous reports of adverse effects. It brings together periodically National Centres for Adverse Drug Reactions Monitoring so that common problems can be discussed, and assists countries in establishing national programmes.

The programme, through its collaborating centre, acts as the guardian of the standardized terminology of adverse reactions used in computerized systems. It is used by almost all participating countries and by a large number of pharmaceutical companies. Currently efforts are taking place to arrive at a medical terminology which addresses the needs of drug regulatory authorities with regard to other areas in drug regulation, including premarketing data, clinical data, and medical and social history data.

To complete the terminology, definitions of the terms are needed. The Council for Organizations of International Medical Science, an intergovernmental organization in official collaboration with WHO, started to convene meetings of experts from regulatory agencies and the pharmaceutical industry to define the most frequently used terms in the context of the WHO programme.

Drug regulation

International activities

As described earlier, drug regulation in its modern form started in the 1960s, as a consequence of the thalidomide tragedy. International collaboration started a few years later. In 1965 the European Community adopted a directive that formed the basis for the current close and complex structure of European collaboration in the area of control and regulation of pharmaceutical products.

However, the first practically active international joint effort in drug control manifested itself in the countries of the Benelux – Belgium, Netherlands and Luxemburg. In the now defunct Benelux Committee were represented equal numbers from each of the three countries for the three disciplines relevant for evaluation of an application for registration: pharmacy, preclinical pharmacology and toxicology, and clinical pharmacology. The Committee tried to establish common standards for the three countries involved, and it finally achieved a high level of mutual understanding between them.

At the end of the 1970s drug regulation, in particular drug evaluation and registration, had become quite complex and the need for more intensive cooperation was felt more strongly than before. As a consequence the drug regulatory activities by the European Community increased, and its scientific body, the Committee on Proprietary Medicinal Products (CPMP) was given a much higher profile.

The need for increased international collaboration in drug regulatory affairs resulted in 1990 in the start of a project that brings together the regulatory authorities of Europe, the USA and Japan, and experts of the pharmaceutical industry in the three regions. The purpose of this International Conference on Harmonization (ICH) of technical requirements for registration of pharmaceuticals is to achieve greater harmonization in the interpretation and application of technical guidelines and to save on human, animal and material resources. It also seeks to eliminate delay in the global availability of valuable new medicines. The activities of ICH have so far resulted in several guidelines accepted in the three regions, and some 20 under way, in various areas of drug registration from stability testing to clinical trials in geriatric patients.

WHO and international drug registration
WHO's involvement in drug registration has developed along lines parallel to those in other communities. It started with the programme on international exchange of information between drug regulators, which resulted in a network of focal points in drug regulatory agencies, the information officers.

As from 1980 WHO has brought together senior representatives from drug regulatory authorities in the biennial International Conference of Drug Regulatory Authorities. These conferences, attended by some 150 participants from over 100 countries, have demonstrated that WHO has an important role to play in the provision of a forum where *all* countries of the world may discuss their problems.

An initiative such as ICH, however invaluable in harmonizing scientific standards of drug regulation, by its very nature tends to concentrate on issues of importance in the highly industrialized countries participating in the project. WHO is an observer at ICH and acts as a liaison between ICH and member states that are not participating in the conference. It ensures that the interest of these countries is properly represented and that products that become available from ICH will be accessible to them. ICH in its turn may also benefit from activities by WHO and collaborate with the Organization in the preparation of guidelines.

Two examples of both procedures are described here:

1 A draft guideline on the detection of toxicity to reproduction for medicinal products was prepared under the auspices of ICH in 1990. The
   text was circulated through WHO's network of information officers to
   all member states and comments were received from some 30 countries,
   most of them outside the ICH sphere. The guideline has now been
   finalized and implemented in all three regions of ICH. At the same time
   it is at the disposal of WHO's member countries, who may adopt the
   guideline if they wish.

2 Studies to investigate activities of pharmaceutical compounds in
   human subjects need a maximum of care and caution. Risk of undue
   harm, although impossible to exclude with complete certainty, must
   be kept at an absolute minimum. Ethical issues, including confidentiality of personal data and informed consent, are of major concern.
   Several institutions, including the European Community and the
   Nordic Council, had prepared guidelines addressing clinical trials.
   WHO decided that there was a perceived need for more general guidelines that would have global validity and started a series of consultations
   to discuss the draft text, based on existing ones, of guidelines for good
   clinical trial practices. This text was offered to ICH and is now subject
   to further discussion in its expert working groups.

   Finally, WHO has recognized that a well-functioning drug regulatory
   system, essential for the availability of safe and effective drugs of good
   quality, is absent or weak in many developing countries. To assist these
   countries in establishing regulatory organizations the *Guiding Principles
   for Small Drug Regulatory Authorities* (1990) identify basic requirements
   and give a step-up approach for organizing a drug regulatory agency. As
   a background to these principals WHO is also preparing model texts for
   legislation on drug control.

Herbal medicines have been used for thousands of years. Over the last 10
years they have been taking up an increasing proportion of the drug market
in industrialized countries. However, herbal medicines are also of great
importance to the health of the individual and community in developing
countries.

   In national programme development, WHO collaborates with its
member states in the review of national policies, legislation and decisions
on the nature and use of herbal medicines, and it promotes the incorporation of proven traditional remedies into national drug policies.

   To assist national drug regulatory authorities in the evaluation of herbal
remedies WHO has issued *Guidelines for the Assessment of Herbal Medicines*
(1995c). These guidelines formulate general principles that ensure a scientifically valid approach to the registration of these products.

   The need for greater precision in preparation and evaluation, and for
increased research have stimulated WHO's regional office for the Western

Pacific, which has a rich tradition of use of herbal drugs, to develop criteria and general principles to guide research work on evaluating herbal medicines. In these *Research Guidelines for Evaluating the Safety and Efficacy of Herbal Medicines* (1993) basic scientific principles as well as any special requirements related to the use of herbal medicines in traditional practice have been incorporated.

Assurance of good quality is one of the aspects of this scientific approach. WHO's document *Quality Control Methods for Medicinal Plant Materials* (1996) lists a collection of test procedures, primarily intended for use within national drug quality control laboratories in developing countries, to complement the *International Pharmacopoeia*. Additionally some suggestions regarding general limits for contaminants are also included, as a basis for establishing national limits. The document is further complemented by the *Guidelines for the Manufacture of Herbal Medicinal Products* (1995), as part of the GMP guidelines for pharmaceutical products.

Collaboration with other institutions

In the framework of its activities in the drug field WHO works closely together with many other organizations, including the pharmaceutical industry. The latter is vital to maintain WHO's programmes on training of experts for drug regulation and quality control. Close collaboration also exists in the coordination of efforts to curb the availability of counterfeit and spurious and substandard drugs. This resulted in a joint workshop of the WHO and IFPMA, which identified many important issues and suggested approaches on how to proceed.

Other non-government organizations with which WHO collaborates include the International Union of Pharmacology (IUPHAR) and the pharmacy professionals' organizations, comprising the International Pharmaceutical Federation (FIP) and the Commonwealth Pharmaceutical Association (CPA).

Development agencies such as the German Foundation for International Development, and German Technical Cooperation have also been most constructively collaborating with WHO in various areas of drug control.

Conclusions

This chapter attempts to provide a demonstration of WHO's commitment to normative activities in general. Of necessity this overview is far from being exhaustive: from its inception, now almost 50 years ago, the Organization has been issuing guidelines, standards and reference values in almost all areas of public health.

WHO does its work using experts – human experts. As a consequence, sometimes the results of the deliberations of these experts meet with

controversy, or even criticism. Sometimes conclusions or recommendations appear to be flawed, unrealistic, or even wrong. However, they are
being made by dedicated people, who try to do the best they can. Generally
normative values issued by WHO are regarded as objective, scientifically
sound and prestigious, and it is in this area of work that the Organization
has gained its reputation for being a technically competent, international
secretariat for matters relating to public health at large.

References

International Nonproprietary Names (INN) for Pharmaceutical Substances
(1992) Cumulative list no. 8.

WHO. *The International Pharmacopoeia. Vol. 1: General Methods of Analysis
(1979); Vol. 2: Quality Specifications (1981); Vol. 3: Quality Specifications
(1988); Vol. 4: Tests, Methods, and General Requirements, Quality Specifications for Pharmaceutical Substances, Excipients and Dosage Forms.*
Geneva: WHO.

WHO (1986) *Basic Tests for Pharmaceutical Substances*. Geneva: WHO.

WHO (1990) *Technical Report Series (TRS), 790 (Thirty-first report of the
WHO Expert Committee on Specifications for Pharmaceutical Preparations).
Annex 6: Guiding Principles for Small Regulatory Authorities.*

WHO (1991) *Basic Tests for Pharmaceutical Substances*. Geneva: WHO.

WHO (1992a) *Technical Report Series (TRS), 823 (Thirty-second report of the
WHO Expert Committee on Specifications for Pharmaceutical Preparations).
Annex 1: Good Manufacturing Practices for Pharmaceutical Products.*

WHO (1992b) *Technical Report Series (TRS), 823 (Thirty-second report of the
WHO Expert Committee on Specifications for Pharmaceutical Preparations).
Annex 3: Proposed Guidelines for the Implementation of the WHO
Certification Scheme on the Quality of Pharmaceutical Products Moving in
International Commerce.*

WHO (1993) *Research Guidelines for Evaluating the Safety and Efficacy of
Herbal Medicines.* Manila: WHO.

WHO (1995a) *Certification Scheme on the Quality of Pharmaceutical Products
Moving in International Commerce. WHO/Pharm/82.4Rev.4.*

WHO (1995b) *Technical Report Series (TRS) (Thirty-fourth report of the
WHO Expert Committee on Specifications for Pharmaceutical Preparations).
Annex 7: Supplementary Guidelines for the Manufacture of Herbal Medicinal
Products.*

WHO (1995c) *Technical Report Series (TRS) (Thirty-fourth report of the
WHO Expert Committee on Specifications for Pharmaceutical Preparations).
Annex 10: Guidelines for the Assessment of Herbal Medicines.*

WHO (1996) *Quality Control Methods for Medicinal Plant Materials* (in
print).

23 Reflections on good clinical practice and medicine regulation

D S Freestone

Introduction

Good clinical practice (GCP) has contributed to the overall improvement in the quality of clinical research. However, the costs are high. Many more monitoring, data handling and quality assurance staff have been employed by the pharmaceutical industry to ensure that studies are protocol-compliant. Regulatory authorities are faced with larger licence applications which inevitably take more time to process. GCP does not necessarily provide for good-quality clinical research. With finite financial resources available, fewer studies can be conducted with full GCP applied. Thus, society may not be best served. The challenge is to refine GCP to provide acceptable – not absolute – clinical research standards while containing costs.

Although GCP started in different countries at different times, and despite differences in medical practice, culture and local circumstances, a high level of commonality exists between Europe and North America. This chapter aims to provide a few reflections on GCP and medicines regulation mainly from a UK perspective.

Purpose of GCP

European GCP guidelines (1990) specify that 'pre-established systematic written procedures for the organisation, conduct, data collection, documentation and verification of clinical trials are necessary to ensure that the rights and integrity of the trial subjects are thoroughly protected and to establish the credibility of data and to improve the ethical, scientific and technical quality of trials'. In the USA, the aims are similar: to 'provide greater protection of the rights and safety of subjects involved in clinical investigations and help assure the quality and integrity of the data filed with the Agency pursuant to the Federal Food Drug and Cosmetic Act and the Public Health Service Act' (Department of Health Education and Welfare,

Food and Drug Administration, 1977). GCP has embraced some objectives which were already recognized as important before GCP as a concept was introduced. Moves towards international harmonization of GCP standards are in progress (International Conference on Harmonization 1993, 1994) and the European Commission has heralded as part of its future work, the development of a clinical trials directive setting out more detailed GCP requirements (Donnelly, 1994).

Clinical trials, GCP and regulators

At present in the UK there are no statutory controls over the conduct of phase I clinical trials of unlicensed medicines in healthy volunteers where there is no potential for benefit to participants. Most other pre-licensing clinical trials in patient sponsored by pharmaceutical companies are conducted under the clinical trial exemption (CTX) regulations. Summarized data on chemistry and pharmacy, the results of preclinical studies, any clinical results and the protocol for the proposed clinical trials are submitted to the Medicines Control Agency. Under the CTX scheme, a medically qualified person, either a staff member of a sponsoring organization or an independent, warrants that the summaries are accurate, that the data support the proposed study, which is itself medically, ethically and scientifically valid. If an ethics committee refuses to approve the study, the Agency must be advised. Sponsors are free to proceed with the trial in 35 days in the absence of any objection. The doctor and dentist clinical trial (DDX) scheme is applicable to studies of unlicensed medicines initiated by prescribers and without a commercial sponsor. In 1993–94 some 145 new, 140 abridge and 499 DDX applications were reviewed and there were 2519 clinical trial variations (Medicines Control Agency, 1994). All new clinical trials should be conducted to GCP standards. However, the regulator's opportunity and ability to influence or to apply in process GCP controls to clinical studies is small. While many clinical trials and variations are filed annually, in 1993–94 product licence applications were made for only 38 new active substances and some 100 complex abridged licence applications (referred to section IV committees: Committee on Safety of Medicines, Committee on Dental and Surgical Materials) relating mostly to new indications and/or formulations. In these circumstances, available resources at present are focused properly on product licence applications.

Clinical data included in UK product licence applications

It is a requirement that all pertinent data, whether published or unpublished, be included in product licence applications. It is for applicants to make the best case possible based on the data available. At this time not all studies reported in product licence applications will have been conducted to GCP standards. Thus, licensing authority medical assessors (assessors) may be faced with an application consisting of reports of studies carried out to full or to part GCP standards, published reports from the literature, or various mixtures. Again, published reports vary in their level of GCP compliance, depending amongst other factors on the dates when studies were initiated. Reports from the literature are more likely to be included in abridged applications where a new active substance has already been previously licensed for a different indication and clinical investigators able to access drug have conducted studies independently of the company. Assessors review applications submitted to arrive at a judgement as to whether acceptable effectiveness and safety have been demonstrated, their judgements in the UK as appropriate being subjected to review by advisory committees. This work is complex; requiring judgements on the extent, quality and appropriateness of the data submitted and risk–benefit assessments. Delays in making important new medicines available to patients are also to be avoided. Thus, for example, evidence of effectiveness and safety for the treatment of a life-threatening condition for which existing treatments are of marginal benefit might more readily be accepted than that of similar extent, quality and appropriateness for the treatment of a minor, non life-threatening condition.

Assessment of quality of applications

Assessment of quality is not straightforward. Inevitably, applications vary from being generally inadequate to excellent. Even now everything seems possible, including lack of definition of end-points, absence of adequate dose finding, no kinetics, inadequate analysis of laboratory data, inadequate/absent details of statistical analysis, investigators not identified, numbers not adding up and so on. Deficiencies need to be balanced against the importance of the new indication/medicine and the company's proposed claims. Faults in clinical development can result in individual studies being excellently executed and reported but with gaps in the information needed to support licensure. Alternatively, it may be apparent that not only have individual studies been very well-performed to full GCP standards but that they are part of a carefully designed and executed clinical development plan. The primary clinical assessment concerns effectiveness and safety. Nevertheless, naturally assessors would not wish to recommend products for licensure where there were doubts concerning the authenticity, veracity, precision or reproducibility of the submitted data, the adequacy of data handling and statistical analysis or where the report of a study did not reflect the results obtained. Clearly, there would also be concerns about recommending for licensure products supported by studies about which there were ethical reservations – adequacy of ethics committee approval and informed consent procedure.

Good clinical practice versus good clinical research

At the opposite ends of the spectrum, acceptable effectiveness and safety might be demonstrated by two multicentre studies conducted to full GCP standards or alternatively derived from a number of published reports conducted independently of a commercial sponsor and published in peer-reviewed journals (the product being already licensed for another indication). Reports of, say, five or six studies by reputable clinical investigators in various parts of the world carried out independent of company, yielding similar results, and published in peer-reviewed journals which are not followed in the journals correspondence by divergent views, are significant. One might take the view that such evidence is at least as compelling as that derived from one or two multicentre, multinational studies, tightly controlled by the commercial sponsor and licence applicant. Although such studies are vetted and signed off by a number of specialists, for example, depending on company style, medical advisor, monitor, data handler, statistician and their managers, it is not usual for any person outside the company's employ to be a signatory, including even the principal investigator. Thus, although the accurate movement of data points from their first recording to incorporation into data listings is of a high order, there is a serious risk of such reports lacking clinical reality as well as usually being dull, repetitive and voluminous. Such reports, albeit fully compliant with good clinical practice, are not necessarily good science or medicine. For example, multicentre studies conducted to GCP lay great emphasis on protocol inclusion and exclusion criteria with significant percentages of patients excluded from analysis because of violations. It might be that the criteria were relaxed some way through studies to allow the planned rate of patient recruitment to be obtained (and therefore to avoid delays to the company's project development plan). All this is properly documented. However, in contrast to this GCP approach, good clinical research would have identified problems in advance, ensured that investigators rarely, if ever, entered protocol violators, and that an acceptable rate of entry was assured. Thus, GCP can be used to paper over procedural problems that should not have arisen.

GCP and size of final medical report

A consequence of GCP is that much is done by routine, whether or not it is relevant, and comments that are demanded by results may not get made. A typical final medical report of, say, 150 patients with appendices of protocol, data-collection form, investigators' names, affiliations and curricula vitae, with data listings for the patients, can easily run to 4000 pages in a product licence application. This is equivalent to over 25 pages per patient and excludes the 150 completed data collection records of 100–200 pages each, usually available on request or supplied separately.

Repetition

Licence applications are highly repetitive, for example, the 10-page introduction stated in the final medical report to the first study reported in the application is valuable but its inclusion in all subsequent study reports and in each of the relevant protocols is highly repetitive. The same comment can be made in relation to the description of the classification and handling of adverse events. Nevertheless, despite GCP compliance it can still be difficult to disentangle adverse events leading to withdrawal from the study, serious adverse events, and other adverse events, particularly if they are segregated into occurrence by geography, and whether they were labelled (documented as occurring in the investigator's manual). This can result in breakdown into many categories, without any overall summation of adverse event occurrence. Furthermore, presentation of adverse events by body systems alone may also obscure the precise nature of the adverse events that occurred.

Withdrawals

Multicentre studies often have high withdrawal rates. Withdrawal rates of 50% or greater are by no means unusual and comments on the acceptability of such high levels of withdrawals are unusual. The final medical report will have attempted to give some reasons for the withdrawals, for example failures in effectiveness, adverse events, administrative reasons, lost to follow-up, but these are often poorly detailed and it may be difficult to compare the true causes of withdrawals between treatment groups.

Statistical analyses

A final medical report of a placebo-controlled trial of an acute therapy with two after treatment follow-ups might contain several hundred P values, most of which had no clinical relevance and were calculated simply because the figures were there, even though with very small numbers in subgroups the probability of statistical significance was remote.

Assessors in a large regulatory authority may have less pressure on their time but increasingly, as regulatory authorities strive to minimize delays in reviewing applications, and with the time limits under which applications made to the European Medicines Evaluation Agency are to be processed, the time available is in practice finite. The final medical report provides a detailed definitive record of a study of a company for posterity and by no means least for the regulatory authority. Clearly, final medical reports that are user-friendly to regulators have great advantages, to both the regulators and to the applicant.

Credibility of data

It is an aim of GCP that data credibility be improved. The authorities, in stating this aim, were concerned to ensure that data were not falsified and specifically that data were not presented for patients who did not exist, or that measurements were not submitted which were never made, albeit the patients did exist. Overt fraud is uncommon and is clearly unacceptable. More common is sloppy clinical research. GCP procedures, monitoring, source document verification and programmes for data checks are clearly of considerable importance in prevention and detection. Obviously, the first line of defence against such irregularities lies with company staff who must take responsibility for the veracity and the quality of the data that they submit. While regulators may maintain formal or informal lists of investigators whose standards have not been found to be satisfactory and will inevitably treat results from further studies from these investigators with circumspection, the prime responsibilities must lie with companies. In the future, an increasing number of regulatory authorities will establish clinical inspectorates. It is likely that different regulators will employ clinical inspectors in different ways but there can be few assessors who have not been faced with a report of a study with suspicious results which are critical to the approval of an application. Such results might be suspicious because they look too good or because they are contrary to the results obtained elsewhere with similar agents. While the report itself may contain information which allows the assessor to make a judgement as to whether or not the report can be accepted at face value, this is not always the case. In these circumstances a report of a field clinical inspection for GCP compliance may be of vital importance.

Ethics

No regulatory authority will wish to license a product on the basis of an unethical study and most protocols, final medical reports and published papers will declare that ethics committee or institutional review board approval is to be or has been obtained. However, regulators rarely see copies or conditions of ethical approval. Other difficulties are the considerable differences of opinion between individual ethics committee members and between committees when a specific research project is assessed (Pearn, 1995). It seems doubtful that differences in opinion between committees should be attributed to purely local issues, and difficult to accept that a project which is unethical in one place is ethical elsewhere. An assessor of a product licence application might not be made aware of ethical reservations but regulatory authority inspectors, in examining clinical trial and clinical development files for evidence of satisfactory ethics committee approval, should detect and clarify concerns.

General comments

GCP has both beneficial and undesirable effects. Because of the infrastructure required to support GCP, it has resulted in much of the processing of clinical research results being transferred from individual clinical investigators to commercial organizations and data-processing units. Naturally, commercial organizations aim to present results in the most favourable light, presenting the assessor with a further consideration – the detection of 'spin'. However, GCP has undoubtedly done much to raise standards of what would have been poor-quality clinical research but has probably occasionally reduced the standards of some high-quality clinical research. However, costs are high to industry, to regulators, and to society since GCP costs inevitably reduce the numbers of projects that can be run by commercial organizations. A time has been reached when refinement is needed to ensure satisfactory standards of clinical research but at the same time containing costs.

Note and acknowledgement

The views expressed are those of the author and do not necessarily represent those of Wellcome PLC, or the Medicines Control Agency.

I am very grateful to Kathryn Dee for typing this manuscript.

References

Department of Health Education and Welfare, Food and Drug Administration (1977) Clinical investigations, proposed establishment of regulations on obligations of sponsors and monitors. *Federal Register* **42:** 49612–49627.

Donnelly, M. (1994) The second European Conference on Medicines Research. Perspectives in clinical trials.

European Commission (1990) *Committee on Proprietary Medicinal Products guidelines on Good Clinical Practice*. III 3976/89. Brussels: European Commission.

International Conference on Harmonisation of Technical Requirements for the Registration of Pharmaceuticals for Human Use (1993) *Good Clinical Practices: Addenda on Investigations Brochure and Essential Documents*. MCA Euro direct publication no. ICH4.

International Conference on Harmonisation of Technical Requirements for Registration of Pharmaceuticals for Human Use (1994) *Proposed Guideline for Good Clinical Practice*. MCA Euro direct publication no. 5085/94 (ICH4).

Medicines Control Agency (1994) *Annual Report and Accounts* 1993/4. London: HMSO.

Pearn, J. (1995) Publication on ethical imperative. *British Medical Journal* **310:** 1313–1315.

24 An updated situation of the current compliance within Hungary and other Eastern and Central European countries

T L Paál

Introduction

As suggested by the title, the aim of this chapter is mainly to update certain overviews on good practices (good manufacturing practice (GMP), good laboratory practice (GLP) and good clinical practice (GCP); further on GxPs previously published (Paál, 1993, 1994). The target area is Central and Eastern Europe, a specific one, comprising developed countries with underdeveloped (or rather misdeveloped) economies but also with a high level of pharmaceutical science and great traditions of the pharmaceutical industry. The aim of this chapter is not only to indicate the development of GxPs in the given countries but also to analyse the reasons for it as well as to point out the main problems and possible future trends. Both rapid changes and further developments, surprisingly slow to take hold in the region, deserve careful analysis.

Before starting any discussion the author is obliged to note that, as a consequence of the rapid changes in the target area, certain information may be outdated at the time of publication. This may be true in spite of the fact that the author officially visited about half of the target countries in recent years as well as having the opportunity to discuss relevant issues with professionals of most of the remaining ones. Thus, with the exception of some central Asian post-soviet newly independent states (NIS), first-hand information is communicated to the reader.

The target area: Eastern and Central Europe

One may think that the definition of this area will not be difficult. However, both terms Central and Eastern need some explanation.

Apart from the past, when the political term Eastern bloc (including the former DDR; Greece belonged to western Europe) excluded the possibility of any geographically sound categorization, the Centre of Europe is used to mean different things even today. (The author witnessed its use for Brussels, Berlin and Vienna in opening addresses of congresses held in each city.) Rejecting the plausible compromise of a multicentred Europe and applying for advice to international organizations, however, creates more problems than solutions.

According to the regional office for Europe of the World Health Organization (WHO, its activity covers geographical Europe plus Israel plus all the former soviet republics, including the central Asian ones such as Uzbekistan. For Israel the reason is obvious, for the former soviet republics the explanation is that originally all of the Soviet Union (with more Asian than European territory) had belonged to the European part of WHO, partition should not mean losing any former soviet republics, which are now independent countries.

At the same time, the relevant WHO European programme bears the title of CCEE/NIS – the countries of Central and Eastern Europe and(/or?) the newly independent states. This does not specify what belongs where.

It may be noted that the United Nations Economic Council for Europe (ECE), which also includes the central Asian former soviet republics in its activities, uses the term countries with economies in transition for the whole region, thus avoiding any geographical trap.

According to a Swiss drug regulator, central Europe represents land-locked European countries. Thus, this term would cover Switzerland, Austria, the Czech and Slovak republics, Hungary, Moldavia and Belarussia.

Geographically, since Europe's eastern border lies at the Ural mountains and it goes without saying that Iceland belongs to Europe together with Lapland and Cyprus, the centre of the continent may be found in Poland, near the Czech frontier.

From the point of view of this chapter countries of the Eurasian continent, indicated on Figure 24.1, will be discussed, although less emphasis will be given to the Central Asian NIS.

The problems of the definition of the term Central and Eastern Europe give rise to the question of whether this region, as a homogeneous one, has ever existed at all?

The wrong Eastern bloc approach

The answer to this question is a definite no! Countries of Central and Eastern Europe or European economies in transition never created a homogeneous bloc of countries. After analysing their historic situation, at least the following major regions, which are also important from the point of view of the introduction of GxPs, can be identified:

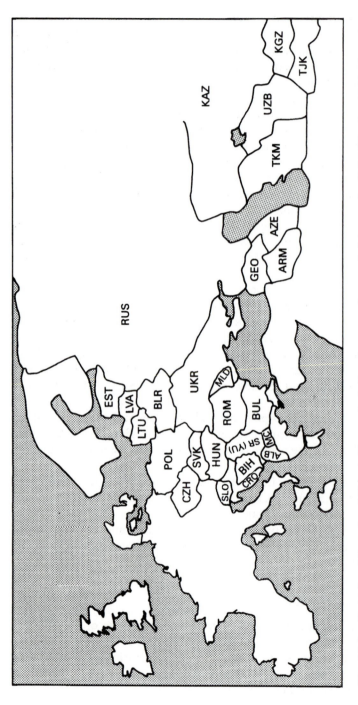

Fig. 24.1   Countries of Central and Eastern Europe (including the post-soviet central Asian ones). ALB=Albania; ARM=Armenia; AZE=Azerbaijan; BIH=Bosnia-Hercegovina; BLR=Belarussia; BUL=Bulgaria; CRO=Croatia; CZH=Czech republic; EST=Estonia; GEO=Georgia;   HUN=Hungary;   KAZ=Kazakhstan;   KGZ=Kirgizistan;   LVA=Latvia;   LTU=Lithuania;   MC=Macedonia; MLD=Moldavia;   POL=Poland;   ROM=Romania;   RUS=Russia;   SR(YU)=Serbia/Yugoslavia;   SLO=Slovenia;   SVK=Slovakia; TJK=Tadjikistan, TKM=Turkmenistan; UKR=Ukraine; UZB=Uzbekistan.

1 The former CMEA (Council of Mutual Economic Assistance; COMECON) member states, participating in a common drug investigation collaboration – Bulgaria, Czechoslovakia, the former DDR, Hungary, Poland and the former Soviet Union.
2 Romania and the former Yugoslavia as non-CMEA collaborators with eastern and western orientations, respectively.
3 Albania (with almost no professional connection to the others).

Moreover, these regions of themselves were not homogeneous, particularly the CMEA group.

The CMEA and GxPs

CMEA collaborations in most Central and Eastern European countries covered manufacturing (with a highly developed international distribution of work, e.g. that of the rights of manufacturing certain goods for the whole CMEA, among member states), international (within CMEA) trade and research.

While certain CMEA drug investigation collaborations between regulatory bodies dated back to the late fifties, they were strengthened in the mid-seventies and have been coordinated by the Hungarian National Institute of Pharmacy from 1981.

It should be emphasized that the CMEA could never take on a supranational character like that of the European Community (EC). In spite of all efforts to the contrary, the CMEA developed guidelines that were only strong suggestions for regulating drug affairs between the member states. They were not mandatory and carried no legal force. The national regulatory bodies, however, should take the guidelines into account when preparing national legislation. This character of the CMEA may be understood by the fact that it was not only a professional but also partly a political organization including both moderately developed European countries and, at the same time, more or less developing ones such as Cuba, Mongolia and Vietnam. This fact made it impossible to develop mutually binding directives or standards (Paál, 1993). For this reason, the development of a working common CMEA drug evaluation system or any standardized system of drug registration, although begun, never succeeded.

The structure of the former CMEA drug investigation and registration collaboration is not discussed here in detail. It should be mentioned, however, that it covered the development of common published guidelines for preclinical and clinical testing requirements. It did not cover any kind of inspection, let alone any concept for their mutual recognition.

From the point of view of GxPs, the CMEA collaboration had both advantages and disadvantages.

Looking at the advantages, the CMEA collaboration introduced the idea to Central and Eastern Europe that drug evaluation and registration could be an international business. Moreover, it had definite professional merits. First, there was a continuous international development of drug investigational guidelines, the results of which were recognized and their use encouraged by health ministers. Naturally, when developing guidelines, every expert tried to be in line with the EC and the USA. This is why there were surprisingly few differences between western and eastern European professional standards (e.g. toxicological, clinical trial guidelines). Western European standards were always taken into account during the development of eastern European versions.

On the other hand, the CMEA collaboration was originally created to exclude, as far as possible, imported western medicine from the market. It aimed not only to facilitate registration of drugs invented within the CMEA but also distributed the manufacture of given medicinal preparations between member states. This philosophy, together with the economical difficulties of the region, was in contrast to the overall introduction of G*x*Ps. It can thus be understood that even countries which were in the position of introducing GMP, GLP or GCP were not keen to do it if it did not cover the medicines they were forced to import from other CMEA countries (i.e. to introduce them for the exclusive benefit of local manufacturers and investigators). Thus, during the CMEA era, only GMP was introduced and then only in Hungary.

Moreover, the CMEA preclinical and clinical guidelines hindered the recognition of, for example, the test guidelines developed by the Organization for Economical Cooperation and Development (OECD), referred to in, and necessary for, GLP. Similar problems arose with the introduction of GCP. It was also not by chance that Hungary, a member of the Pharmaceutical Inspection Convention (PIC), developed by the European Free Trade Association (EFTA) since 1976, joined the other open EFTA collaboration, the Pharmaceutical Evaluation Report (PER) scheme, and introduced GLP only after the CMEA collaboration ceased to exist.

By 1987, the Eastern European drug collaboration was no longer under CMEA control. It survived as a multilateral agreement between the contracting states until 1990, when it terminated its activity.

Similarities in Central and Eastern Europe

Because of economic problems, hidden by political will, the working system of the region was born in a quantitative approach, which dismissed quality in the 1950s (Paál, 1993). As a consequence, GMP was often considered a non-productive activity by ministries and manufacturers, even in the seventies. At the same time, the artificially forbidden unemployment, did not facilitate the introduction of strict documentation and the use of standard operating procedures (SOPs), which from the basis of any G*x*Ps.

In drug production, auditing of the supplier and vendor rating cannot be strong in an economic system where there is generally one supplier (importer, wholesaler, etc.), and both parties are state-owned.

The position of the internal quality assurance units was weakened by the above-mentioned quantitative approach in drug factories. They did not exist in most research centres, clinics and hospitals. There was no tradition of auditing by the sponsor in drug research units; all were state-owned enterprises. This fact, combined with efforts to eliminate the competition totally meant that there developed an integral part of the former CMEA philosophy that research data are confidential and, during experiments, anyone not involved is *persona non grata*. As far as clinics are concerned, sponsors' efforts at looking at details greatly surprised doctors, even in the eighties in some countries.

Differences in Central and Eastern Europe

The drug regulatory environment, important for the development of governmental G*x*P inspectorates, varied in our target countries.

In Hungary, the National Institute of Pharmacy (NIP) was established to mirror the US Food and Drug Administration drug control and registration authority and to work under the supervision of, but independently from, the Ministry of Health (now Welfare). Thus, all kinds of professional inspectorates could be situated here. The same is basically valid for Romania and, quite recently, to Bulgaria and Slovakia.

In the former Yugoslavia and Soviet Union as well as in Bulgaria and Poland, in the past drug registration was governed by the ministries – the administrative decision-makers. The drug institutes with quality assurance professionals mostly participated by performing quality analyses exclusively. The real decision-makers were professional bodies comprising members of the Academies of Sciences who made the toxicological and clinical evaluations. Where to place practical GMP, GLP and GCP inspectorates in this three-pole system was a delicate question (Hansen, 1993).

The former Czechoslovakia also had this system, with the speciality of having everything doubled (e.g. a Czech and a Slovakian one), with close collaboration and some responsibilities also covering the other part of the former country.

After disbandment, countries of the former Soviet Union in particular but also, to a certain extent, those of the former Yugoslavia experienced the results of the former Yugoslavia experienced the results of the former centralized system: almost every drug regulatory institution remained in Moscow (and Belgrade). Moreover, the newly emerging countries have not been in a position to create their own drug regulatory system that would create further new differences, civil wars in certain parts of the region caused further drawbacks (e.g. Baltic states versus central Asian NIS, Slovenia versus Bosnia, etc.).

It is interesting to note that most of the newly emerging states tried to copy the drug regulatory system of their parent country, which gave rise to further differences. For example, drug institutes existed in Ukraine but not in Central Asian NIS. The Baltic countries, especially Estonia, established a registration system similar to the Finnish one within a few years (Rägo, 1994). A Drug regulatory agency was also established in Kirgizistan (but not in neighbouring countries).

None of these problems arose in the successor states of the former Czechoslovakia. This may be explained by the formerly doubled drug regulatory system, discussed before.

There were also differences in the organization of the pharmaceutical industries. In most countries, all factories were organized to create one national trust (Polfa in Poland, Pharmachim in Bulgaria, etc.). In Hungary, however, the six big state-owned pharmaceutical manufacturers were always individual profit centres and governmental control was only exerted through taxation.

Further differences in the political openness of the target countries may explain why Hungary could join the (EFTA) PIC in 1976. By contrast, the CMEA Adverse Drug Reaction Monitoring Centre (situated in Prague, Czechoslovakia) was not allowed to send data to the World Health Organization.

Another problem arose in countries which were emerging by splitting away from larger predecessors (the Soviet Union, Czechoslovakia, Yugoslavia). This was lack of proper national legislation, particularly a comprehensive Drug Act. Moreover, the mandatory introduction of any G*x*P has required the issue of supporting legislation first. These did not apply to Poland where the new Drug Act was issued in 1991 or to Hungary, where the introduction of GLP and GCP was possible using a proper legal technique (see under the country analyses, below).

All of these similarities and differences should be taken into consideration when discussing the implementation of G*x*Ps in Central and Eastern Europe.

Implementation of G*x*Ps in Central and Eastern Europe – country analyses

It should be noted that seminars and discussions with the participation of drug regulators from Central and Eastern Europe (e.g. the Pre-ICDRA Workshop for registration officers from countries of Central and Eastern Europe attending the 7th International Conference of Drug Regulatory Authorities (ICDRA), organized by the WHO regional office for Europe,

14–16 April 1993 in Hillerod and the Eastern Europe – Regulatory Challenges in the Pharmaceutical Market Seminar of the IBC Technical Services, 5 and 6 December, 1994 in London) greatly facilitated the updating of this section.

Good manufacturing practice

Hungary

As mentioned previously, Hungary was the first country to join the EFTA PIC as a non-signatory to the Convention.

Why was Hungary first? The explanation is that the Hungarian pharmaceutical industry, on the one hand, has always been strong and export-oriented. On the other hand, Hungarian drug control traditions (e.g. introduction of regulatory drug control in 1927, that of compulsory drug registration in 1933) helped many people in drug production; they became accustomed to visits by empowered drug control bodies from both inside and outside the factory. This did not mean that introduction of GMP was an easy task and that all decision-makers in the pharmaceutical industry were convinced about its necessity. However, from the seventies to the eighties, the Hungarian pharmaceutical industry generally acknowledged the PIC and made great efforts to obey its requirements.

Because the GMP was required by a decree of law (Paál, 1990), the Hungarian drug control authority, NIP, was empowered to take the measures necessary. Being also the drug registration authority, the NIP integrated the GMP into drug registration very soon.

The milestones of the implementation of GMP in Hungary have been discussed in more detail elsewhere (Lipták, 1990).

Inspectors with industrial experience and a good command of English were recruited to form a division of the NIP.

A number of national seminars on GMP were held, mostly by Hungarian inspectors but, in some cases, foreign consultants were also hired. Training and refresher courses on GMP have also become an integral part of post-graduate education for pharmacists.

Apart from corrective measures that were occasionally necessary, the Hungarian GMP inspectorate was able to celebrate its 15th anniversary during the 1991 PIC seminar held in Hungary knowing that the need for GMP had not been the subject of discussion for years and generally no critical deficiencies had been observed during inspections in the past years.

Because of their interesting (non-EFTA, non-EU) position, Hungarian inspectors have generally been requested to participate in various PIC working groups, including the harmonization of the EFTA GMP with the EC one. Moreover, their skill has been utilized by WHO (for example, when its new GMP guidelines were drafted in 1991).

The Czech and Slovak republics

The introduction of GMP began soon after in the former Czechoslovakia, which had also developed a pharmaceutical industry. The shortcoming was, however, the doubled system, mentioned previously: two drug control institutes, two registration bodies, two Ministries of Health, one for the Czech and one for the Slovakian part, but without federal health authorities and drug law.

First an internal GMP standard was issued by the Spofa United Pharmaceutical Association in 1974. Later, decrees of the Czech and Slovakian vice ministers of health began the implementation of GMP. In the mid-eighties, there were already two working GMP inspectorates in the drug control institutes, and Czechoslovakia has become a PIC candidate country.

The doubled authorities, however, were originally not accepted by the EFTA PIC, which required one appointed authority per country. Although solving this problem with a compromise, Czechoslovakia still waited to join the PIC.

In 1990, both the Czech and the Slovak Ministries of Health issued new legislation on governing the quality of human drugs and of products of medicinal and packaging technology, including GMP, based on resolution WHA 28.65 of the World Health Assembly in 1975. These sources of law formed the legal basis of GMP inspections in the Czech and Slovak republics after their division at the beginning of 1993 until the new Drug Bills, which are in preparation in both republics, will be issued.

According to recent findings, GMP was obeyed in more than 90% of pharmaceutical factories in both the Czech and Slovak republics at the end of 1994.

Poland

In order to strengthen its control over the local pharmaceutical industry, the Ministry of Health and Social Welfare (MHSW) issued an Act on Pharmaceutical Products, Wholesale Outlets and Pharmaceutical Inspections in 1991. The chief inspector is one of the deputy ministers of the MHSW and supervises 49 regional inspectors. In addition, 25 professionals were trained in GMP in the Institute of Drugs in Warsaw.

The question is whether regional inspectors, dealing with inspection as part-time officials, can perform the same task as is required by a PIC inspector. Moreoever, although GMP compliance was also endorsed by foreign (e.g. Hungarian) inspectors, certain old Polish drug production facilities do not comply with GMP. According to regulations issued by the MHSW, GMP must be fulfilled by the end of 1996. This plan, was recently openly referred to as unrealistic by a Polish industrial expert.

Nevertheless, Polish authorities, especially professionals working in the

Institute of Drugs, do their utmost to implement GMP in drug manufacture and Poland became a candidate country for the PIC in 1992.

Romania
This country joined the EFTA PIC a few years later than Hungary, in 1981. The reason was its export orientation and the fact that Romania never took part in the CMEA drug investigation collaboration.

The GMP inspectorate was developed in the drug institute ISCDPR, Bucharest. The requests of PIC member states for inspection reports have always been answered, proving that the system and the inspectorate are working. At present, GMP compliance is obligatory for newly established manufacturing sites but it could not be made mandatory for all the pharmaceutical factories.

Slovenia
In this country, the introduction of GMP proceeds in a different way from those mentioned previously. After the Yugoslavian federal state broke apart, the two big export-oriented Slovenian drug manufacturers, Krka and Lek, succeeded in the introduction of GMP; the proper legislation and inspection system is still incomplete. The Ministry of Health, which performs the drug regulatory tasks, is still waiting for the new Drug Act that is expected to cover GMP also.

Croatia
Not all, but some Croatian drug manufacturers have implemented GMP. Sources of law (ministerial decrees) covering GMP also have been drafted. The Ministry of Health, working as the drug regulatory authority, is waiting for this to come into force and a step-by-step introduction of GMP is expected.

Bulgaria
Although GMP is not yet required by law and the pharmaceutical industry mostly cannot obey it, a GMP inspectorate started its working in the National Drug Institute in Sofia. A step-by-step introduction may be expected.

Estonia
This country, establishing a new drug regulatory authority, comprising a GMP inspectorate, the State Agency of Medicines in Tartu, has a leading role in introducing GMP among Baltic countries. Since 1992, three new GMP-compliant manufacturing sites were established while GMP has just begun in an old pharmaceutical factory (Rägo, 1994). The local inspectors have been trained in Sweden. Estonia wants to be a member of the PIC. A draft Medicines bill, also covering GMP, was finalized in 1994.

Other Baltic countries

Although development in Latvia and Lithuania has been slower as far as GMP is concerned, than Estonia, its establishment, especially in newer manufacturing sites, has begun.

Russia

Although some industrial manufacturing control did exist in the former Soviet Union (and it was called inspection), GMP has not been required in general and only some pharmaceutical firms would be able to obey it. This situation has been slowly changing in Russia. The control of drugs belongs to the State Inspection of Quality Control of the Ministry of Health which, using the State Institute of Standardization, mostly requires quality analyses and the activities are focused on the *Pharmacopoeia* instead of GMP inspections. The registration of drugs is governed by another ministerial division, the Pharmacological Committee and the State Institute of Drug Expertise. In recent years, the level of import of medicines increased but demand could not be met. This did not facilitate understanding of the importance of GMP.

Introduction of western skills and capital, however, started to open the doors to GMP. The example of a western joint venture with Akrihin company, near Moscow, showed that GMP could gradually be implemented even in a country where no traditions of such control had existed.

European NIS (Ukraine, Belarussia, Moldavia)

As concerns CIS (Commonwealth of Independent States) member states, at the moment of independence the main problem had been that almost all of the drug control institutions of the former Soviet Union were inherited by Russia. For this reason, together with the shortage of medicines, sophisticated quality assurance systems such as GMP have not been given priority until now.

The author, reinforced by experience gained, for example, in Belarussia, is of the opinion that even in countries where GMP has been heard of, interest (as expressed in seminars organized by WHO or the International Federation of Pharmaceutical Manufacturers Associations – IFPMA) is growing among professionals, but implementation is delayed.

Central Asian post-soviet countries

As industrialization is less advanced here, the situation as regards GMP is even less promising than in the European NIS. Some elements of GMP are applied, even if unwittingly. (The author of this chapter saw that in Turkmenistan less favourable manufacturing sites were improved by campaigning, basic documentation was kept, samples were sent to Moscow for analysis but the release was made locally, etc.)

Good laboratory practices

Specifics and misconceptions

It should be noted that the term GLP is often used in a broader meaning in the literature to cover the organization of work of routine hospital, quality control and laboratories. In this chapter the term is used as specified by the OECD – the safety characterization of new chemicals (comprising toxicological and physicochemical studies). Although some elements of GLP, an effective laboratory organization, may well also be used in laboratories performing other tests, this term is exclusively used in its OECD meaning in this chapter.

The other danger, especially in regions where the introduction of GLP is subject to discussion, such as Central and Eastern Europe, is that GLP is confused with laboratory accreditation. In order to clarify these terms according to what was said in an OECD GLP panel meeting recently, let us accept that accreditation is directed to the technical and personnel qualification suitability of a laboratory to carry out certain types of studies (e.g. melting point measurements, chronic or ecotoxicological studies, etc.). By contrast, GLP-compliance monitoring is focused on establishing whether a given study was performed according to GLP principles.

Moroever, it is worth pointing out that GLP, compared to GMP and GCP, has certain characteristics that should be mentioned here. This means that a number of special questions should be answered when assessing the trends of implementation of GLP in Central and Eastern Europe.

It is very important that GLP should cover not only pharmaceuticals but all the new chemicals, i.e. pesticides and industrial chemicals, involving a number of ministries responsible for health, industry, environment, agriculture, etc. Thus:

1 Is it worthwhile introducing GLP in one sector (e.g. for the registration of pharmaceuticals), at least temporarily?
2 How many GLP inspectorates should be established (e.g. for the inspections of studies of new chemicals, each belonging to different ministries)?

For this reason the introduction of GLP is a more complex issue than that of GMP and GCP and the correct answers to the following questions are even more important:

1 May the publication of GLP in the local language be enough to introduce it without regulatory measures?
2 What kind of legislation should support the steps of its introduction?

3   May the introduction of GLP be satisfactory without the establishment of a governmental inspectorate for regular compliance monitoring?

The implementation of GLP in Central and Eastern Europe has been facilitated by the efforts of the ECE and the OECD. The assistance of these international organizations will be discussed first.

The help of the ECE and OECD

In September 1991, an *ad hoc* meeting on chemicals management was held by the United Nations ECE with the collaboration of the OECD secretariat in order to popularize the chemicals programme, including GLP, and the mutual acceptance of data, for the countries of Central and Eastern Europe.

During this meeting, the Hungarian experiences were recognized and Hungary was offered observer status in the OECD GLP panel.

This joint meeting recommended in its report that the countries of Central and Eastern Europe should be involved in the environmental collaborations of the OECD, among others on GLP. A workshop would be held on the implementation of OECD GLP and the concept of assurance at compliance with GLP for countries of Central and Eastern Europe, to assist them. It would be held under the auspices of the senior advisers on environmental and water problems of the ECE in cooperation with the OECD in Hungary, the only target country with a working GLP inspectorate at that time.

The workshop was held in October 1992 in Balatonfüred, Hungary, with representatives of nine countries of Central and Eastern Europe and a number of experts from western Europe and the USA.

Among other general topics of information about GLP, there were also lectures on the Hungarian experience in its implementation and compliance monitoring, on environment protection and the need for implementation of GLP. Roundtable discussions and an *in situ* demonstration of a GLP inspection on the premises of the Toxicological Research Centre, Veszprém, Hungary, by Austrian and Hungarian inspectors were also organized.

The report of the workshop emphasized, among other things, that:

1   The participants held the view that the introduction and application of the OECD GLP principles on testing laboratories would facilitate the mutual acceptance of data, generated either in OECD member countries or in those in Central and Eastern Europe, in compliance with GLP, in physicochemical, toxicological and ecotoxicological laboratories for the safety testing and characterization of new chemicals. The

mutual acceptance of data may avoid repetition of studies done in other countries, saving time, staff and money, increasing the export possibilities as well as reducing the number of animal experiments.

2   It was pointed out that introducing GLP is more than performing studies at a high scientific level of laboratories and study audits. It required proper organization of work according to GLP principles, available in the local language, and regular inspections by an empowered authority (GLP monitoring authority).

3   The workshop recommended a step-by-step approach to the application of GLP and implementation of compliance monitoring procedures, based upon the experiences gained in OECD member countries and in Hungary.

4   The workshop noted with appreciation that the GLP documentation had already been translated into German, Czech, Hungarian and Polish. The delegate of Ukraine expressed his readiness to explore the possibility for the translation of the GLP documentation into Russian.

5   The workshop recommended that the ECE member countries should be encouraged to explore the possibility of organizing follow-up workshops of this kind, in order to provide an exchange of experience related to the implementation of GLP and thus promoting the environmentally sound management of chemicals in the target countries.

The follow-up of the 1991 ECE–OECD joint meeting was held in October 1994, also in Vienna. On that occasion representatives from 19 Central and Eastern European countries (including those from Central Asian NIS) participated. Among others, the Hungarian experiences in implementing GLP principles and compliance monitoring to achieve mutual acceptance of safety data were presented in a lecture, requested by the organizers (held by this author – its content is mostly reproduced in this chapter). After detailed discussion of the results and difficulties in the countries, the meeting in its recommendations emphasized the benefits of introduction of GLP in Central and Eastern Europe.

Hungary
In the early 1980s, the Hungarian Pharmacological Society published the GLP developed by the US Food and Drug Administration in a methodological letter. The pharmaceutical industry and the toxicological research centres, however, debated the need for of its overall introduction at that time. The reason was that certain centres were in the position of introducing GLP, while others felt they would not. Until 1990, when the CMEA drug investigation collaboration was terminated, this situation was accepted by the regulatory drug control authority.

In 1990, however, the NIP, also establishing a GLP inspectorate, after careful discussions with the Hungarian pharmaceutical industry issued the Hungarian translation of the OECD (i.e. the EC) GLP. It was taken as a discussion paper, planned not to be mandatory until 1993, but the NIP's inspectorate announced its readiness to perform GLP inspections on a voluntary basis and to certify the results during this intended training period.

The NIP inspectorate worked with inspectors (from the GMP inspectorate) as generalists accompanied by toxicological experts.

Like the introduction of GMP in Hungary, training courses on GLP were organized with both Hungarian and foreign lecturers. Joint inspections with western specialists facilitated the training of Hungarian investigators and inspectors.

It is worth noting that all the first inspections gave negative results: although very experienced toxicology laboratories with scientifically high reputable staff were inspected, no compliance with GLP could be established. After there had been substantial reorganizations, taking the inspection reports into consideration, the first laboratory complying with GLP was found in March 1991.

During the 1991 ECE–OECD *ad hoc* meeting, the Hungarian experiences were recognized and Hungary was offered observer status in the OECD GLP panel. Hungarian representatives have been participating in panel meetings since 1992.

In the meantime, in addition to the NIP GLP inspectorate for pharmaceuticals, another one working in the agricultural field was also established in late 1991 in Hungary. The Ministry of Agriculture and the Ministry of Welfare started discussions about the joint operation of these two GLP inspectorates in 1992.

A great impetus to these discussions was given when the international GLP workshop was held in 1992 in Balatonfüred, Hungary.

In 1993, the OECD environmental committee, on the recommendation of the joint meeting of the management committee of the special programme on the control of chemicals and the chemicals group, proposed that the group of the council on non-member economies be asked to consider inviting Hungary to participate as a full member of that part of the chemicals programme involving GLP and mutual acceptance of data.

Full membership was granted in Spring 1994.

As has been noted before, Hungarian representatives have been participating in the work of the OECD GLP panel and OECD GLP training courses and seminars since 1992.

Since 1 January 1993 the application of GLP has been mandatory for studies intended for use for drug registration purposes in Hungary. The interministerial discussions, mentioned before, were crowned by the establishment of the common national GLP board of the Ministries of Agriculture and Welfare, with the agreement of ministers responsible for environment protection, foreign economical relations, industry and trade. The board consists of members delegated by the participating ministries while the main GLP inspectorate, which is entitled to issue GLP-compliance certificates to foreign authorities, is situated in the NIP. Whenever inspection of laboratories, supervised by a ministry, different from the Ministry of Welfare, is necessary, experts delegated from the other ministry accompany the NIP inspector. The work of the inspectorate is controlled by the national GLP board.

It should be emphasized that the introduction of GLP into drug registration did not require a new source of law in Hungary. An Act of Parliament empowered the Minister of Health (now Welfare) to regulate drug registration and the Minister delegated this task to the NIP that might issue requirements and guidelines on drug evaluation and registration. Thus, GLP has been made mandatory. The nationwide, overall introduction, however, needed a stronger legal background. For this reason, a ministerial decree, also reproducing certain relevant OECD texts, was issued in 1994.

The activity of the Hungarian GLP inspectorate as well as those laboratories complying with GLP are indicated in Table 24.1.

Table 24.1 *Good laboratory practice inspections executed in Hungary*

Year	Number of inspections			Results of inspections	
	Total	Domestic	Joint	IC	NC
1990	3	3	0	0	3
1991	6	5	1	3	3
1992	4	4	0	4	0
1993	7	6*	1	7	0
1994	4	3*	1	3	1

Executed by the NIP GPL inspectors, together with agricultural experts in 1993 and 1994, respectively.

Joint = Together with a foreign inspector; IC = in compliance; NC = non-compliance.

The Czech and Slovak republics

In the former Czechoslovakia, the importance of GLP was soon recognized. The US Food and Drug Administration GLP was translated by Spofa United Pharmaceutical Association in the early 1980s. In 1986, the Drug Research Institute translated GLP and adopted to its own conditions.

In 1988, the Czech and Slovak drug control institutes in Prague and in Bratislava elaborated a locally applicable GLP document that was discussed in a state seminar. The first official document on GLP was issued as working material of the committees on new drugs of the Ministries of Health of the Czech and Slovak republics in 1990.

In the Czech republic, the State Institute for Drug Control in Prague was entrusted by the Czech Ministry of Health with the task of organizing GLP inspections in 1991.

In Slovakia, the State Institute for Drug Control in Bratislava was appointed by the Slovak Ministry of Health to act as a state inspection body for GLP covering both drugs and chemical substances, also in 1991.

Until the end of 1992, inspectors from the Czech republic took part in inspections in Slovakia and vice versa.

However, no written sources of law required compliance with GLP. For this reason, the Czech and Slovak drug institutes drafted a guideline on the basis of the OECD GLP principles and EC directives and submitted it to their ministries for approval in 1992.

After the federal Czechoslovakian state divided, the new Drugs Acts (as well as the new Chemical Acts for agricultural and industrial chemicals) are expected to incorporate it in the legislation in both countries.

At present, GLP is 'recommended' and (pharmaceutical) GLP inspectorates are available in both Czech and Slovak republics.

Poland

A GLP inspectorate in the Drug Institute in Warsaw was established in 1992 as the first step towards introducing GLP in the country. Inspection services are available.

At present, GLP is not required by law in any industrial sector.

Slovenia

The situation is similar to that of GMP. Drug manufacturers introduced GLP on a voluntary basis. No local inspectorate has been established yet; the laboratories, performing studies on a contract basis, are subject to foreign inspection. A new law has recently been drafted which would require GLP compliance in the pharmaceutical, pesticide and biochemical industries. It is not expected, however, to cover other industrial chemicals.

Croatia

GLP principles are issued by the Ministry of Health in a bylaw. Since it is not based on an Act of Parliament, the mandatory introduction of GLP still needs legislative support. It is planned to be obligatory for pharmaceuticals, pesticides and biocides but not for veterinary preparations and industrial chemicals.

A governmental inspectorate has not yet been established. Still certain pharmaceutical factory laboratories are able to perform GLP-compliant studies and these are carried out for foreign sponsors on a contract basis; foreign GLP inspectors are welcome in Croatia.

Bulgaria
Organization of a GLP inspectorate within the National Drug Institute is under consideration. However, no local inspections have been available until now.

Russia
GLP is not yet obeyed. There are a few laboratories that could comply with GLP, particularly physicochemical ones.

Ecotoxicological studies, at least at the required level, are not available. Toxicological testing is controlled, and results of the studies approved or rejected by the chief state hygienic inspector; however, this inspectorate does not work on the basis of GLP.

Other countries of Central and Eastern Europe
Although toxicological studies were rarely repeated during drug registration (thus, foreign data were accepted) and certain laboratories really work under conditions close to GLP conformity, no formal GLP inspectorates exist and no national GLP guidelines were issued.

While the laboratory environmental research and monitoring programmes are well-organized in the Baltic states, Romania, etc. and, for example, in Lithuania, a methodological guideline *Control Systems of Measurements, Results, Precision*, containing some elements of the quality assurance of generating data, was issued by the Environmental Protection Department in 1987. GLP *per se* is not yet recognized. Moreover, discussion with professionals and policy makers of these countries revealed that GLP will be given hardly any priority in the near future. These countries intend to organize global environmental protection and drug control systems without formally recognizing GLP.

Good clinical practices

GCP is the kind of G*x*Ps where the situation has been changing dramatically in Central and Eastern Europe. GCP-compliant trials are available in almost every country (Statuch, 1994). The interest in GCP has been recognized by western European professionals (Gerlis, 1992). Contract research organizations (CROs) established local representations and hired clinical trial (CT) field monitors in a number of them (Pozsonyi, 1994; Anonymous, 1992).

It should be borne in mind that GCP is similar to *Brahma*, the supreme god of Hindu mythology, who has four faces. Speaking about GCP you may find that, besides the sponsor, the investigator and the monitor, discussed in detail in the literature, there is also the 'fourth face' – the governmental GCP inspector, who plays an important role in the acceptance of trials in a number of countries. The GCP situation in Central and Eastern Europe is discussed here, also evaluating the possibility of establishment of a local governmental inspectorate.

Hungary

The (EC) GCP text was translated, completed with references to the relevant local sources of law and issued in 1992. Since 1 January 1994 it has been obligatory in CTs that are regularly inspected by NIP GCP inspectors.

These are the facts. The issue of introduction, however, is worth more detailed discussion.

GCP was already widely known by Hungarian investigators in the eighties. In 1987, the Helsinki Declaration and the role of new drug investigation by ethical committees were incorporated in modern sources of law on drug registration and biomedical research. For instance, the Hungarian central ethical committee that gave approval for studies on new medicines comprised not only doctors but also clergymen, representatives of non-professional societies, etc., even in the 1980s. The Hungarian GCP was issued as a NIP guideline in 1992, declaring that studies not complying with GCP will simply not be accepted from 1994. Between 1992 and 1994 the GCP was proposed but not mandatory. During this period, the NIP was ready to perform GCP inspections and to certify its results on a voluntary basis. Moreover, clinical trial or GCP monitors sent or hired by the sponsors (Pozsnyi, 1994) were already acknowledged in Hungary (Paál, 1994).

As has been discussed previously, both GMP and GLP became mandatory in 1994. Thus, with these GxPs as prerequisites for GCP on the one hand, the mandatory introduction on the other hand created a satisfactory surrounding to GCP. Mandatory introduction meant that GCP was not thought of by clinicians and paramedical staff as if it were some strange attitude of foreign sponsors, obeyed if well-paid but not taken seriously – which is always the danger when different requirements apply for foreign contract and local research CTs! This is the benefit of having the fourth face, too! At the same time, the above-mentioned training period permitted the correction of defects, revealed by the application, without regulatory consquences.

Besides the measures mentioned before, the step-by-step introduction was provided, following introduction of the GMP and GLP, also by training courses for clinical investigators. Such courses have been organized regularly by the Imre Haynal University of Health Sciences, Budapest. Moreover, a number of sponsors, having developed their CT monitor network in Hungary (Pozsonyi, 1994) organized GCP courses, mostly inviting both foreign experts and NIP professionals. The NIP inspectors underwent an international training course in Vienna. As previously noted, the Hungarian GCP is based on the EC GCP, but the Hungarian one is more than a simple translation. It has been adjusted to the Hungarian legal situation, which is stricter than the European average. For instance, not only the informed and witnessed consent but the written, signed consent of patients to be involved in clinical trials is required by law (the Health Act of Parliament). Second, all CTs are to be authorized at the outset and the approval of a central ethical body is also a prerequisite for the trial (Paál, 1994).

The route of CT applications and their approval have recently been discussed (together with those in the Czech republic and Poland) in the literature (Statuch, 1994). Thus, it is not reproduced here. It is admitted, however, that the disadvantage of the present Hungarian CT approval system is what was its advantage in the past: the monopoly of the central ethics committee (affiliated to the Scientific Health Council, SHC) in the approval of human phase I and II trials. Since this ethics committee applies first for advice to the committee for clinical pharmacology of the SHC, then the ethical opinion is sent to the SHC presidium, then to the NIP, the whole approval process is rarely shorter than 3 months – rather long for an international multicentre trial.

In spite of this, mostly balanced by mandatory GCP compliance, the recognition of Hungarian efforts to introduce GCP into clinical research may be proved by the number of foreign CTs in Hungary (Table 24.2). Since local CTs are not a prerequisite for drug registration in Hungary if a good clinical dossier is available (except in cases of bioequivalence studies with reference preparations marketed only in Hungary), the CTs shown in

Table 24.2   *Authorized clinical trials in Hungary*

Type of trial	Number of protocols		
	1992	1993	1994
Human phase I	3	3	0
Human phase II	1	6	14
Human phase III	57	69	83
Bioequivalence	4	3	4
Human phase IV	2	31	24
Total	67	112	125

Table 23.2 were mostly contract research ones. It was pointed out in the literature (Anonymous, 1992) that Hungarian CTs had been successfully included into EC applications.

Moreover, the well-known Swedish company Astra established its clinical research centre for Central Europe in 1993 in Budapest.

The Czech and Slovak republics

In Czechoslovakia, GCP was first recommended by medical symposia in 1965 and in 1975. In 1986, a *Recommendations for Standardization of Clinical Pharmacological Studies* were issued by the Clinical Pharmacological Centre in Bratislava.

At present, both in the Czech and Slovak republics all the clinical trials have to be authorized and supervised by the drug registration committees of the Ministries of Health. The trial protocols were, however, only advised by the committees to fulfil the criteria of the EC (Dzúrik, 1992). In Slovakia, where new recommendation for CTs were issued by the Ministry of Health in 1993, the compliance with GCP was first controlled by the Clinical Pharmacological Centre of the Institute for Preventive and Clinical Medicine; then a GCP inspectorate was established in the Institute of Drug Control. The Czech republic has a similar situation. Since GCP is not required by law, however, this control does not involve regulatory consequences.

The drafted GCP decrees and the new Drug Bills, also incorporating requirements for GCP compliance, are under preparation in the Czech republic. Contract research trials complying with GCP are widely available in both countries (Pozsonyi, 1994). In Slovakia, the drug act, issued in 1996, requires GCP.

Poland

Regional ethical committees for clinical trials, comprising medical professionals as well as laypersons, clergy, etc., were established more than 15 years ago. In addition, the Chamber of Physicians possesses an ethics committee to which appeals can be directed.

There is a difference between clinical trials for drug registration purposes and those of purely scientific character, although all CTs have to be registered (Statuch, 1994). While the former are to be authorized by the Drug Commission of the Ministry of Health and Social Welfare, the latter only need to be approved by the local ethics committee. For this reason, the approval of a research trial is fast and possibly most western CTs in Central and Eastern Europe are performed in Poland (Pozsonyi, 1994).

According to the Act on Pharmaceutical Products, Medicinal Materials, Pharmacies, Wholesale Outlets and Pharmaceutical Inspections, issued in

1991, there is an obligation to obey GCP during conducting CTs. Foreign and locally hired Firms' monitors are welcome (Pozsonyi, 1994). At present, however, no official GCP inspection is mandatory. When discussing Polish drug registration requirements, the GCP compliance is generally not mentioned.

Slovenia

All the local the clinical trials have to be approved by the Drug Committee of the Ministry of Health. This Committee also supervises the conduct of the trials.

In 1991, regulations were issued that strongly recommended the application of GCP during CTs. However, no local government inspectorate works and the compliance with GCP is not a prerequisite yet, although its basic documentation is required. The new Drug Bill is drafted, that is expected to settle the issue.

At present, according to local professionals, because of the lack of any requirement for GCP compliance only a limited number of contract research CTs are performed in Slovenia. The two big pharmaceutical factories, Krka and Lek, however, organized certain CTs where GCP was required to be met.

Croatia

Ethics committees work in hospitals. Their basic responsibility is to decide ethical aspects of clinical trials as well as the adequacy of local conditions.

Sponsors and investigators should notify the Ministry of Health about human phase IV trials while other CTs may be started after the written approval of the Ministry has been granted. In these cases the trials are authorized by the central drug committee.

Several ministerial decrees, also covering GCP, have already been drafted. The investigator and sponsor are obliged to conduct the CT according to the GCP (the notification/application sent to the ministry should contain a reference to it) but no official GCP inspection is performed.

Patient consent to a clinical trial is required by law only for early human trials of drugs which are not registered in the country of origin. In the past, it was very complicated to obtain a written patient consent; it might be taken as proof that an adverse event was almost inevitable. The situation and patients' understanding have improved greatly in the last few years. Ministerial regulations require GCP, the drug act is under preparation.

Estonia

Like other post-soviet republics, GCP is a new phenomenon, which was not required at all in Estonia in the past. Since 1990, clinical pharmacological graduate courses have also incorporated the basic principles of GCP in the Medical University of Estonia.

In 1990, its essence was issued as a compulsory appendix to the Act on clinical trial ethics committees. In 1991, mirroring the Nordic guidelines, the whole GCP text was issued (Rägo, 1994). International research CTs have already been performed in Estonia (Pozsonyi, 1994; Rägo, 1994).

Russia

The pharmacological committee, in collaboration with the state centre for drug expertise, approves and supervises CTs. Trials with healthy volunteers, according to local traditions, may be taken as unethical and not approved (Anonymous, 1992).

There are only a few standing real ethical committees. According to local professionals, in order to fulfil the needs of foreign firms, unexperienced *ad hoc* committees have been convened in certain hospitals. (It should be noted that in the former Soviet Union the central All-Union Pharmacological Committee, comprising only physicians, approved the clinical trial protocols 'also from the ethical point of view'.) Moreover, patient consent is only required by law for surgery at present; thus, it may rarely be given for new drug CTs (Anonymous, 1992). Because of former Soviet traditions, patients may believe that their consent may mean that there is a definite risk connected with the trial.

At present, GCP is only recommended by the committee. This does not mean, however, that GCP-compliant trials are not available at certain leading clinics and hospitals. Moreover, sponsors may attend and monitor clinical trials in Russia. (It should be emphasized that this *per se* is vastly different from former soviet rules.)

All this means that, without formal GCP requirements and recognition, more and more CTs complying with GCP are performed in Russia and the interest of foreign CROs is growing (Pozsonyi, 1994).

Romania

At present, GCP is not a prerequisite for conducting CTs but a source of law specifying this is under approval.

Other countries

As regards the GCP situation in other countries of Central and Eastern Europe, naturally certain pronounced differences may be found between them. (For example, the Serbian situation is very similar to the Croatian one, that in the other Baltic countries to the Estonian one, GCP is well-known in Bulgaria, even required by the recent drug act issued in 1996 while, as a local expert has said, Ukrainian investigators work according to 'their own GCP'. At the same time, Central Asian NIS were only involved in CTs as part of multicentre trials during the Soviet era; consequently, no priority is given to GCP there nowadays.) It is generally true, however, that although GCP-compliant trials may be available in certain clinics, they are not required by law and no standing inspectorates work.

Assessment of the current situation of GxPs in Central and Eastern Europe

In the introduction to this chapter certain general features of countries of Central and Eastern Europe were presented. Following that, country analyses were then made. In conclusion, general trends will be discussed.

General GxP trends

GMP
In order to understand the problems of introducing GMP, it should be acknowledged that it is very difficult in countries where medicine is in short supply. The problems caused by poor (or unstable) quality are balanced by the constant demand that prefers 'anything to nothing'. Under such circumstances, building quality assurance measures in production becomes easier only when the pharmaceutical industry is also interested in export.

In the introduction to this chapter the quantity approach and the CMEA collaboration, intended to eliminate competition, were outlined. In spite of the strong pharmaceutical industry in certain countries, drug selection was kept at a low level (much fewer than 1000 brands and about 1200 different strengths were available in the mid-eighties in Hungary). The local pharmaceutical companies worked for the domestic and the rouble-based CMEA market where GMP was not required.

On the other hand, in other countries with weaker connections with the CMEA market where pharmaceutical research was governed by the process patent law, the export possibilities to western Europe were automatically limited.

It is not by chance that Hungary, which had traditionally been the most research-based pharmaceutical industry in Central and Eastern Europe, having the chance to export (although, as a rule, via joint research, production, etc.) to western Europe, introduced GMP first. (It is interesting to note that joining the PIC meant the 100% introduction of GMP, required by law, in 1976 in Hungary but not in 1981 – and still not yet – in Romania.)

After the political and economical changes, certain countries possessing quite a strong pharmaceutical industry found themselves 'too strong' for the domestic market while the former huge foreign markets (particularly the former soviet one) could not pay in hard currency. This time, however, all the countries in the region had financial limitations and even updating the rundown production facilities and equipment caused problems, let alone the (sometimes considerable, sometimes minimal) reconstructions required by the introduction of GMP.

Thus, it is not by chance that financial limitations are usually mentioned, from Poland to Russia, when the lack of GMP is discussed although *per se* this is a misinterpretation. GMP is more than building new or reconstructing old manufacturing sites. It is a concept of disciplined, organized and documented work. Many of its elements might be introduced without vast investment.

Consulting the map of GMP compliance of our target region shown in Figure 24.2 (in which Central Asian NIS were left out because of the general lack of GMP), one can see that Romania (PIC member) and especially the Czech and Slovak republics and Poland (PIC candidates) are close to the situation in Hungary. Their pharmaceutical industry has also been productive, with export possibilities. In the southern and Baltic regions considerable development can also be found. The post-Yugoslavian countries, particularly Slovenia and, to some extent, Bulgaria, with mostly cheap generics and the Baltic states having enormous help from the Nordic countries, have taken enormous steps towards GMP. (Among the Baltic States, the leading position of Estonia in this respect may be explained by the establishment of the independent drug regulatory authority which always facilitates the introduction of inspections.)

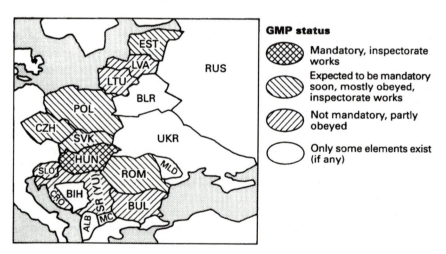

GMP status

Mandatory, inspectorate works

Expected to be mandatory soon, mostly obeyed, inspectorate works

Not mandatory, partly obeyed

Only some elements exist (if any)

Fig. 24.2   *The good manufacturing practice (GMP) compliance map of Central and Eastern Europe. See Figure 24.1 for abbreviations.*

The shortage of medicine in Russia and the European NIS, as has been pointed out previously, continues to hinder GMP. In the Central Asian NIS, moreover, only limited drug manufacture (if any) took place in the past; medicines (including parenterals) were compounded in hospital and community pharmacies.

GCP

It is easier to discuss the GCP situation, also related to one ministerial sector, than GLP after GMP. It could also be (and has been) related to the role of the research-based pharmaceutical industry, producing new chemical entities for clinical research, but it is far from being the case.

In the CMEA era practically all drug preparations were, as a rule, subjected to human phase III-like local clinical trials. Even the CMEA collaboration did not give exemption (although the CTs were, in some cases, formal, covering only 25–50 patients). However, it gave investigators the feeling of clinical research with results to be published.

Although this practice (of questionable scientifical value) was gradually given up from the mid-eighties, Central and Eastern Europe was then 'discovered' by western European sponsors. The literature agrees (Anonymous 1992; Pozsonyi, 1994) that CTs here are of high quality and patient enrolment is faster than in western Europe. Thus, with the exception of some NIS, where the orthodox 'one registration means one CT' principle has been mostly reserved (as in Ukraine, performing local CTs connected with paracetamol registration recently), CTs are mostly research ones for western sponsors in Central and Eastern Europe.

Particular problems in some countries, such as caused by the central authorization and supervision system, when no GCP honorarium could be paid, were overcome (in the given case donations of hospital equipments and reagents were acknowledged). GCP was soon obeyed, as it was pointed out by western Firm representatives; the investigators had been very surprised at first, but they obeyed at last. Changing the rule of free-of-charge CTs to CT fees to be (at least partially) earned by the investigators, which was impossible in the former Soviet Union, facilitated the understanding. The substantial differences between hospitals and even clinics were overcome, before selecting investigators, by consultation with the local authorities; they were especially fruitful for sponsors without local representation (Dzurik, 1992).

The present GCP compliance monitoring situation is indicated in Figure 24.3 It can be seen that the western part of Central and Eastern Europe with the possibly higher developed pharmaceutical industries is closer to the introduction of GCP (Hungary has already introduced it) than others.

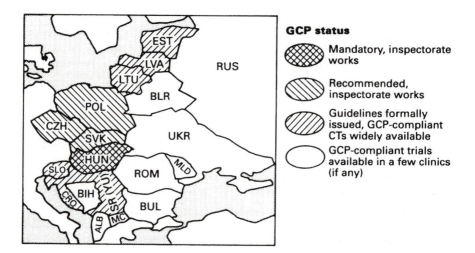

Fig. 24.3   *The good clinical practice (GCP) compliance map of Central and Eastern Europe. See Figure 24.1 for abbreviations. CT=Clinical trials.*

Compliance with GCP and the establishment of GCP inspectorates are far from being uniform in Central and Eastern Europe; however, this is not always reflected by the number of trials placed by foreign sponsors to a given country. Sponsors are more interested in fast trial approval and sending foreign or hiring their own local CT monitors than relying on the inspections of the local authorities. This point will be referred to again later. In the experience of this author, the misconceptions and deficiencies of GCP in Central and Eastern Europe do not differ considerably from those in other countries.

It is interesting to note that, like GLP, the concept of GCP was confused with that of accreditation at first. Thus, requests were sent to the NIP from trial sites 'to accredit them according to GCP on the basis of retrospective CT data exclusively'. They were, of course, refused but inspections of running trials were offered.

The workload of GCP-compliant trials has often been underestimated by investigators who are unexperienced in GCP, stating that 'they always worked according to GCP without knowing it'. It resulted, for example, in Hungary, in a number of initial GCP inspections with negative results, as in the introduction of GLP.

The main reported deficiencies were mostly violations of protocol (fewer or more patients enrolled than specified), use of very detailed protocols instead of specific SOPs (e.g. for delivery and dispensing of investigational medicines, etc.), use of non-specific SOPs for doctors and paramedical staff, descriptions of their general spheres of activity within the hospital ward rather than those in the given trial and lack of an investigators' brochure ('this drug is well-known to us').

All the above-mentioned is important from the point of view of the Hungarian experience, showing that the sponsors' and CRO's CT monitors, both foreign and locally hired, have generally been more lax than NIP inspectors in the evaluation of the GCP defects, especially 'small' (?) violations of protocol. Studying the spheres of interest, this may be understood but by no means acknowledged. This phenomenon raises the question again of whether the 'GCP-compliant clinical trial business' could be directed exclusively, to foreign contracts, neglecting the need for its overall introduction and inspection.

GLP

It is interesting to note that, while pharmacologists and toxicologists soon became acquainted with GLP, the level of its formal recognition differs considerably in the countries of Central and Eastern Europe. In most of these countries even less priority was given to GLP than to GMP and GCP. Moreover, in countries where steps have already been taken towards it, both GMP and GLP preceded GLP, with the exception of Hungary.

The reason may be that, in the pharmaceutical sector, GLP is needed by only a research-based (focused to new chemical entities) local industry with export possibilities. In the past, it was most characteristic for Hungary; consequently, several Hungarian industrial and research toxicological laboratories had developed to such a level that achieving GLP needed only a few more steps. Some of these laboratories have already been privatized.

In the other, mostly Central European countries toxicological studies were often performed in universities that have not had enough financial resources to reorganize themselves. Moreover, in the countries of the former Soviet Union the physicochemical and toxicological characterization of new chemicals, including pharmaceuticals, was (mostly has been) centralized into state-owned research institutes. Thus, neither sponsors nor investigators belonging to the state, whether monitoring or auditing, have had a tradition.

Quality assurance measures such as GLP were even less common, or even unheard of, in sectors outside pharmaceuticals (industrial chemicals, pesticides, etc., let alone environment protection) in Central and Eastern Europe.

As shown in Figure 24.4, only the 'most western part' of the target countries is in the position of possible GLP compliance, at least in certain laboratories in one industrial sector.

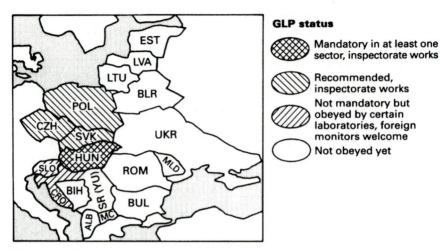

Fig. 24.4   *The good laboratory practice (GLP) compliance map of Central and Eastern Europe. See Figure 24.1 for abbreviations.*

Although the overall introduction of GLP is less developed than that of GMP and GCP in the countries of Central and Eastern Europe, some conclusions may be drawn and the questions raised in the previous section on GLP may be answered, mostly on the basis of the Hungarian example. The publication of the GLP principles in the local language is a prerequisite but it is far from being enough.

'Self-qualification' by scientifically minded investigators can well be misleading. A governmental inspectorate for continuous compliance monitoring is necessary.

The GLP can be introduced, even on a mandatory basis, in only one ministerial sector with a view to showing a convincing example for the other branches of industry that they may follow suit later. This finding is of great importance in a region where, as was discussed previously, the former CMEA (and soviet) 'distribution of activities' principle has created differences between countries in the level of development of various industrial branches. (For example, it is not impossible that in certain NIS, because of the strong 'supportive' industry, GLP would be worthy of introduction into the pesticide and not the pharmaceutical sector!)

Before implementation, however, careful discussions are needed with the laboratories concerned.

Special emphasis should be given to the possible misinterpretations of GLP (e.g. 'it is simple, being identical to the scientific execution of the study' or 'it is unnecessary, meaning money and effort for nothing' are two extremes, but misinterpretations may include anything between them). Initiatives of the ECE as well as professional help (written guidelines, GLP panel, etc.) of the OECD may and should be exploited.

As for GLP and accreditation, apply for both as far as possible. (GLP-compliant studies should be executed in laboratories, previously accredited for the given type of the study. It is up to the accreditation and the GLP compliance monitoring authorities to identify where they can collaborate.)

The general question of lacking financial resources must not be overestimated but compared with the benefit of avoiding unnecessary repetition of studies (such as staffing and resources needed, environmental and animal protection) as well as the greater chance of introducing innovative products to foreign markets.

No Eastern bloc but formation of regions

Consulting Figures 23.2–23.4, it can be seen that, as far as G*x*Ps are concerned, the formation of certain regions can be identified in Central and Eastern Europe.

Region 1

Hungary is the only country where all three G*x*Ps have been mandatory and governmental inspectors monitor their compliance.

Moreover, Hungary applied a logical approach to its introduction of G*x*Ps. Its first element was a logical order – first GMP (mandatory since 1976), then GLP (since 1993), finally GCP (since 1994). The second element was how it was introduced. At the beginning, the requirements and guidelines were issued, establishing the corresponding governmental inspectorate which was ready to perform inspections, on a voluntary basis. After a specified training period (2–3 years), this became the G*x*P obligatory.

Why first in Hungary? The author of the present chapter, in spite of his patriotic feelings, must admit that Hungary and Hungarians do not differ from their neighbouring countries so significantly that this could answer the question. The explanation may originate from other reasons.

1   The local pharmaceutical industry, highly research-based, was not historically centralized into one national trust. Consequently, it was already interested in import and was, even in the past, competitive under certain conditions.

2   Clever legislation: as was pointed out previously, unlike in other Central and Eastern European countries, the introduction of GLP and GCP and outdating of GMP did not require new laws in Hungary. The Minister of Welfare was empowered by an Act of Parliament to regulate

the introduction and marketing of pharmaceuticals and the NIP was empowered by the Minister to register drugs, including accepting internationally established professional requirements and issuing guidelines.

It is very important to note since, in the countries of Central and Eastern Europe, an overall reconstruction of legislation has been taking place with fewer priorities given to more professional than economical sources of law. In order to avoid delays, the simplest legal technique should be identified that may be supported later by a higher and more sophisticated source of law.

3   The simplest drug regulatory system: as for the development of inspectorates of governmental agencies, Hungary has been in a unique position. While in other Central and Eastern European countries drug registration and clinical trial authorization belonged to ministries and/or to scientific drug evaluation committees with the involvement of drug institutes – to organizations not always adequate to incorporate practical inspectorates – in Hungary, the NIP has been the sole drug control and registration authority working, although with scientific bodies of advisory character, under the general supervision of, but independently from, the Ministry of Welfare. Thus, all kinds of professional inspectorates could well be situated here.

Region 2

The Czech and Slovak republics and Poland had already approached Hungary, although they started the introduction of GxPs much later. The reason for this later start may be explained by their pharmaceutical industry, which was highly centralized in the past, and their drug regulatory system, which is more complicated than the Hungarian one.

It should be noted that, because of the special 'doubled' regulatory system, the disintegration of federal Czechoslovakia did not greatly affect the introduction of GxPs in the Czech and Slovak republics.

Region 3

Two other regions, in almost the same position, should be found in the south-western (Slovenia, Croatia and, possibly, Serbia after the termination of the civil war in the region) as well as in the north-western part of Central and Eastern Europe (the Baltic countries). Both started their independence only a few years ago (newly established institutions, legislation, etc.). The rapid development of the former may be explained by its fairly developed pharmaceutical industry. The close collaboration of Nordic and Baltic countries, although they had much worse conditions, helped the Baltics to develop their own industries during the former Soviet era.

Region 4
Bulgaria and Romania will be mentioned next, with their highly developed drug regulatory systems. All their intentions to introduce all three GxPs were hindered by the conditions of the industry and, in some cases, political priorities (or lack of priorities, failing to respect quality assurance measures). It is not by chance that GMP, promising some possible financial benefits when introduced, is in the most developed state.

Region 5
Classifying Russia and the remaining European NIS (Ukraine, Belarussia and Moldavia) as one region is not quite correct since Russia, with GCP-compliant trials available and some GMP elements, could well be a region in itself. This author is convinced that GCP can also be achieved in certain Ukrainian clinics. GMP is more problematic and no intention to introduce GLP could be identified until now.

Region 6
The central Asian post-soviet countries also form a region with smaller differences and great financial and economic problems. In some of these countries the establishment of the national drug regulatory system is underway. Where it has been established, mostly mirroring the former complicated system, the shortage of financial resources hinders its effective introduction.

GxPs have been mostly unheard of.

Albania cannot be placed in a geographical GxP region. From this point of view, the situation, in the opinion of the present author, is only slightly better than in the Central Asian NIS.

Conclusions

Crossing the frontiers, there are no abrupt cultural or traditional differences between western and eastern parts of Europe. Such differences do exist when remote countries are compared but the changes are continuous. Consequently, after abolishing political barriers, industrial and economical differences govern the speed of implementation of GMP, GLP and GCP. It is certain that, sooner or later, they will find their way to all regions of Central and Eastern Europe.

Recent developments showed that the author of this chapter was right almost 3 years ago (Paál, 1993): as far as GxPs are concerned, the target countries cannot be taken as a homogenous Eastern bloc. These differences may be explained and related to various factors discussed in detail in this chapter.

However, Central and Eastern Europe is no longer a dark horse for western professionals and firms seeking a drug market, joint production and investigation possibilities, attracted by the relatively low costs, high professional standards and spare capacities. Thus, more and more Central and Eastern European countries may be taken as a promising area to be involved in multinational drug production and research.

References

Anonymous (1992) Russia: ideal for the adventuresome. *World Pharmaceutical Report* **1:** 5.

Dzúrik, R. (1992) How to organize clinical trials in Czechoslovakia. *Applied Clinical Trials* **1:** 42–44.

Gerlis, G. (1992) Good clinical practice in Europe. *BIRA Journal* **11:** 8.

Hansen, J. (1993) Regulatory authority – proposed Belgian institute of drugs. *Regulatory Affairs Journal* **4:** 582.

Kot, T. and Czarnecki, A. (1995) Registration in Poland. *Regulatory Affairs Journal* **6:** 14–21.

Lipták, J. J. (1990) Good manufacturing practice (GMP's) inspection systems: Hungarian policy and practice. *Regulatory Affairs* **2:** 57–68.

Paál, T. L. (1990) East European perspectives on the European Economic Community's registration procedures. *Regulatory Affairs* **2:** 85–114.

Paál, T. L. (1993) Implementation of 'good practices' in Eastern Europe. In: *Implementing International Good Practices*, Dent, N. J. (ed.), pp. 235–248. Interpharm.

Paál, T. L. (1994) GCP – current events in Eastern Europe. In: *Good Clinical Practice and Ethics in European Drug Research*, Bennett, P. (ed.), pp. 37–47. Bath: Bath University Press.

Pozsonyi, S. (1994) Decentralized management of clinical research in Central and Eastern Europe. *Applied Clinical Trials* **4:** 50–53.

Rägo, L. (1994) Regulatory affairs in Estonia. *Regulatory Affairs Journal* **5:** 1004–1008.

Statuch, C. (1994) Clinical trial approval in Poland, Czech republic and Hungary. *ESRA Rapp.* **1:** 22–23.

PART NINE

Reporting research and development findings and statistics

25 Good statistical practice in clinical research

S W Cummings

Introduction

The application of good statistical practice (GSP) to the design, analysis and reporting of clinical trials is fundamental to successful and effective drug development. The wide choice of acceptable statistical methods, the constant evolution of new methodologies and variations in statistical philosophy have, however, created difficulties in providing a standard definition of GSP. Most advice offered is to be found in biostatistical guidelines issued by a few regulatory authorities or in some cases by industry statistical associations. Many pharmaceutical companies have also developed their own internal statistical standard operating procedures (SOPs). The guidelines issued by regulatory authorities have emerged as the standard statistical references for drug development. In general, these guidelines are not prescriptive but offer advice and direction to both drug developers and regulatory authorities on the biostatistical principles of study planning and clinical trial methodology.

Biostatistical guidelines

The guidelines which describe GSP serve three main purposes. First, they define the broad statistical framework for the overall clinical development of new compounds; second, they define the relevant principles of study design and analysis; and third, they describe generally acceptable approaches in accordance with these definitions as well as advising against approaches which are not acceptable. Many clinical trials have some unique statistical issues for which existing methodologies may be either inadequate or ambiguous. In such cases, the principles of GSP as outlined in the guideline documents can often be helpful and instructive in evaluating alternative strategies and selecting an appropriate study design or method of analysis. The guidelines also emphasize the role and underline the importance of access to qualified statisticians and to statistical expertise throughout the planning, conduct, evaluation and reporting of clinical trials.

Since 1988, several regulatory authorities have issued guidance on the design, conduct and analysis of clinical trials and in particular on the statistical methodology that applies. The Food and Drug Administration (FDA) division Center for Drug Evaluation and Research (CDER) in the USA was the first regulatory authority to issue specific statistical guidance in a report entitled *Guideline for the Format and Content of the Clinical and Statistical Sections of New Drug Applications* (1988); however, this report does not provide in-depth discussion on design issues and methodology. The Nordic Council on Medicines *Good Clinical Practice* guidelines for Scandinavia, which were issued in 1989, contain an excellent summary of the statistical principles governing clinical trials. One year later, in 1990, the Committee on Proprietary Medicinal Products (CPMP) working party on efficacy published their directive on *Good Clinical Practice for Trials on Medicinal Products in the European Community*. The CPMP directive emphasizes the importance of statistics and of access to biostatistical expertise throughout a drug development programme.

In 1992, Koseisho, the drug review department of the Japanese Ministry of Health and Welfare, issued its *Guidelines on the Statistical Analysis of Clinical Studies*. In contrast with other guidelines, the Japanese proposals are arguably more stringent and provide detailed advice on what primary measures, data summaries and specific methods of analysis are acceptable. In 1992, a more specific European guideline on statistical methodology entitled *Note for Guidance on Biostatistical Methodology in Clinical Trials in Applications for Marketing Authorisations for Medicinal Products* was commissioned by the CPMP working party on efficacy and, after wide public debate within the European statistical community, the final guideline was released in December 1994.

The statements contained within the statistical section of the FDA guideline and the Japanese and CPMP biostatistical guidelines are generally compatible across the three regions and provide a common understanding of what is uniformly acceptable and what is not. This degree of consensus has helped to define a universal statistical basis for the assessment of evidence and decision-making in drug regulation amongst sponsors, regulatory agencies and experts. Conversely, differences of opinion or emphasis across the three regions have stimulated fresh debate in the hope that further agreement may be reached. It is important to stress that the guidelines themselves and the extent to which further commonality can be achieved should not serve to limit the development of new, and the refinement of old, statistical methodologies to the benefit of both industry and regulatory authorities.

Internal pressures to reduce costs and accelerate drug development schedules continue to encourage the development of more efficient study designs and more powerful analytical methods. While these developments are likely to incur increased short-term costs as both industry and agencies modify their practices in line with more demanding guidelines, over the long term, costs are likely to decrease or at least remain constant as greater cross-industry and cross-agency harmonization is achieved.

Biostatistical staffing levels

The development of innovative treatments for indications which were previously untreated; the pressures to accelerate drug development time-lines through more efficient study designs; advances in computing, telecommunications and related technologies; and increased scrutiny of the statistical aspects of new drug applications by some regulatory agencies have combined to challenge and extend traditional statistical thinking and to enhance the role and contribution of the biostatistician. As a consequence the pharmaceutical industry has experienced significant growth in the number of qualified statisticians working in drug development during the past decade. The industry figure worldwide is estimated to exceed 2500, while in Europe this estimate is close to 800. In many countries, professional biostatistical groups have been established both to promote debate on statistical issues and standards pertaining to drug development and to assert the professional identity of statisticians working in this area. The growth of statisticians working in drug development in the pharmaceutical industry has not, however, been mirrored by a corresponding increase in the number of statistical staff employed directly by regulatory authorities. With the notable exception of the FDA in the USA, which employs a large biostatistical staff, only three other national regulatory authorities (UK, Sweden and Germany) employ a full-time statistician while in other countries, e.g. France and Holland, statistical experts are included as full-time members of a drug regulatory advisory committee.

International Conference on Harmonization

A major force in achieving even greater consensus on statistical issues in the reporting of clinical trials has been the International Conference on Harmonization (ICH) whose purpose is to harmonize regulatory requirements from each of the three major pharmaceutical markets – USA, Europe and Japan. The ICH report on the *Structure and Content of Clinical Study Reports* (1995) underlines the progress that has been made in defining common ground for the discussion on clinical trial methodology and has also found a useful purpose as a vehicle for presenting common views on statistical issues.

Interactions between industry and regulatory statisticians

FDA statisticians review new drug applications (NDAs) with particular emphasis on the statistical evaluation of efficacy and safety. They are also generally available for both formal and informal discussion with industry statisticians on matters of design, analysis plans and presentation of results. Opportunities for both formal and informal discussion between industry and FDA statisticians have encouraged debate on some issues which otherwise would have stayed dormant and have been instrumental in progressing the development of new approaches in clinical trial design and analysis.

In the USA sponsors may meet with the FDA review staff on several occasions during the development of a new drug. Key to these activities is the end of phase II meeting and the pre-NDA meeting. The end of phase II meeting is where decisions are taken as to how efficacy will be evaluated in phase III, what measurements will be taken and what statistical techniques will be applied. This meeting offers an opportunity for the sponsor to modify its approach consistent with FDA advice. The pre-NDA meeting offers the sponsor the opportunity to present prototype analysis proposals to both statistical and medical reviewers and to present and justify any major changes to the clinical development and statistical analysis plans arising from new information. A good example of this approach occurred in the analysis of angiographic studies. Initially, it was thought that change in mean per cent stenosis was the best measure of the effect of intervention on atherosclerosis. In 1991, following a National Institute of Health (NIH) workshop on atherosclerosis and a consultants' meeting, the consensus changed in favour of minimum lumen diameter. For several angiographic end-point studies which were underway, the primary end-point was changed and the data analysis section of the protocol revised. Sponsors of these trials were able to present the new consensus view, to explain how this would be presented within the report and to evaluate the impact of this change on power and sample size calculations.

Outside the USA, there have traditionally been only limited opportunities for dialogue on statistical issues between national regulatory agencies and industry during the preparation and pre-review stages of the drug development plan. In practice, it has rarely been possible to gain prior review and approval to modify trial assumptions or study design and analysis plans based on new or accumulating evidence. At least in Europe, it would appear that this situation is likely to continue as the number of agency statisticians remains small and their activity focuses on the review and approval of new drug applications. As a consequence, it may continue to be difficult to incorporate international regulatory statistical review comments into the planning phase of a drug development programme.

Standard operating procedures for good statistical practice

As noted earlier, the divergence of philosophy and operating practices amongst industry statisticians, regulatory statisticians and external experts has made it difficult to produce specific SOPs for GSP. This difficulty was highlighted in an article published by the Statisticians in the Pharmaceutical Industry (PSI) professional standards working party entitled *Good Statistical Practice in Clinical Research: Guideline Standard Operating Procedures* (1994). The objective of the PSI paper was 'to provide guidance in the writing of SOPs which could then be adapted by companies and agencies consistent with their own operating procedures'. The authors point out that guideline SOPs governing statistics should not be applied in isolation but as part of a total quality management system to improve efficiency, speed and precision in drug development. The guideline SOPs discuss the design, planning, conduct, evaluation and reporting of clinical trials and the decision-making process which rests on the evidence produced by these trials. In discussing GSP, it is altogether appropriate to follow the guidance of the PSI working party, which is to avoid writing multipurpose SOPs but to propose guidelines which, if followed, would be beneficial in helping to establish organization-specific SOPs.

The principles of GSP will be discussed here primarily in the context of phase III trials and for a selected number of topics. The focus on phase III trials reflects the phase of drug development where guidance has been most widely developed and where the diversity of trial designs and statistical methodologies leads to most debate. The selection of the topics below highlights those areas which in some cases are not only the most critical but also the most demanding.

Clinical development plans

Each clinical trial should be undertaken for scientific or ethical reasons and be part of an overall clinical development plan (CDP). The CDP should clearly distinguish between exploratory trials and confirmatory trials since the interpretation of results and of future actions based on the results from these trials will differ. In planning a drug development programme, an attempt should be made to minimize both the total number of trials and the total number of patients included in each trial. In designing a clinical programme one must therefore seek to minimize the number of trials and patients required to provide convincing evidence that the drug works while protecting against the undesirable risk of exposing too many patients to an experimental drug for which we do not generally have any clear picture of efficacy or safety. The design of each trial in the CDP must be appropriate to the study hypothesis and be based on valid statistical arguments. For example, it is not appropriate to evaluate two antihypertensive therapies by designing a study in which all patients simply switch from the same starting therapy to the other, since time and treatment effect would then be confounded. Only in a crossover design, where the treatment sequence is randomly allocated, can the treatment effect be distinguished from the time (or period) effect. Two-treatment, two-period crossover trials do, however, create an additional problem in that the carry-over effect from period 1 to period 2 introduces a bias in the estimation of the treatment effect and, moreover, the carry-over effect itself cannot be precisely estimated. In principle, design considerations should be balanced with regard to the difficulties in providing unbiased estimates of treatment and other effects of interest.

Another example of incorrect trial design would be a comparison of treatment responses to different doses based on the final dose given in a dose titration study. Since the decision to titrate a patient to the next dose level is based on the patient's response to the current dose, the allocation of patients to final dose is not a random process but is a deterministic event; hence the estimates of treatment effects will be biased and difficult to interpret.

The advice provided by the statistician for each protocol includes determination of sample size, validation of the study design, assistance in the selection and prioritization of efficacy variables, and the definition of the statistical framework within which hypothesis testing will be conducted. Statistical design issues should not be limited to individual protocols nor to what each protocol will uniquely contribute to the plan, but should also take into account a broad perspective across all trials. The CDP should consider if, how, and when data may be combined across studies and describe the methodology which will be used to pool data or results across different trials. In deciding to combine studies, it is important to avoid trial selection bias and to specify which studies will be combined as part of the CDP. If the decision regarding which trials will be combined cannot be made immediately, then it is important that the final selection be made prior to the unblinding of any individual trial that could potentially be included in the combined analysis. Sometimes this will be through a formal meta-analysis but other summarization methods are equally acceptable. Finally, the overall analysis strategy should be detailed in a statistical analysis plan which provides a complete description of the variables to be analysed and the methodology that will be used both for individual protocols and across protocols.

Number of confirmatory trials

The possibility that a large, single clinical trial can produce convincing evidence that a drug works in a particular indication is in contrast to the long-standing regulatory requirement that a minimum of two positive confirmatory trials is needed. Lewis (1995) has recently challenged this requirement, claiming that if the purpose of a phase III trial is to generalize the study results to a broader population, then a single well-controlled trial should be sufficient both to permit such generalization and to confirm work that has gone before. The decision to initiate more than one confirmatory trial as part of a CDP should therefore be taken in relation to the true need to confirm a new finding as opposed to reconfirming the evidence from earlier studies. In some cases, e.g. in life-threatening diseases, conducting more than more trial is unethical even if the evidence suggests that replication of the trial would be helpful. In the situation where only one trial is possible, it has been argued that the significance level may have to be redefined to be 0.05^2 or 0.0025, consistent with the overall risk of a false-positive result that would arise from two independent trials, each at the 0.05 level of significance. On the other hand, the replication of important studies can greatly add to the interpretation of evidence and the confidence in the decision taken. Until further debate has occurred and a consensus view is reached, it may be difficult to reach a clear recommendation for or against two or more confirmatory trials.

Sample size estimation

The inclusion of a sample size statement in the protocol gives assurance to the reader that the trial was designed with due diligence. The sample size estimate should ideally be based on a single primary efficacy variable and on evidence about this variable obtained from earlier studies or from the literature. Sometimes, there may be two or more primary efficacy variables, in which case the sample size calculation will depend on how these will be analysed, adjusting or not for multiplicity. In some cases, historical data may not be available or are limited in value, and an independent expert opinion may either supplement current evidence or be the sole source for determining parameter estimates for the sample size calculation. In most clinical trials, the sample size calculation depends on estimates of the expected response in the control group, the size of the difference to detect and on certain risks that we are prepared to take in falsely concluding whether the drug works or not (the Type I and Type II errors respectively). In the case of a binary variable, these estimates are sufficient to permit sample size calculation while in the case of a continuous variable the calculation depends on estimates of the magnitude of the (mean) treatment difference to detect and the variability (standard deviation) of the difference to be detected. Not only must the evidence on which sample size calculations are based be supported by appropriate estimates, references and assumptions, the magnitude of the treatment effect must also be clinically relevant. If, for example, the primary variable is a surrogate variable, the sponsor should be able to demonstrate a link between the surrogate measure and the clinical end-point under investigation. In some clinical trials where the main focus is on safety, sample size may be calculated based not on efficacy but on adverse experience rates. In such trials, if the estimate of the underlying incidence of adverse experiences in the control group is very low, there is a risk that too few patients will be included in the trial and power will also be low. On the other hand, when the estimate of the response rate in the control group is too high, sample size may be over-estimated and studies may be overpowered.

If, during the course of a trial, results from other studies are published which suggest a different control response rate or a different estimate of variability, it seems reasonable that these revised estimates could be used to evaluate possible design changes or to re-estimate the sample size for ongoing trials. Indeed, the CPMP guidelines on *Biostatistical Methodology* suggest that reassessment of the variability of the primary variable based on a blinded review of the trial at some interim time point is acceptable. Any specific actions in this regard must be documented as formal protocol amendments and the design consequences fully investigated.

Interim analysis

One common approach which has gained wide acceptance in recent years and is included as a matter of routine in large long-term end-point trials (mega-trials) is that of interim analysis. Formal interim analysis with appro-priate adjustments for controlling the Type I error may be stated as part of the protocol and the methodology specified as part of an interim analysis plan. It is essential that *all* interim analyses, whether for regulatory, ethical, scientific or administrative purposes are indicated in the protocol.

In addition to the range of statistical issues discussed in a CDP, reference should also be made to the procedures and systems which will be used to collect, monitor and process the trial data. Precise statements covering these topics can be helpful in illustrating how consistency in measurement techniques, data review and data preparation has been accomplished. This can be included as part of the CDP but can also, perhaps, be best expressed as part of a data management plan which provides a high-level overview of the various data types, data collection tools, review tasks and review tools applicable to the program as well as detailed overview of how data review will be accomplished.

Protocol review and approval

The study protocol should include a detailed and comprehensive statement of the trial objectives and statistical methodology to be employed to meet these objectives. Careful consideration should be given to the choice of study design and to the treatment comparisons to be made. A loosely worded objective can create uncertainty regarding the choice of primary variable(s), the timepoints at which analysis will be conducted and the treatment comparisons to be made. Imprecise or ambiguous statistical methodology may permit multiple – and sometimes incorrect – approaches to be made to the analysis and the potential for bias regarding which results will be selected for presentation. A precise statement of objectives, treatment comparisons and statistical methods is required to ensure that the study design is correct and that the trial will be successful in producing unbiased estimates of treatment effects on which conclusions will be based.

The project statistician must acquire sufficient knowledge of the underlying therapeutic area, an awareness of the relevant background material and of the results from earlier or related trials in order to bring precision and order to the protocol review process. Statistical design considerations enter into many aspects of trial protocol development, including the choice of run-in period, type of study design, specification of inclusion/exclusion criteria, definition of the primary variable, estimation of sample size, data analysis methods, patient recruitment and randomization, and procedures for the blinding and unblinding of results and individuals. Most of these topics are discussed elsewhere in this chapter but two topics specific to the planning phase of a trial merit further discussion below – the impact of inclusion/exclusion criteria and the definition of the primary variable.

Inclusion/exclusion criteria

The study population for a clinical trial should be based on well-defined inclusion and exclusion criteria and patients selected for inclusion in a trial should strictly match these criteria. The inclusion of patients from a homogeneous population minimizes between-patient variability and hence maximizes the power of the trial. Loosely-defined entrance criteria can inflate variability and reduce power. While good study design should encourage the use of narrowly defined exclusion/inclusion criteria, this may lead to restrictive results and sometimes to difficulties in extrapolating study results to the population at large. For some studies – particularly in new therapeutic areas – some relaxation of the entrance criteria may be desirable. On the other hand, over-relaxation of the entrance criteria can increase between-patient variability and hence the patients included in the trial may not be representative of the population for whom the treatment is being evaluated. Sometimes, entrance criteria must have to be relaxed either to increase the pool of eligible patients or to accelerate patient recruitment. Such changes should be documented as formal protocol amendments and the statistical, clinical and economic consequences of these changes should be evaluated.

Primary variables

The protocol should make a clear distinction between primary and secondary variables to be analysed and focus on a single primary variable of interest whenever possible. The role of secondary variables, however, should not be discounted since formal analysis of these variables may be mandated by regulatory agencies. If more than one primary variable is included, then the rules used to combine several end-points and other multiplicity considerations must be specified and the effect on the overall Type I error must be explained. The primary variable on which the main study hypothesis will be tested will normally be the variable on which the sample size calculation is based. The choice of primary variable should represent the accepted norm in the field of research under investigation, must have been validated in previous trials or determined from previously published data and should be reliable. Evidence should be provided to demonstrate that the primary variable is indeed sensitive to clinically relevant treatment effects in the population under study. In evaluating a new drug application, considerable weight is attached to a clear and unambiguous definition of the primary variable and on the conclusions based on this variable. A *post hoc* definition of the primary variable is rarely acceptable and must be fully justified as a formal protocol amendment together with an appropriate evaluation of the impact of this new definition on the study objectives and hypotheses to be tested.

The statistician should review the study protocol with particular reference to the data being collected *vis-à-vis* the study objectives to ensure that there are no potential conflicts. For example, if an efficacy parameter will be derived from other data items, it is important to ensure that these items are recorded in accordance with the study objectives. In confirmatory studies, it is also important to ensure that the effect size to be detected is of clinical significance. Formal protocol approval must include the signature of the project statistician as a key member of the project team. Any protocol amendments must also receive critical statistical review and also receive formal statistical approval. The impact of protocol changes on design assumptions, sample size and trial conduct should be investigated by the project statistician, documented, signed and dated, and entered into the project folder.

Statistical analysis plans

Only a few years ago, it was not unusual that the only statistical statement that appeared in a protocol consisted of a power calculation and a sample size estimation for the trial. All other statistical documentation, including descriptions of the analysis strategy and decisions regarding the choice of primary variable and patient inclusion, tended to be made at the end of the trial, and often after the trial was unblinded. This approach was clearly unsatisfactory and had the potential to introduce multiple forms of bias since decisions made during the statistical analysis will have a significant impact on the trial results and their interpretation. As statistical guidelines became established, pre-specification of primary variables in the protocol and of the ground rules for analysis prior to unblinding became routine and reflected a desire for increased statistical rigour. Even so, changes to the study protocol were still generally not well-documented nor subject to any formal protocol amendments and the impact of such changes was rarely explored. Today, the statistical aspects of study design generally follow the advice contained in regulatory guidelines and the analytic approach and presentation of results are documented in a formal statistical analysis plan (SAP). A SAP should be approved not only by the statistical department but also by their regulatory and clinical colleagues. Aspects of the statistical analysis which transcend protocols or which are concerned with the analysis of data across protocols should be summarized as part of the program SAP, while separate SAPs will normally exist for each protocol. The widespread adoption of formal SAPs reflects an increased sensitivity to statistical issues in clinical development, a more rigorous approach by statisticians themselves and increased statistical critique of submissions by some regulatory agencies.

The SAP may be listed as an appendix to the trial protocol or as a separate study document. Both approaches are acceptable. Although it is clearly desirable to define the SAP early in the planning process, the dynamic nature of most clinical programmes lead to changes in scope and leads to duration, often making it difficult to fix this plan well in advance. It is important that all decisions regarding the SAP are made before unblinding of the study so that the potential influence of statistical decision-making on the trial results based on knowledge of treatment assignments is neutralized. If changes to the SAP after unblinding are necessary, then all decisions, actions and timings must be clearly documented and signed. In this case, it may be advisable also to present the results according to the original plan and to explain any differences between the planned and final analyses. A more pragmatic approach is to modify the SAP to take account of decisions taken during the conduct of the trial and only to finalize the plan immediately prior to unblinding of the study; or at least before the analysis begins. Any changes to the SAP should be justified, approved and fully documented in the statistical report.

All decisions concerning the inclusion/exclusion of protocol violators and the statistical methods for dealing with these occurrences must be documented prior to study unblinding and the same rules should be seen to apply to all protocols within the same clinical development plan where possible. Examples of protocol violators are patients who fail to meet the eligibility criteria, those who take prohibited concomitant medication during the trial and those who discontinue the trial. Decisions regarding the management of data from these patients must be taken before the blind is broken and methods for dealing with these occurrences dealt with in the SAP.

The specific areas to be addressed as part of an SAP are:

- Trial objectives, hypotheses to be tested and/or parameters to be estimated.
- Procedures for handling withdrawals and protocol deviations.
- The statistical analysis strategy – per-protocol or intention-to-treat (ITT).
- Procedures for handling missing data.
- Multiplicity.
- Levels of statistical and clinical significance to be used.
- The statistical model to be used and alternative strategies to be adopted if the model assumptions are not met.
- Influence of baseline data or covariates.
- Plans for interim analyses and the stopping rules.

Two of the points listed above will be further discussed here – the choice of statistical analysis strategy and multiplicity.

Statistical analysis strategy

The choice of analysis approach – per-protocol or ITT – is confusing, if not controversial. The per-protocol approach aims to exclude all patients from the analysis who are considered protocol violators. Valid data from patients who drop out of the study are included only up until the time that the drop-out occurs. In the ITT approach, data from all patients who were randomized to treatment are included in the analysis irrespective of whether they are protocol violators or have recorded invalid data. Moreover, ITT analyses will normally include information on patients who dropped out of the study beyond the point of drop-out by adopting a number of different analytical techniques designed to take account of missing data. The per-protocol approach aims to answer the scientific question posed in the protocol, whereas the ITT approach gives estimates of treatment effects which are more likely to correspond to those seen in subsequent practice.

The data used in a per-protocol analysis should be supported by a precise accounting and analysis of which patients, selections of data and timepoints have been eliminated and the reasons for their exclusion. By the same token, the appropriateness of the ITT approach should also be investigated and justified in relation to the choice of approach to handle incomplete or missing data patterns. The per-protocol analysis is more vulnerable to introducing biased estimates of treatment effects compared to the ITT approach. However, there are some particular cases where the ITT approach is clearly the method of choice, e.g. in mortality trials which compare an active agent with a negative control. Whichever approach is adopted (per-protocol or ITT), the principle should be to include as many patients and as many data points as possible and to restrict exclusions only to those patients who have the wrong indication or whose information could bias the estimation of treatment effects. The difficulty in understanding the adopted usage of ITT in the regulatory environment in contrast to the original intent of this term is further discussed by Lewis (1995).

Multiplicity

Multiplicity is a phenomenon which occurs in every clinical trial and can arise in the following ways:

● Multiple treatment comparisons.
● Multiple efficacy end-points.
● Multiple timepoints.
● Multiple subpopulations.
● Multiple interim analyses.

Since multiplicity cannot be eliminated, consideration should be given to minimizing multiplicity at the design stage. The SAP should discuss multiplicity in some detail and describe the statistical procedures that will be applied. The adjustment of P values (Type I error adjustment) should always be considered and the use of adjustment procedures (or not) explained. The influence of multiple analyses on the overall significance level is illustrated in Table 25.1.

Table 25.1 *Effect of multiple analyses on the significance level*

Number of independent tests	Significance level
1	5.0%
2	9.8%
3	14.3%
4	18.5%
5	22.6%
10	40.1%
100	99.4%

The first column in Table 25.1 lists the number of independent tests that are performed and the second column illustrates how the overall P value increases as the number of tests increases. In other words, as we increase the number of analyses from 1 through 10, the overall significance level – the probability of falsely concluding that there is a difference between the treatments – increases from 5 to 40%. As the number of tests approaches 100 (which is not uncommon in some trials with multiple variables, observations and time points), the overall Type I error rate has almost reached 100%, making it virtually certain that we would observe at least one significant difference by chance alone. In practice, multiple analyses are rarely independent and the significance levels quoted in Table 25.1 should be viewed as an upper bound on the Type I error rate, at least in the case where the results are positively correlated.

Evaluability of patients for analysis

The selection of patients and data to be excluded from the analysis depends on the statistical analysis strategy and on the selection procedures to be applied. Many factors contribute to the definition of the analysis dataset, including compliance to therapy and to the protocol, the nature and quality of the data submitted for analysis, disease history and concomitant therapy. It is important that any possible bias in the selection process is minimized, and hence, that all decisions regarding the selection procedures which will exclude patients and data are made prior to the unblinding of the study.

The criteria for patient inclusion/exclusion should be precisely documented in the SAP. Responsibility for determining patient selection criteria should be clearly specified and will normally be a shared responsibility involving project team members from the clinical, statistics and data management groups. During the course of a trial, the original entrance criteria may turn out to be too rigid either with regard to patient availability or the rate at which patients can be recruited into the trial. Rather than risking an incomplete or inconclusive study because of a failure to reach the recruitment target, an assessment of patients who fail to enter the study may suggest a relaxation of some of the inclusion/exclusion criteria in order to attain the desired sample size, albeit with respect to a slightly different study population. The effect of all losses of patients and data and of decisions to exclude observations and the reasons for exclusion from the per-protocol analysis must be carefully examined and explained as part of the statistical report or in a separate reference document.

In accordance with the SAP the statistical report should specify all important deviations related to study inclusion or exclusion criteria, patient management or patient assessment, together with a description as to how all protocol violators will be summarized. It may also be helpful to group protocol violators and other discrepancies into appropriate categories, such as:

- Violation of inclusion/exclusion criteria.
- Patients taking prohibited concomitant therapies.
- Patients receiving the wrong dose of test drug.
- Patients who discontinue the trial.
- Patients who were not compliant with study procedures.
- Patients with missing or incomplete data.

In principle, only *major* protocol violations should mandate the exclusion of patients or selected patient data from the per-protocol analysis. A major violation is one which is likely to affect the validity of the data from the patient.

For example, consider a clinical trial where the objective is to evaluate treatments for congestive heart failure (CHF) based on exercise tolerance testing. To be eligible for inclusion in the study, patients were required to demonstrate that they had stable CHF as determined by two successive baseline exercise tolerance times within 60 second of each other. This rule was not strictly applied and several patients were randomized whose exercise times differed by more than 60 seconds. In this case data from such patients were deemed unreliable and patients were classed as major protocol violators.

Another common situation arising in clinical trials leading to a major protocol violation is where the patient visit does not take place in accordance with the protocol. Here, some licence is granted and observations are still considered valid if the visit occurs within a window around the scheduled visit date. If, however, the visit occurs outside of this window, then the data collected cannot be regarded as representative of data for the time-point in question and such data will be excluded from the per-protocol analysis. Other examples of major protocol violations associated with the exclusion of data at certain time-points include failure to take study medication or intake of prohibited medication at, or immediately prior to, the clinic visit.

In some cases, entrance criteria are specified to reflect more of a safety concern rather than in terms of defining a strict study population (e.g. reference ranges for some biochemical parameters) and violation of these 'soft' criteria will not normally lead to patient exclusions.

A special case occurs where entry into the study is dependent on attaining an extreme (high or low) value of the primary efficacy measurement at baseline. For example, in an antihypertensive trial where patients must have a baseline sitting diastolic blood pressure (SDBP) of

>90 mmHg, patient selection will inevitably favour those who appear to have the more severe disease. The consequence is that subsequent treatment values will tend to be less extreme due solely to the phenomenon known as regression to the mean and the within-group treatment effect may be inflated. However, since the regression to the mean phenomenon will affect both the active and control groups similarly, the between-treatment differences should not be affected.

Drop-outs have a major influence on the power of the study and this effect is more severe for the ITT approach compared to the per-protocol approach. If, for example, we assume that the effect of drop-outs is immediate and complete, then for a trial with n patients per group and for a fixed drop-out rate (p), the reduction in power in the per-protocol case (assuming that the per-protocol analysis is influenced by drop-outs only and not by other types of protocol violators) is due solely to the fewer patients who will be included in the analysis, i.e. $(1-p)n$. In ITT analysis, we assume that, on average, patients who drop out of the study do not benefit from the treatment, i.e. they have zero benefit and hence the magnitude of the planned difference to detect (Δ) is reduced by a factor of $1-p$. Since power is a function of $\Delta\sqrt{n}$, i.e., it is monotonically increasing as the quantity $\Delta\sqrt{n}$, increases, a drop-out rate (p) will always have a more severe effect on the ITT analysis where power is a function of $\Delta(1-p)\sqrt{n}$, compared to the per-protocol analysis where power is a function of $\Delta\sqrt{(1-p)n}$ since $(1-p) \le \sqrt{(1-p)}$ for $0 \le p \le 1$. Table 25.2 illustrates how the power of the study decreases as the drop-out rate increases for both the per-protocol and ITT strategies.

Table 25.2   *Impact of protocol violators and drop-outs on power*

	Original power		
Drop-out rate	95%	90%	80%
Per-protocol approach			
5%	94.0%	88.5%	77.9%
10%	92.7%	86.7%	75.7%
15%	91.3%	84.8%	73.3%
20%	89.6%	82.6%	70.7%
Intention-to-treat approach			
5%	92.8%	86.8%	75.8%
10%	90.0%	83.1%	71.2%
15%	86.5%	78.6%	66.3%
20%	82.2%	73.6%	61.0%

In the per-protocol approach, for an original power of 95%, the effect of drop-outs ranging from 5 to 20% results in a corresponding loss of power ranging from 1 to 6%. As the original power decreases, so the loss in power approximates almost three percentage points per 5% increase in the drop-out rate.

A similar pattern is seen for the ITT approach where protocol violators and drop-outs are included. Here, the magnitude of the power decrease for the same drop-out rate and original power is almost double for each entry compared to the per-protocol approach. In this case, the greater loss in power is due partly to the fact that the difference to detect is smaller since estimates of treatment effects are more conservative.

Randomization and blinding

The randomized, double-blind clinical trial is the clearly established gold standard in the evaluation of new therapies. The assignment of patients to treatment according to a randomization schedule and the preservation of the blind with respect to treatment during the conduct of the trial avoids the possibility of systematic bias in patient evaluation and treatment and in the selection for data for analysis.

By contrast non-randomized and/or open-label studies may introduce serious bias and lead to inconclusive results. Results from any open study having as its primary variable a 'soft' end-point, e.g. a subjective evaluation of therapy or an intervention based on a subjective decision to send a patient to surgery, are likely to be viewed with great scepticism. Even when a trial is conducted as an open-label study, randomization should always be applied and should be done in a blinded manner. If the randomization is not blinded, the treatment groups will most likely end up with different selections of patients on average and treatment comparisons will be biased or at worst invalidated. Treatment comparisons may also be biased if patients having prohibited concomitant diseases or taking prohibited concomitant medication are included in the analysis. This was an important issue in the primary prevention study on mortality (1992) conducted as part of the SOLVD (Studies of Left Ventricular Dysfunction)program comparing enalapril, an angiotensin-converting enzyme (ACE) inhibitor, with placebo in patients with an acute myocardial infarction. As the trial progressed, the administration of ACE inhibitors became accepted as the standard therapy for patients with CHF and more and more patients in the study, particularly in the placebo group, began to take this prohibited therapy. The increasing use of open-label ACE inhibitors in the placebo group could be interpreted as diluting the treatment difference between enalapril and placebo and possibly contributing to the non-significant difference in mortality seen in the prevention part of the trial. In this case, since the conclusions were based on a hard end-point, they were perhaps less sensitive to bias.

A variety of randomization methods exists to assist in efficient trial design with the objective of maintaining power while minimizing the number of patients to be randomized. Procedures describing responsibilities for the creation, distribution and storage of randomization schedules should be clearly documented such that the minimum number of personnel involved in the trial have access to this list. The only individuals having access should be those who are responsible for treating trial patients in the case of a medical emergency and those responsible for interim analysis. At the conclusion of the trial, the administration of treatments to patients should be verified against the randomization schedule for each centre and any gaps or other suggestions that the planned randomization schedule was not followed should be documented and discussed with regard to any impact on the analysis.

The procedure for generating the randomization schedule should be capable of being reproduced (if the need arises) through the use of the same random number table or the same computer routine and seed. The choice of randomization technique reflects the study design and is selected to improve efficiency, for example in multicentre trials, stratification by centre is more efficient.

In addition to patients and investigators remaining blind to treatment, it is now common for *all* individuals who are involved in trial conduct, patient management, data processing, analysis or interpretation to remain blind until the conclusion of the trial. This approach ensures that any potential bias concerned with setting data management conventions and statistical analysis ground rules will be minimized. For example, if the statistician or clinical staff know the patient's treatment when determining the study inclusion and exclusion rules, it is possible, either consciously or unconsciously, that the rules could affect the results. The blinding procedures should be specified in the study protocol, including the emergency circumstances under which the code may be broken for individual patients. Documenting these procedures is important since blinded decisions carry greater weight.

Another possible means of unblinding occurs when one or more of the patient measurements can be predictive of which treatment the patient is taking. For example, in placebo-controlled trials assessing the incidence of fractures in patients with osteoporosis, knowledge of bone mineral density values could potentially unblind the trial investigator to treatment. Similarly, in placebo-controlled mortality trials evaluating the effects of lipid-lowering therapy, the lipid values themselves will be predictive of treatment. At the design stage of a clinical trial, careful consideration should be given to all measurements that could potentially be predictive of trial therapy and efforts made to process these data in a blinded fashion. The simplest way to process laboratory samples of this type is to employ a central laboratory and to retain test results at the central facility until they are required for interim or final analysis. This approach also reduces measurement variability since all samples will be processed using the same assay methodology.

The only individuals who may be unblinded during the course of the trial are those responsible for performing the interim analysis and, in some cases, members of a safety monitoring committee whose role is to assess the interim analysis results and advise the steering committee as to decisions concerning early trial termination. Strictly, the safety monitoring committee members need only be unblinded with respect to group results and a smaller number of individual cases with serious adverse experiences. When such analyses are performed, the integrity of the blinding of the trial must be preserved with respect to all staff involved in the conduct of the trial and in taking decisions based on the outcome of the trial.

Interim analysis and stopping rules

An interim analysis includes any evaluation of the efficacy or safety data during a trial which compares results from one or more treatment groups. The integrity of interim analyses procedures can be strengthened if the presentation and interpretation of interim results are the responsibility of an independent safety monitoring committee whose members are not directly involved with the day-to-day management of patients or involved in the conduct of the trial. An interim analysis may be requested for one of several reasons – scientific, ethical, regulatory or administrative. Whatever the reason, an interim analysis plan should be written which fully describes the purpose, frequency, methods of analysis and presentation of results. Particular consideration should be given to the hypothesis to be tested at the interim stage and whether the study will have sufficient power to give clinical meaning to the interim results. If the intention of the interim analysis is to stop the trial prematurely, then the stopping rule should also be described in detail. The three principal reasons for early trial termination are:

- An unexpected safety concern.
- Overwhelming efficacy.
- Lack of efficacy.

An interim analysis plan should also specify the procedures governing data access, define statistical responsibility for performing the analysis and list those who will be exposed to the results. The statistician performing the interim analysis should be independent of the project statistician responsible for defining the final SAP and for setting statistical ground rules. In long-term, end-point trials it is not uncommon for several interim analyses to be proposed. The execution of interim analysis plans must be performed against clearly predefined procedures such that the integrity of the trial and the final statistical analysis are preserved. All staff involved in the conduct of the trial and in taking decisions based on the outcome of the trial should remain blind to the results of the interim analysis and the results from an interim analysis must not be used to alter the conduct of the trial. Another possibility in presenting the results of interim analysis is to assign labels, e.g. A and B, to the different treatment groups rather than formally unblinding the treatment codes for interim analyses. This approach could allow wider dissemination of interim results without compromising the study blind.

In long-term trials the interim analysis plan may include several planned analyses with appropriate adjustments for multiplicity. The time-points for these analyses could be based on calendar time, observation of a fixed number of study events or on a fixed number of patients completing a minimum exposure to therapy. Whatever the rationale, the number of analyses, the end-points to be evaluated, the level of significance and the stopping rule in force should be clearly specified in the interim analysis plan. The impact of the interim analyses on the overall Type I error, i.e. the risk of falsely concluding that the treatments are different, should also be explored. Unexplained or inappropriate interim analysis can lead to spurious results, weaken confidence in the conclusions drawn from the study and lead to wrong decisions. The impact of an interim analysis on the original sample size calculation and on the future conduct of the trial and any such influences should be documented while continuing to preserve the blind as much as possible.

For clinical trials that are not subject to a formal interim analysis plan and for which there is no external review committee, an unplanned interim analysis may be requested for a number of reasons. Such analyses should still be based on written analysis plan which clearly describes the circumstances leading to the request and the extent to which blindness will be preserved. In particular, the results from an unplanned interim analysis should not independently lead to premature termination of the trial.

A special category of unplanned interim analysis is the so-called administrative analyses which should be undertaken only to provide data for management decision-making, e.g. in providing data to guide the design of future trials, to assess future resource allocations or to assess new system requirements. In principle, administrative interim analyses must be distinguishable from other types of interim analyses, should ideally be performed on blinded data or with respect to treatment group labels only and exclude the possibility of early stopping or major design changes.

Statistical reports

The statistical report is prepared by the project statistician and describes the results of the study and the statistical interpretation of those results. The statistical report should correspond and give priority to the schedule of analyses pre-specified in the SAP. Should other analysis be required, this should be justified and documented before unblinding the study. While some variations in the presentation of results exist, the main elements of the report should include:

- A synopsis of the trial.
- A description of design issues.
- A description of the data management procedures and conventions used in the trial.
- The statistical methodology.
- The study population analysed based on this methodology.
- The trial results.
- The conclusions.

The statistical report is also where any deviations from the protocol will be recorded and any design, data management or statistical deviations will be discussed. The statistical report should also explore the influence of demographic factors and differing medical practice. The results of a study may be presented either in an independent statistical report authored by the project statistician or in the form of a joint clinical/statistical report jointly authored by the statistician and the clinical monitor. Both approaches are valid, although the joint approach perhaps offers more possibilities for ensuring that any clinical interpretation is consistent with the statistical findings. The statistical report (or the statistical contribution to the joint statistical/clinical report) should be reviewed by a second, independent statistician before issue. Finally, statistical judgement should always be brought to bear on the presentation and interpretation of results presented in the clinical study report.

It is not uncommon for statistical and clinical interpretation and conclusions based on the same results to differ and care must be taken to ensure that the final report is balanced with respect to both views. Two common areas of possible contention between statistical and clinical staff are the interpretation of multiplicity issues and (unplanned) subgroup analyses. In such circumstances, interpretation of results and conclusions must be carefully negotiated to reach a compromise solution. Only subgroup analyses pre-specified in the protocol or in the SAP carry high weight and may be considered confirmatory, although in practice most subgroup analyses tend to have low power and should be regarded as exploratory. It is important to distinguish between those analyses that are confirmatory and those that are exploratory, since exploratory analysis cannot form the basis for formal proof of efficacy.

The results for the primary variable should be discussed in relation to what are considered to be clinically relevant treatment effects in the population under study. One common finding in very large trials which are overpowered is that a highly statistically significant result may not have any clinical relevance. Of course, the converse is also frequently true, where a clinically meaningful difference may fail to reach statistical significance due to too small a sample size or higher than expected variability.

The results of a trial should also provide appropriate data summaries on patients who were screened but not randomized. The effect of all losses of patients and data must be explained. A descriptive analysis should be performed on patients lost to follow-up or withdrawn from treatment including a summary of the reason for loss, relationship to treatment and outcome. Unplanned analyses of baseline measures which are imbalanced between treatments should be investigated and the effect of these imbalances on the conclusions should be quantified.

Statistical reports do not usually contain a statement on the underlying quality of the data being analysed. In preparing a statistical analysis, a data management report can be a helpful document in providing a summary of not only the underlying quality of the database *vis-à-vis* the protocol and data-handling guidelines but also stating the degree of review conducted across the database and a listing of discrepancies which will not be resolved.

Data management

The data resulting from a clinical trial programme represent the key company asset to support product development and registration. The study databases on which the statistical analysis will be performed should be complete, accurate and validated and be a true representation of the source data. All data management activities should be based on thorough and effective SOPs. The procedures describing the various data management processes which govern the collection, processing and reporting of data from a clinical programme and for individual protocols can most conveniently be documented in a data management plan (DMP). This document is usually authored by the project data coordinator but relies on input from all project team personnel. It is important for the integrity of the trial that all decisions regarding data management conduct are made prior to the unblinding of the trial. This applies equally to data-handling guidelines and coding conventions. The DMP is also where the data review plan is specified. The statistician should review and if appropriate approve all key data management documents and procedures.

Data management plan

The scope of a DMP includes, but is not limited to, a description of the data flow corresponding to each data source, an overview of the data to be collected by data type and protocol, data-handling guidelines, coding conventions, data reporting requirements and a data review plan (DRP). The DRP describes the data review strategy, the data review tools to be used, the degree of review to be applied to each data type and the review responsibility. A summary of the DMP should be included either as an appendix to the trial protocol or as a separate study document. In the same way that decisions regarding the inclusion of patients in the analysis should be made prior to study unblinding it is desirable that all decisions regarding data management conventions are made prior to finalization of the study database. It is important that the creation of the electronic database be done in accordance with the procedures described in the DMP. The project statistician should carefully and critically review and approve the data collection tools, data flow procedures, transformation programs and change control systems which will be used to create the study databases from the source data.

Data management report

At the conclusion of each trial a data management report (DMR), authored by the project data coordinator, should be delivered to the project statistician and the clinical monitor. The DMR describes the procedures that were followed and comments on any deviations from what is stated in the DMP. The report provides an overview of the quality and content of the final study database, describes any outstanding or unresolved questions and provides estimates of the error rates associated with different data types. Any subsequent errors or database inconsistencies discovered by the statistician should be documented in the statistical report.

Database transformations

In most clinical trials data will be transformed from the entry database or file structure into datasets that are more suitable for reporting purposes. These transformation programs may be executed in the creation of the final database or they may be run against the final database to provide specific datasets for statistical analysis. Transformation programs and other programs used for data entry and data review must be fully tested against documented test plans and the appropriate validation procedures should be documented. Moreover, the statistical analysis procedures and programs must be validated. In the past, the statistician was uniquely responsible for all programming of datasets from which analysis would be performed.

There was little, or usually no, peer review of these programmes. No formal validation was required and for most programs the need for validation of entry systems, query programming, analysis datasets, data summaries and listings was not subject to any formal plan. Today, software validation is a major area of research and a formal step not only in system development but in the reporting of data. This has given rise to a role for a statistical programmer and for independent verification of analysis programs.

Database changes

Once data have been entered into the entry database, errors may also be identified during subsequent review by data management, clinical and statistical staff. For each trial, an audit trial should be available to allow both internal and external auditing staff to track data from its source to the final database. Procedures should be introduced to ensure that all such changes are documented in accordance with good clinical practice.

Archiving

At the conclusion of a trial, all original study documentation, including all data and reports, should be retained in a project folder and archived for future reference. In addition, the project folder should contain a chronological account of all significant events occurring during the project from which the programme history may be constructed. Specifically, the information contained in the project folder should be sufficient to allow the statistical analysis to be reconstructed from the final study database. The statistical contribution to the project folder includes, but is not limited to:

- Statistical documentation not held in other formal study documents.
- Final protocol, amendments and statistical consequences of amendments.
- Randomization lists (including the randomization table or seed used to generate the allocation schedule).
- Statistical Analysis Plan.
- Statistical report.
- Statistical program source code.
- Test plans and validation routines for statistical programs.

With the recent development of electronic archiving tools and the integration of office software, consideration should always be given to holding an electronic version of the project folder for both internal and potentially external use.

Acknowledgements

I am grateful to my statistical colleagues at Merck for providing several of the examples quoted in this chapter; to Dr Steven Snapinn for the tables illustrating the various power calculations and the examples on incorrect trial design and on the evaluability of patients for analysis; to Tom Cook for comments on the Japanese guidelines and the atheroscelerosis example and to Drs William Malbecq, Leonard Oppenheimer and Steven Snapinn for their critical review of the draft manuscript.

References

CPMP Working Party on Efficacy on Medicinal Products (1990) Good clinical practice for trials on medicinal products in the European Community. *Pharmacology and Toxicology* **67**: 361-372.

CPMP working party on efficacy on medicinal products (1994), *Biostatistical Methodology in Clinical Trials in Applications for Marketing Authorisations for Medicinal Products (Final)*. Brussels, Belgium: Commission of the European Communities.

Food and Drug Administration (1988). *Guideline for the Format and Content of the Clinical and Statistical Sections of New Drug Applications*. Rockville, MD: FDA, US Department of Health and Human Services.

PSI professional standards working party (1994). *Good Statistical Practice in Clinical Research: Guideline Standard Operating Procedures. Drug Information Journal* **28**: 615-627.

International Conference on Harmonization (1995) *Structure and Content of Clinical Study Reports*. ICH efficacy topic 3. Draft 11. International Conference on Harmonization.

Koseisho (1992) *Guidelines on the Statistical Analysis of Clinical Studies*. PAB-NDD #20. Tokyo: Koseisho (Japanese Ministry of Health and Welfare).

Lewis, J. A. (1995) Statistical issues in the regulation of medicines. *Statistics in Medicine* **14**: 127-136.

Nordic Council on Medicines (1989,) *Good Clinical Trial Practice: Nordic Guidelines*. NLN publication no. 28. Uppsala: Nordic Council of Medicines.

Studies of Left Ventricular Dysfunction (SOLVD) investigators (1989) Effect of enalapril on survival in patients with reduced ventricular ejection fractions and congestive heart failure. *New England Journal of Medicine* **325**: 293–302.

26 Good laboratory practice and preclinical expert reports

R W James

Introduction

In European Union (EU) member states the documentation which is submitted to support applications for authorizations to market human and veterinary medicines must include expert reports on the pharmaceutical, preclinical and clinical sections of the dossier (Directive 75/319/EEC). The preclinical expert report should provide the assessor with a critical evaluation and interpretation of the pharmacodynamic, pharmacokinetic and toxicological data. One of the key responsibilities of the preclinical expert is specifically to comment on the quality and conduct of the studies included in the application dossier. Compliance with good laboratory practice (GLP) is an integral part of the assessment and quality of studies and the preclinical expert must be familiar not only with the principles and practice of GLP but also be able to recognize and define the circumstances when studies which may lack certification of GLP-compliance can still be used to support an application. Before discussing the emphasis which the preclinical expert should place on certification of studies for GLP-compliance, it may be helpful to explain that the amount of preclinical information required to approve a new product differs depending upon whether the application is for a product containing a new active substance or for one which contains a previously licensed active substance.

Applications for new active substances

A new active substance is one which has not been previously assessed by the regulatory authority to which an application for a marketing authorization (product licence) is being made. It is important to note that active substances approved in other territories will be regulated as a new active. Novel excipients (non-active ingredients) may be treated in the same way as a new active ingredient in terms of data requirements. New salts, esters or molecular compounds of known active substances may also be treated as new actives. The toxicology and pharmacology requirements for a new active substance clearly depend upon the nature and proposed clinical use of the product and the data package presented to support the application should be individually tailored to the product.

Applications for established active substances

The circumstances when it may not be necessary to provide the systematic results of animal toxicology studies are as follows:

1   The new product is 'essentially similar' to the original product, authorized in the country concerned with the application, and the person responsible for marketing the original product has consented to the preclinical documentation, used in the original filing, being used for the purpose of assessing a subsequent application.
2   It can be established using published scientific literature, presented in accordance with the second paragraph of article 1 of Directive 75/318/EEC, that the active constituent or constituents of the product have a well-established medical use, with recognized efficacy, and an acceptable level of safety.
3   The new product is 'essentially similar' to a product which has previously been licensed in one or more member states. Exceptions occur, requiring the provision of results of appropriate preclinical documentation, when the application is for a different therapeutic use, or the product is to be administered by different routes, or in different doses to those previously authorized.

The term abridged application is used for applications for which the results of the preclinical (animal toxicology and pharmacology) and clinical studies may not have to be provided. The existence of this route for the approval of copy products prevents unnecessary testing on humans and animals. When the abridged route is followed, it may be possible to justify the complete omission of preclincal data. However, it is more often the case that some preclinical data will be required because of differences in impurity profile due to variations in the manufacturing process.

Irrespective of whether the expert is dealing with an application to market a new active substance or with an abridged application, the GLP status of all the studies which are included in the preclinical dossier must always be evaluated. There are, however, two distinct classes of study which are referred to as pivotal and non-pivotal. The distinction between pivotal and non-pivotal studies is very important since this has direct relevance as to how both the expert and the assessor evaluate the file.

Good laboratory practice and pivotal studies

The following study types, which provide information upon which toxicological risk assessments are based, are defined as pivotal:

1   Single-dose toxicity.
2   Repeated-dose toxicity (subacute or chronic).
3   Reproduction toxicity.
4   Genotoxicity.
5   Carcinogenicity.
6   Local (toxicity) tolerance.
7   Toxicokinetics (pharmacokinetic studies which provide systemic exposure data for studies 1–6 above).
8   Pharmacodynamic studies designed to test the potential for adverse effects (i.e. general (safety) pharmacology studies).

Studies, in addition to those mentioned above, which provide general or specific information which is essential for safety assessment, e.g. validation of virus removal or inactivation for biological/biotechnological products, should also be carried out in accordance with GLP.

The preclinical expert report must clearly indicate whether or not the pivotal studies included with the documentation were conducted in compliance with GLP. It greatly helps the assessor if the expert report contains a tabular overview (see Table 26.1) of the preclinical documentation as this facilitates a general check and overview, including conformity with GLP, of the studies. It is important to note that pivotal studies which lack certification of GLP-compliance and which commenced before 30 June 1988 (before the implementation of Directive 87/18/EEC) can be included with the application dossier. However, the expert is expected to assemble a cogent and defensible argument when commenting favourably on reports of pivotal studies which are not certified as complying with GLP.

There is no requirement for pharmacodynamic studies related to the mode of action (i.e. primary pharmacology studies) or pharmacokinetic studies (other than those providing systemic exposure data for study types 1–6 listed above) to be certified as GLP-compliant. Although these non-pivotal studies need not be certified as GLP-compliant, the expert must be satisfied that the study reports constitute a true and accurate record of the data generated during the experiments.

A summary table for each individual pharmacodynamic, pharmacokinetic and toxicological study should be prepared and appended to the preclinical expert report. The GLP status (GLP-compliant, non-compliant or GLP not applicable) must be clearly indicated in the case of each study report. It is not uncommon for these tables to be prepared by someone rather than the expert but it is the responsibility of the expert to ensure that

Table 26.1 *Suggested format for a tabular overview, to be included in expert reports, of studies included in the preclinical dossier*

Type of study	Species	Route	Duration of treatment	Doses (as mg/kg body weight per day) administered as substance/salt (specify)	Conformity to GLP: yes/no
IIIF: Pharmacodynamics					
IIIG: Pharmacokinetics/toxicokinetics					
IIIA: Single-dose toxicity					
IIIB: Repeated-dose toxicity					
IIIC: Reproduction					
IIID: Mutagenic potential					
IIIE: Oncogenic/carcinogenic potential					
IIIH: Local tolerance					
IIIQ: Special toxicity					

these tables have been compiled accurately and that they do not contain any misleading information or statements. The expert should therefore review these summary tables against the original reports to verify the study design and GLP status and to check that the results have been correctly transposed.

Expert's evaluation of GLP-compliant studies

Even though the studies included with the preclinical dossier may all be certified as GLP-compliant, experts are advised to carry out independent assessments of critical information, contained in study reports, which may have an impact on the suitability of studies for evaluation in support of applications for marketing authorizations. In particular the expert should be concerned about deviations from study protocols; the circumstances surrounding the reissue of amendment of final reports; and the verification of study conclusions.

Deviations from study protocols

It is inevitable that minor deviations from the study protocol will occur, even in the best managed facilities, during the conduct of preclinical studies. Such deviations must be clearly identified in the study records and commented upon by the study director. It is usual for deviations from study protocols to be identified in the final report, either in the body of the report or preferably, as a separate annex to the report. It is important that the expert is able to obtain a clear overview of study conduct including the nature and consequences of any deviations from the study protocol. Whenever possible, experts are advised to check that reports are written in a manner which allows an independent reviewer to identify clearly and evaluate the significance of any protocol deviations which may have occurred during the study.

Typical examples of protocol deviations include occasional missed doses; variations of temperature and humidity outside the ranges specified in the protocol; the need to change or include additional injection sites; failure to record clinical observations; incorrect recording of body weights; failure to record food consumption; the need to repeat blood-sampling procedures to verify abnormal results or due to sample inadequacy; variations in the time of water and food deprivation before and during urine collection; and failure to obtain and preserve tissues at necropsy. In the great majority of instances, protocol deviations will involve only occasional animals and will not have a significant impact on study interpretation. Even when protocol deviations are minor, and do not have an adverse impact on study validity and interpretation, the frequency of occurrence should also be examined.

A high frequency of even trivial deviations from the study protocol indicates poor overall standards of study supervision and facility management and creates an unfavourable perception of the testing facility in the eyes of both the expert and the assessor.

The expert must be completely satisfied that there are no differences of opinion with the study director as to the impact of protocol deviations on study interpretation. If, in the opinion of the expert, a protocol deviation has occurred which is of such magnitude that the conduct and/or interpretation of the study have become questionable, then the expert may have to conclude that the documentation provided with the application does not support the granting of a marketing authorization. Applicants will of course be reluctant to submit an unfavourable expert report. For this reason it is highly desirable to involve the expert in the planning and evaluation of studies prior to finalization of study reports, otherwise there is always a risk that the expert will form an unfavourable impression of deviations from study protocols.

Working with amended or reissued reports

Even after the final report of a study has been issued, it is still possible that it will subsequently be amended or even reissued after incorporation of revisions. The expert should carefully check the information provided with each study report since it is a GLP requirement that amended or reissued reports should be clearly identified as such. An amended or reissued report should also contain a detailed justification, signed by the study director, as to why it became necessary to issue amended pages or to reissue a revised study report.

The possible reasons for amending or reissuing a study report are many and varied. The normal practice, which is followed when a report is changed after issue of the final report, is to prepare amended pages. Occasionally it may be more appropriate to reissue a report which has undergone significant revision since issue of the final report. In this author's experience the commonest reasons for reissuing or amending study reports involve the re-evaluation of the terminology and diagnostic criteria used to describe treatment-related histopathological effects; the statistical analysis of data; and the interpretation of data, particularly with respect to the definition of no observable adverse effect levels (NOAELs). The decision to amend or reissue a report usually reflects a perception that the original study report was in some way scientifically inadequate, even though its compliance with GLP was never in question. The expert must however carefully consider the circumstances and reasons which have led to the amending or complete reissue of a finalized report and formulate an independent view of the justifications for so doing before evaluating the impact on the perception of safety of the test material.

Verification of study conclusions

It is usual for each preclinical study report to contain a summary of results and conclusions prepared by the study director. The expert is expected to form an opinion as to whether or not the conclusions given in each study report are in fact supported by the data. Experts should therefore not base their opinion upon study summaries without first independently verifying the study conclusions. This involves not only consideration of the impact of protocol deviations and any circumstances which may have led to the issue of amended pages or even the reissue of a final report, but also the study director's perception of the nature of the intended biological actions of the test material and their influence on the results obtained.

The study director may place undue emphasis on the results of statistical comparisons, rather than scientific judgement, to identify treatment-related effects. Statistically significant differences between control and treated animals may simply reflect a predictable or intended pharmacological effect. Judgement is necessary to determine whether or not such effects should be classified as adverse (i.e. toxicologically significant) effects. Interpretation of statistical output without reference to historical control data may also result in incorrect conclusions. Experts should assure themselves that the control data, for any given study, are within the testing facility's historical range and that there are no untypical values which have not been commented upon by the study director.

Thus it is possible, even when a study is certified as GLP-compliant, for the expert to disagree with some or all of the study director's conclusions. Again, as already stated, if the expert is involved during the earlier stages of the development programme then such difficulties can be avoided.

Non-GLP studies

A number of circumstances have been outlined when it is possible to include studies, which are not certified as being GLP-compliant, in an application dossier. The expert needs to give careful consideration to the implications of basing an opinion on such studies particularly with regard to their conduct and reporting in terms of acceptable standards of scientific research.

Pivotal studies

Only those pivotal studies which were commenced before 30 June 1988 can be considered in this category. It is highly desirable that experts ensure that applicants have actually established that the raw data for such studies are still available for inspection and that they will continue to be available for an appropriate length of time (i.e. at least 10 years) after the granting of a first application for authorization to market a product in a EU member state. If the raw data are not longer available then regrettably the studies must be repeated so as to comply with GLP requirements. When the raw data are still available the expert should only proceed to form an opinion as to whether or not the studies support the safe use of the product when the applicant has carried out a fully documented retrospective GLP audit of the studies and confirmed that the study conduct and reporting conforms to GLP standards.

Non-pivotal studies

Non-pivotal studies are discovery pharmacology and pharmacokinetic studies which contribute knowledge about the pharmacological properties of a drug but which are not an integral part of the toxicological hazard identification and risk assessment process and need not be certified as GLP-compliant. None the less, the expert must be satisfied that the reports of these studies properly reflect the raw data and that the studies were conducted to acceptable standards of scientific and research practice. Especially in the case of discovery pharmacology studies, the results from humans will have rapidly superseded those of animal models in importance and there is no need for the expert report to dwell on this aspect of the dossier. Although not forming the basis for risk assessment, the pharmacokinetics and biotransformation section of the preclinical expert report is vital to the validation of toxicity testing. It may also serve to provide interpretation of any adverse effects in animals, in terms of relative exposure to active substances and/or their metabolites, as compared with the anticipated human exposure at efficacious doses. Thus, whilst whose pharmacokinetic studies which are related to primary pharmacological or chemotherapeutic effects may be considered outside the scope of GLP, any kinetic studies which are used either to support or interpret toxicity tests are clearly within the scope of GLP and must be certified for their compliance with GLP.

Expert reports based on published data

Abridged applications based on submission of papers published in scientific journals to demonstrate that the active constituent or constituents have an acceptable level of safety are sometimes known as bibliographic applications. In general such applications can only be successful in the case of very well-established ingredients which have an established medical use and recognized efficacy. Data which are published in scientific journals are not easily adapted for incorporation into regulatory dossiers and seemingly trivial, but important, details about the composition and purity of test compounds, the sources and quality of the test animals, and the quality control of diets and drinking water are often omitted. The expert is usually unable to form any view as to whether or not the studies were conducted to GLP standards in GLP-compliant facilities. It has also been made clear that use of the summary basis of approval (SBA) documentation, produced by Food and Drug Administration reviewers, will not usually be regarded as an acceptable means of supporting abridged applications for approval of products containing active constituents which have not been previously approved in EU member states. It is also common for papers published in scientific journals to question rather than support the safe use of established active ingredients. The papers often describe results of experiments which are either irrelevant to the therapeutic use of the compound or the route of exposure and/or the extent of exposure is not appropriate for the identification and quantification of human hazards. When such publications are included with the documentation they can cause considerable problems unless the expert is able to explain why the results should not be regarded as toxicologically important.

Scientific validity of studies

Certification that a study has been conducted in compliance with GLP is based on the performance of audits, which are intended to confirm:

1   That the testing facility has an adequate number of qualified personnel and that the organizational structure is appropriate to ensure that GLP standards are maintained.
2   That a functional quality assurance unit (QAU) exists to assure the testing facility management that studies are conducted in accordance with GLP standards.
3   That the design, environmental control and procedures for pest control and the cleansing of testing facilities are consistent with the conduct of studies to GLP standards.
4   That the testing facility has appropriate and adequate equipment to perform studies and that the inspection and maintenance schedules ensure the validity of results.
5   That reagents and solutions are properly labelled and suitably stored.
6   That the testing facility has written standard operating procedures (SOPs) which are relevant to the studies undertaken.
7   That standards of animal care preclude the occurrence of circumstances which might interfere with the purpose or conduct of studies.
8   That procedures designed to ensure that test and control materials are administered at the doses specified in protocols.
9   That the protocol and study conduct are in accordance with GLP standards.

10 That final reports are prepared to GLP standards and that records and specimens are appropriately stored.
11 That computerized data collection systems are appropriately located and operated and maintained according to GLP requirements.

Even when all of the above criteria are deemed to be satisfactory and the study is certifiable as GLP-compliant, there are a number of other issues, which are beyond the scope of GLP, but which should be addressed in the preclinical expert report. These include:

1 The physicochemical characteristics of the drug (particle size, lipophilicity, low solubility) and whether these were adequately controlled in batches of test compound used in the preclinical studies.
2 The impurity profiles of the batches used for preclinical testing as compared with the impurity profile of the material to be marketed.
3 The implications of any differences of the chirality and chemical form of the material used for preclinical testing and that intended for marketing.
4 Drawing attention to any deficiencies in the design (i.e. selection of parameters, choice of dosages, study durations) of studies *vis-à-vis* the proposed clinical usage of the product.
5 Justification for the omission of particular studies (e.g. oncogenicity/carcinogenicity studies, reproduction toxicity studies) and identifying the need for any additional studies.
6 What target organ toxicity was observed in animals and what monitoring of those organs was included in humans during the clinical studies.

Conclusions

The preparation of a preclinical expert report is a complex task requiring a detailed review and analysis of the scientific basis and validity of the studies which form the basis of the application. Even though all of the studies included with an application may have been certified as GLP-compliant, this constitutes but one aspect of the production of the preclinical expert report. Compliance with GLP is mandatory for pivotal studies (i.e. those studies which are used as a basis for toxicological hazard and risk assessment) which were commenced after 30 June 1988. There is no requirement for non-pivotal studies (i.e. discovery pharmacology and pharmacokinetic investigations which provide information relevant to the pharmacological rather than toxicological evaluation of drugs) to be certified as GLP-compliant. When dealing with applications which include pivotal studies which were commenced before 30 June 1988 but which are not certified as

GLP-complaint, the expert has to form a view as to whether or not this precludes meaningful evaluation of such studies. The requirements for preclinical studies to support abridged applications to market new or copy products are variable. The preclinical expert therefore has to be able to formulate a view both as to the necessity of providing preclinical data and the need for GLP-compliance when selected preclinical studies are included with abridged applications.

27 Production of the expert report for good clinical practice

D B Jefferys

Introduction

This chapter will seek to explore the interrelationship between the clinical expert report and the approach to good clinical practice (GCP) within Europe. The requirements for expert reports were introduced in 1995 by Directive 75/319. The original concepts for the report came from the expert Agré system operating in France. Although the legal requirement was set out in 1975, the reports were introduced by the European Community (EC) member states in a rather slow manner over the next 13 years. In the UK, expert reports were required for new active substance applications from October 1985 and abridged applications from April 1986. The development of the clinical expert report will be described in detail later in this chapter.

In mid 1980s the concept of GCP was becoming established within Europe and at that stage there were a series of local and national guidelines. In the late 1980s the issue was taken up by the Committee for Proprietary Medicinal Products (the CPMP) and under the auspices of its efficacy working party, the EC guidelines were produced. The European guideline was issued for extensive consultation and comment during 1990 and was issued in its final form in July 1991, coming into effect on 1 January 1992 through Commission Directive 91/507/EEC. In retrospect it can be seen that both concepts were pursuing a similar objective from different angles. The EC GCP document had as its major theme education and self-regulation with the point of control being the sponsor. Thus, the document is directed towards sponsor audit and the obligations upon the sponsor to fulfil those responsibilities. This closely parallels the way in which the clinical expert report has widened to become regarded by some as the clinical expert report process. The common objective is to produce reliable, well-authenticated, high-quality clinical research brought together in a well-presented dossier which validates the proposed summary of product characteristics. GCP might be regarded as a critical appraisal of the procedure of the research, while the expert report is concerned with the critical appraisal of the development programme itself.

A third, perhaps complementary element which is now coming to the fore is good regulatory practice. These two or three concepts should be harnessed together to drive forward the successful development of a new drug and to speed its introduction into the market.

The development of the clinical expert report will now be considered further and its evolution into the expert report process alongside GCP presented. Inevitably, this will be considered from the perspective of a regulatory authority, but this may be appropriate since the regulatory authority is arguably the end customer for both GCP and the expert report.

The concepts of the European GCP guideline

Before considering the evolution of the clinical export report, it may be helpful to summarize the approach and concept behind the European GCP guideline. The GCP guideline seeks to set out the responsibilities of the sponsor and the responsibilities of the investigator (Jefferys, 1992). It is very much written as a guideline of best practice with a major emphasis on the education of the investigator and self-regulation by the sponsor company. The guideline sets out to guarantee a clear audit trial, which is important when one remembers that the clinical expert is meant to familiarize him- or herself with all the clinical data in the submission, including the raw data and the detailed protocols. The overarching thrust of the guideline is to ensure the quality, integrity and the authenticity of the data submitted in the dossier for authorization.

A significant driving force behind the development of the GCP guidelines in Europe was the emerging new regulatory procedures, at that time called the Future System, which came into effect at the beginning of 1995. Therefore, an additional objective of the guideline was to set a common standard whereby there could be an international acceptance of clinical trials undertaken across countries and, in addition, to ensure high quality research with adherence to protocols and appropriate statistical analysis. In Europe it was recognized that for both the centralized and decentralized procedures there needed to be a ready acceptance of studies performed across nations and of multicentre, multinational trials. This is a theme which has been taken further by the International Conference for Harmonization (ICH) which took up GCP as one of its major themes. Thus, if a study has been undertaken to GCP, then the data should be readily acceptable to different regulatory authorities.

GCP was introduced into Europe as a guideline. Subsequently, some of the technical requirements of the guideline were formerly introduced in the Commission Directive 91/507 which was implemented on 1 January 1992.

This guideline enshrines GCP in European law and also introduces the concept of an audit certificate. It does not, however, require GCP inspections to be undertaken across the European Union (EU), nor does it define what is required or indeed meant by an audit certificate. There have been two discussion papers produced by the EC on clinical trials in recent years and, at the end of 1994, the EC Commission indicated that it was considering bringing forward a clinical trials directive. Detailed discussions on this began in 1996. Parallel to this, several member states have been considering or introducing voluntary GCP inspections.

The evolution of the clinical expert report

The requirement for expert reports was set out in Article 2 of Directive 75/319/EEC. This specified that each of the three parts of the dossier should include an expert report. This requirement applied to all types of applications, excluding at that time variations and clinical trial applications. The absence of a properly prepared expert report constituted grounds for refusing the application. The clinical expert report has developed significantly over the intervening 20 years. Its development has paralleled that of GCP. Indeed, many of the concepts behind the clinical expert report have influenced the European GCP guidelines and, similarly, some of the new requirements for GCP have fed back into the expert report process. This should not be surprising since both concepts have the same aim, which is to improve the quality of regulatory submissions and the scientific documentation within the dossier.

The original idea behind the expert report came from the expert Agré system in France. Although the requirement for expert reports was set out in the 1975 Directive, the reports only slowly became mandatory across Europe during the next 14 years. In the UK, expert reports were required for new drug applications from October 1985 and for abridged applications from October 1986.

The original objectives of the expert report were fourfold. First, they were to aid the assessment process by requiring applicants to undertake their own assessment of the dossier. In effect, applicants were being asked to write their own or, perhaps more accurately, a draft assessment report. Thus, many of the detailed requirements of the expert report arose from the assessment requirement of the mid 1980s. Second, it was hoped that by introducing a formal critical assessment document, this would guide and focus the development of the candidate product. Third, the objectives of the report were to improve regulatory submissions by requiring a named independent expert effectively to 'sign-off' the dossier. Within this there was a particular problem in the mid 1980s of premature dossiers and it was believed that the expert report should help reduce the number of such premature applications. Finally, the objectives of the approach were to produce updated reports for the then multistate procedure and, subsequently, for the Concertation procedure which was introduced in July 1987.

During its subsequent evolution, the clinical expert report in particular has centred upon the critical assessment of the dossier and as such has developed into a major element within the quality assurance process within the development of the product. Thus, the links between the clinical expert report and GCP have become more firmly established.

Presentation of the expert report

The clinical expert report is normally less than 25 pages in length. This has posed considerable difficulties over the years, principally because of a misunderstanding over the role of the expert report. Many have complained that it is not possible to summarize the clinical part of the dossier within 25 pages. This has missed the point that the report is not meant to be a summary, but rather a critical assessment of the dossier, only summarizing important issues when it is necessary to produce a free-standing document. This misunderstanding led to very lengthy clinical expert reports being generated in the first few years. These were usually summaries and not critical assessments. The longest clinical expert report received in the UK exceeded 800 pages. With this in mind, the UK regulatory authorities embarked upon a major educational exercise assisted by the Trade Associations. At the same time, in the 1989 edition of the *Notice to Applicants* (Committee for Proprietary Medicinal Products, 1989), it was made clear that the factual written summary was valuable, but that this should be attached as an annex (with appropriate cross-references) to the clinical expert report. In addition, a series of tables were requested. In the 1995 edition of the *Notice to Applicants* this has been taken a stage further with the stipulation of a tabular overview as a more detailed requirement for a written summary which will be used in the development of the new assessment report.

The written summary

The 1995 edition of the *Notice to Applicants* gives considerable guidance on the requirements for the summary. It should be factual, complete and concise. There should be cross-references to the documentation in the relevant part of the dossier and, as appropriate, the summary may include tables, graphs, etc. It is made clear that duplication should be avoided between the summary and the expert report. Wherever possible a tabular presentation should be used.

The written summary is particularly required for:

1 New active substances.
2 Abridged applications with reference to the published literature.
3 Other abridged applications where the volume and complexity indicate that a summary would be helpful.

The summary should be preceded by the overview table which, again, is a new requirement in the 1995 edition of the *Notice to Applicants*. The summary should usually not be longer than 30 pages, although a longer summary of up to 100 pages may be necessary for complex dossiers, multiple indications and/or large numbers of patients evaluable for safety and efficacy. The need for such summaries is to help facilitate mutual recognition and especially to facilitate the secondary assessment, which will be a key feature of the new decentralized system.

The role of the clinical expert

The role of the clinical expert is arguably one of the most important in the development of the new medicine. The expert is meant to analyse the dossier critically and 'to take and defend a clear position on the product'. The expert is meant to consult the current CPMP guidelines and to discuss any deviations from these guidelines which have occurred during the development of the product. The expert is also required to consider the data in the light of the GCP guideline and this will be discussed in greater depth later in this chapter.

The expert is asked to consider carefully the summary of product characteristics and the labelling and the patient information leaflet. The expert is asked to make comments on these documents and to ensure that statements in the product literature accurately reflect the data in the dossier. It can thus be seen that the expert report is a document for critically assessing the dossier and not for summarizing it. The new statements on the summary should help ensure that the expert report is used for its prime purpose. A frequent question is: who should undertake the role of the expert? The legislation simply states that the clinical expert report has to be signed by one person who has a formal qualification in medicine. A brief curriculum vitae is asked for and, in particular, this should record the relevant background of the expert and his or her involvement with the product and its development. The supplementary questions are: should the expert be a company physician or an independent expert? Can additional experts be involved in the production of the report and/or sign the report? Let us explore these issues in a little more depth.

The production of the expert report

The expert report has evolved into a process, rather than a document to be generated as a final element in the compilation of the dossier. It is for this reason that some now refer to the expert report process rather than just the expert report. Four quotations from senior research and development executives are given in answer to the question below.

When to produce the expert report?

'Useless 2 months before the submission'.
'At least 6 months before submission'.
'When the candidate product enters phase II development'.
'A living document reflecting the development of the product and produced during the development of the product'.

These quotations make clear the notion that the expert report should be brought together during the development of the product. Thus, it becomes a key part of the quality assurance programme and will have close links with the European concept of GCP. One approach to the development of the product and the expert report is to draft the putative summary of product characteristics at the beginning of the phase II development and then to develop the critical expert report alongside the clinical studies. Thus, the expert report process should be at the heart of the development of the product. This enables the possible deficiencies in the development of the dossier to be highlighted and new studies to be commissioned or new analyses undertaken. Particular examples where this has been done successfully have included the recognition that additional drug interaction studies were required or the need for specific safety monitoring in the light of signals generated from the preclinical data or the need for additional patients to be studied in particular at-risk groups, such as the elderly or those with renal impairment.

It is clear that if the clinical expert report is written at the end of the development phase, the report can only serve to highlight deficiencies and cannot seek to remedy them with additional information.

The development of a modern medicinal product is a significant undertaking and thus many individuals from different disciplines are likely to be involved in the development of the expert report. For a new active substance, it is likely that there will be a drafting team involving those from a variety of disciplines taking part in the development of the product. Such a drafting team may profitably include external experts who can give a more detached and perhaps critical view of the development of the product. These experts should be involved at an early stage. The drafting group is also likely to include medical writers who may be involved in the production of the report.

There will be a need for an interrelationship between the pharmaceutical/biological expert report, the preclinical expert report and that of the clinical expert. In particular, there are issues which will carry through all three parts of the dossier. These may include issues of bioavailability, stability, impurity profiles and, in the preclinical dossier, issues such as mutagenicity, carcinogenicity, reproductive toxicology, comparator pharmacokinetics and, especially, target organ toxicity. The clinical expert will wish to see that there are appropriate statements in the product details and in the labelling reflecting any bioavailability or stability issues and that there is a reassurance of a lack of any target organ toxicity produced in animals from subsequent human studies. Again, it will be important for the clinical expert to analyse carefully the Summary of Product Characteristic (SPC) to see that preclinical concerns are adequately reflected in the special precautions, warnings and in the statement on use in pregnancy.

For particular applications which involve a niche or novel product, it may be desirable to involve an external expert of considerable standing. In other instances it may be appropriate to list one or two key experts who have contributed to the development of the report. It is, however, a requirement that the final report is signed by one person who takes full responsibility and ownership for the report. This is considered essential in that, whilst it is an expert report process, at the end of that process there needs to be accountability and a clear statement from one individual.

How do regulatory authorities use the expert report?

How should applicants use the expert report process?

The statement below from Dr J C Ritchie given in *ESRA News and Views*, November 1993, clearly captures the expectations of the regulatory authority and the opportunity provided to the industry by the expert report process. This quotation is reproduced in full.

Industry must strive to capture and communicate the picture of the product's development through time to regulators so that they can understand how and why some of the critical decisions were taken during development. In Europe we are extremely fortunate in being able to do this through the provision of Expert Reports. These documents represent a marvellous opportunity for the company to present and explain the rationale for the product's development, as well as being the forum for addressing potential regulatory issues. However, as an assessor I found that all too frequently this opportunity was missed.

Use of the expert report by the regulatory authority

The expert report is a key document for regulatory authorities. It is used by assessors to guide their subsequent work and to give them a clear view of the issues contained within the dossier. A good expert report can greatly reduce the time taken to assessment, perhaps by up to a factor of 3. This is in addition to the benefits produced by the expert report process on the development of the product and the production of the dossier itself. Assessors will usually read the expert report immediately after considering the summary of product characteristics. If the expert report is appropriately cross-referenced, they will then proceed in a hierarchical manner through the dossier, addressing particular issues. In the UK the complete expert report is laid before the Advisory Committees such as the Committee on the Safety of Medicines (CSM). During 1994 a major project undertaken by the countries of the EU was to generate a new assessment report guideline (CPMP, 1994). This guideline is also likely to be accepted as the new guideline for the PER countries (the pharmaceutical evaluation report scheme) which encompasses countries such as Hungary, Australia, South Africa, Canada, as well as those of the EU. This guideline reinforces the importance of the expert report since the expert and the summary will play a major role in the development of the new assessment report, which will be the vehicle transmitted between member states. The assessment report is the vehicle through which the decentralized procedure will operate. The expert report will also be an integral part of the final assessment report. Thus, the new European licensing system will further reinforce the importance of the expert report and its role. It is for this reason that such considerable emphasis has been given by regulatory authorities in seeking to improve the standard of expert reports, not only for new active substance applications, but more recently for abridged applications.

How should companies use the expert report process?

The expert report process is, as Dr Ritchie described, a unique opportunity for applicants to present their document to national and supranational advisory bodies. It is the opportunity to describe the development of the product and the particular issues faced during the development. The document should be used to analyse the dossier critically and to explore any contentious issues. Moreover, it is the vehicle to anticipate issues and to consider any potential deficiencies in the dossier. The expert should look for any weaknesses in the dossier and the data and then seek to argue why these are not of potential concern to regulatory authorities. The expert should seek to justify fully the efficacy of the product and to provide reassurance as to the safe use of the product in normal clinical practice. There is therefore a common way of judging the expert report by both the applicant and by the regulatory authority. It should be that the concerns (if any) raised by regulatory authorities should be those clearly set out as issues in the expert report. It may well be that the regulatory authority perceives these to be of greater significance and to be the provisional grounds for refusing a marketing authorizaton, whereas the applicant considers that the issues are adequately addressed and do not constitute grounds for refusing the authorization. This is ultimately a matter of judgement and different positions may be taken by the regulatory authority and by the applicant. However, if there are issues not set out in the expert report, but raised by the regulatory authority, then there may be only two possible explanations. The first is that the expert has missed the issues, or the second is that the regulatory authority has misunderstood the data in the dossier. If the latter is the case, then this is why assessment reports are now made available to the applicant and there are appeal procedures. Perhaps too frequently the former position is found to occur, with issues inadequately discussed in the expert report. The requirement for a critical analysis is still taken too lightly by some experts who prefer to concentrate on summarizing the data and on highlighting the strengths of a product and the dossier rather than recognizing the potential weaknesses. This is a major missed opportunity and one that is rather short-sighted. A good example of this was provided in a dossier for an antihypertensive product, when the expert report concentrated on the two studies which demonstrated efficacy and failed to describe the third study which did not demonstrate efficacy. It was left to the assessor within the regulatory authority to note that this study was undertaken in patients from a mixed racial background and that this was the reason why efficacy was not adequately demonstrated in the third study.

The expert report and quality assurance

It can be seen that the expert report has developed into a part of the quality assurance programme for both the clinical development phase of the product and for the production of the dossier. Thus, the production of the clinical expert report is now a major task which should lie at the centre of the development programme. Arguably, it is no longer a task that can be undertaken by one individual, but has to be brought together in a final document written and owned by one person. Many of the themes within the European GCP guideline equally apply to the role of the clinical expert. In particular, these are to be found in adherence to the protocol, statistical analyses and the integrity of the data. The clinical expert has, however, been given specific tasks within the role of GCP.

GCP was introduced into Europe through the CPMP guideline and through the requirements in the Commission Directive 91/507. It was originally envisaged that there would be a GCP Directive sitting alongside or, indeed, as a part of a clinical trials directive. This has not yet occurred and therefore in March 1992 it was recognized that there was a difficulty, since GCP had been brought forward but there was no adequate mechanism for implementing it. Therefore, it was decided that as an interim measure there should be a new section within the clinical expert report which would be entitled 'Compliance with GCP'. The expert was therefore asked to ensure that all studies undertaken after 1 January 1992 complied with GCP and, furthermore, the expert was asked to comment on any studies not complying with GCP. In this the expert was asked to state why guidelines (not necessarily the European guidelines) had not been complied with. It was also recognized that many studies may have been commenced, or indeed, undertaken before the new European guideline was adopted. Therefore, the expert was asked to note whether any studies had been undertaken before 1 July 1991, and whether these had been undertaken in accordance with GCP guidelines then operating in other territories or in other areas, and furthermore, to comment on any deficiencies in these studies. At the time of the production of this statement, it was envisaged that this would last for 1 or 2 years. In the event this requirement has remained in force somewhat longer. It is likely to be set out in the revision of Part IIB of the *Notice to Applicants* which is currently being undertaken.

This section has led to significant concerns and requests for clarification. It is not envisaged that the clinical expert will familiarize him- or herself with the entire dossier and act as an independent auditor. Rather, it is intended that this statement should be considered alongside the CPMP *Good Clinical Practice* guideline which clearly lays the obligations for GCP on the sponsor with the requirement for sponsor audit. Thus, it would be envisaged that the clinical expert will seek information from the sponsor as to the procedures which the sponsor has in place to audit the studies and to verify the data. The expert would be required to make comments on the data quality assurance programme within the company and for the arrangements put in place for the audit and quality assurance of the data for the studies and, in particular, the pivotal studies undertaken for the particular product. It would not be envisaged that the clinical expert would go beyond this. The expert would be expected to give a statement as to the procedures which the sponsor has in place to fulfil the requirements of the CPMP guideline. To aid in this, it is likely that most companies will be given audit certificates for particular studies and increasingly these may be augmented by GCP compliance certificates given by EC member states.

Future developments

The expert report has evolved significantly in the last 20 years. The expert report has now become a living document and is often required to be updated both during the initial assessment and with the new European licensing arrangements during the subsequent mutual recognition phase of the decentralized procedure (Jones and Jefferys, 1994). Moreover, the document may well be required to be updated for certain renewal applications and for the more complex type II variations. Thus, the role of the export report is likely to be further enhanced. In all of this, the clinical expert report can be seen as a part of the quality assurance programme alongside the more formal GCP guideline. Both have as their objective the production of a high-quality dossier reporting high-quality science. On its own, GCP is rather sterile; it needs the clinical expert report process to generate the interactive element leading to the high-quality scientifically based development programme. Both these developments will be essential for the health of the industry and to aid the regulatory process move into the next millennium.

References

Cartwright, A. C. and Jefferys, D. B. (1987) Expert Reports for Product Licence Applications in Europe – a Regulatory Review. *Pharmaceutical Medicine* **2:** 229–237.

Committee for Proprietary Medicinal Products (1988) *Good Clinical Practice for Trials on Medicinal Products in the EC.* III/3976/88.

Committee for Proprietary Medicinal Products (1989) *Guidelines on the Quality, Safety and Efficacy of Medicinal Products for Human Use: Notice to Applicants for Marketing Authorisations for Medicinal Products for Human Use in the Member States of the European Community.*

Committee for Proprietary Medicinal Products (1994) *Guideline on the Assessment Report.* III/9447/94.

Directive 75/319 (1993) *The Rules Governing Medicinal Products in the EC,* vol. 1. III/5826/93

Draft Notice to Applicants 1994. III/5944/94.

Jefferys, D. B. (1992) Good clinical practice: EC expectations, education, self-regulation, or imposition? *Drug Information Journal* **26:** 609–613.

Jones, K. and Jefferys, D. (1994) EMEA and the new pharmaceutical procedures for Europe. *Health Trends* **26:** 10–13.

PART TEN

Computers

28   Validation of computer databases for GxP

S H Segalstad

Introduction

Computer systems may be used to replace manual systems partly or fully, or may be used as additions to a complete manual system. These two types of system use have to be treated totally differently in the pharmaceutical industry. The authorities demand heavy documentation for the development and production of our pharmaceutical products. The requirements include both quality assurance (QA) and quality control (QC). Regulatory computer systems which we use have to fulfil the same requirements. Validation of computer systems is an important issue addressed as a demand in all the pharmaceutical standards. Even the development (programming) of the computer system has to follow QA procedures, and the users are responsible for the quality of the systems they use. This chapter will explain how to reach a stadium of a validated database, and has reference to more literature on the issue.

Please note that at the time of writing the author was employed within the pharmaceutical industry and some comments therefore reflect this.

Definitions

Non-regulatory computer systems

Computer systems used as an addition to a complete manual system are not regarded as regulatory systems and do not need to be treated as such. Examples of non-regulatory computer systems are databases or other systems used for collecting and querying information across manual files, for giving better and more accessible overviews, for keeping track of resources like personnel, equipment and workload, and like word-processing systems. Accounting systems are also regarded as non-regulatory systems for the pharmaceutical industry, but may have to comply with other regulatory rules from a business or economic perspective.

Regulatory computer systems

Computer systems used for generating or storing raw data, calculating data, or used instead of manual systems are regarded as regulatory systems. Such systems have to be treated like all other types of equipment, as described in good manufacturing practice (GMP), good laboratory practice (GLP) and good clinical practice (GCP). This involves QA and QC, and includes standard operating procedures (SOPs), control, and validation, in addition to documentation that the procedures have been followed as described.

Validation

Validation is 'establishing documented evidence that provides a high degree of assurance that a specific process will consistently produce a product meeting its predetermined specifications and quality attributes' (Food and Drug Administration, 1987). This definition is used for all types of validation, also for computer systems. It is totally the end-user's responsibility to validate the system as it is used in the user's environment.

Standards and guidelines for compliance, and their enforcement

Most countries have appointed international GMP/GLP/GCP guidelines if they have not established their own national sets. In general there is little difference between the different national/international guidelines of each of the three types – GMP, GLP and GCP. However, most of these guidelines do not include specific descriptions of how to handle computer systems or computerized systems. All describe how to handle equipment, and regulatory computer systems are regarded as equipment. GCP, (GCP: EEC Note for Guidance, 1990) has the strictest approach: 'must use validated, error free data processing programmes'. This means that computer systems cannot be used for GCP, as there as yet is no such thing as an error-free system. To our knowledge the regulatory agencies have not enforced this, but care should be taken to ensure quality in a GCP system, as well as in GMP and GLP systems. Pharmaceutical Inspection Convention (PIC), GMP (1991) includes the requirement: 'Validation should be considered as part of the complete life cycle of a computer system'. This GMP has one chapter focusing on computerized systems. The UK Department of Health (1989) has published an advisory leaflet covering applications of GLP principles to computer systems. The Japanese inspection authorities and Organization for Economic Cooperation and Development (OECD; 1992) have drawn up equivalent documents.

A problem with these guidelines is that they include terms like adequate, enough and high degree of assurance, but they do not define these words. Words like these make it unnecessary to change the guidelines each time the requirements change. But is also makes it difficult for companies to stay in compliance with such guidelines, as these small words can be variously interpreted.

In order to stay in current compliance at any time it is important to keep the knowledge of the demands updated. There are several journals which target these issues.[1, 2] The little words also make it possible for a stricter interpretation to be made each time an inspection is performed, as the inspectors will find that one company has done something well, and then they will add this as a requirement for the next company. This helps to increase demands. If the pharmaceutical companies did more bench-marking in order to stay on the same level, the demands would not accelerate so quickly.

The strictest approach to the *handling* of computer systems is found in the enforcement of GLP, as described in the UK Department of Health advisory leaflet number 1, and as Food and Drug Administration (FDA) inspectors have shown in their audits of computer systems for GLP around 1993. The reports from the FDA audits are available from the FDA[3] under the Freedom of Information Act. The reports include comments on the lack of vendor audits, the lack of system development in a quality environment, as well as lack of standard operation procedures, change control and disaster recovery procedures and lack of documentation of what has been done.

We can safely assume that this approach will also be included for GMP and GCP in the future. As our present systems and development projects for new products hopefully will be used in the future, we will be erring on the side of safety if we apply the strictest approach to all our computer systems now.

ISO 9000 Series

The pharmaceutical industry does not have to comply with the ISO 9000 series or its equivalents. ISO 9000 is an international quality standard which is increasingly used in various industries. However, it is well worth studying the guideline ISO 9000–3 (1991) to ISO 9001, which covers the life cycle of a computer system with emphasis on the development stages. Basically it describes a QA system for the life cycle development of a computer system, but the description can easily be modified to give good ideas for the operation phase of a computer system.

[1]The Gold Sheet, 5550 Friendship Blvd, Suite One, Chevy Chase, MD 20815, USA.
[2]European Federation of Pharmaceutical Industries' Association (EFPIA), Avenue Louise 250, Boîte 91, B-1050, Brussels, Belgium.
[3]Food and Drug Administration, US Department of Health and Human Services, 5600 Fishers Lane, Rockville, MD 20857, USA.

Vendors with an ISO 9000 or equivalent certificate are usually serious vendors. They have built the quality into their system. They have proven that they have QA systems, including QA organization, and QA procedures for development and control. But the certificate does not say anything about the *level* of quality. It is possible to get an ISO 9000 certificate for the manufacture of a small, noisy, gas-consuming car that breaks down after 10,000 miles, if you just state that this is your level of quality!

Roles

Different persons in the organization have different responsibilities for the computer system. These roles must be defined and documented, preferably in an SOP for each system. There are often four or five roles involved for a large computer system, but there might be more, or fewer.

The *application manager* is responsible for implementing the system and suggesting necessary changes. Changes must be made in order to make optimal use of the system, and may be made in the system itself, in the way we work, or in the organization. The application manager is responsible for having SOPs written for the system, for keeping track of all documentation, updating the user handbook, etc, but may not have to perform it himself/herself. Some organizations will want to have the system manager or application manager in the information system (IS) department, whereas others may want to have one of the users as the application manager.

There might be a *superuser* in some or each of the departments where the system is used. He or she acts as a first-hand trouble-shooter for users and relays the problems to the application manager when needed. In a smaller system the application manager might have this role as well. Suggestions for system changes may come from superusers, who may also implement the approved changes.

This *IS person* is responsible for back-ups, hardware, installation of new software and maintenance of the systems.

The *QA department* also has a role, as QA authorizes the SOPs, the validation protocols and reports for the system. QA may also comment on security issues.

The *user* has a role as a user. In complex systems there may be different types of users depending on their type of job in the organization, which should also be reflected in the user access of the system when possible.

In our organization we have three levels of key persons for a large application: the application manager, the superusers in the departments, and the IS person. We think we are better off having a user as the application manager, as the user will know the work which the system is supposed to aid getting done. Today most computer systems are so easy to handle that computer experts are not needed as application managers. There is a superuser in each department where the system is in use. Each system has one IS person assigned, but most IS people are responsible for several systems. Additionally we have QA persons with special responsibilities for computer systems for regulatory GxP use, and of course normal users. Key persons for smaller applications like instrument computers may have one application manager plus some aid from the IS department, in addition to users. Discussions with many application managers have revealed that most organizations prefer users to fill the application manager role to IS persons.

The system may have groups with responsibilities for the system, like a steering committee and a work group.

The *steering committee* (parliament) for a system will make the political decisions on how to proceed, how to prioritize the different jobs to be done with the system, and say yes or no to suggested changes. The committee is definitely needed for a large system with users in various parts of the organization. Members of the committee should come from the upper echelons of the organization where the system is used, and consist of people either from the top management there, or somebody who has been assigned the same authorities. Members of the steering committee do not have to know the technical parts or the use of the system, but must be willing to cooperate with persons in the work group who do.

The *work group* (government) for the system consists of key persons like the application manger, the superusers, and the IS persons – all, or some of them. These are the people who know the system well, and they must be able to communicate with a steering committee which does not have a comprehensive knowledge of the technical parts of the system. This means that they must be able to translate technical issues into everyday language, and may suggest changes for the steering committee, as well as performing the changes suggested or approved by the steering committee.

Validation

GMP, GLP and GCP all have requirements of validated computer systems, but no details on how this can be achieved. The regulatory agencies have no guidelines to validation or computer systems except that they have to be validated. Many consultants claim that validation is so difficult that only experts can do it, and they are the only experts. It is the author's firm belief that we are much better off being part of it ourselves than letting experts do it for us. However, we can use the expertise of the consultants, and do the job together with them. It is most important that the consultants who provide the knowledge also transfer the technology to the user. We may do the job with a consultant or without, but should never let the consultant do it alone.

The reason is that we are the only experts on our use of a system. We are the ones to be audited by the authorities and those who need to know what we have done regarding QA and validation of the system when we are audited. It is not an excuse to say: 'Consultants did the work for us and we don't know anything about this'.

Performing the validation together with a consultant or by ourselves will let us be in charge of what is going on, and will also give us the knowledge of what is done. If we leave it to the consultant, we might get a validation, but not necessarily one which reflects our way of working with the system, and thus not a good one. There are some consultants who write a statement like: 'I have inspected the NN computer system(s) of NN company. As of today they are in compliance with ...'. Changes done after that will not be their responsibility, which makes the statement not even worth the paper it was written on, as we do make continuous changes in the system. If we work with them instead, we know what has been going on, and we can answer questions from the regulatory agencies. We are also then able to keep a change control system, which, if performed well enough, will give us a computer system in a validated state at any given time.

It is up to each organization to define the extent of the validation needed. This is both an advantage and a disadvantage. The disadvantage is that they will have to make the definitions themselves and be able to defend them when authorities audit the systems. This requires a lot of knowledge about the system, the organization and the interpretation of the requirements. The advantage is the freedom of making one's own interpretation, and performing the work one deems necessary.

Validation is much more than having a validation plan or test plan carried through. The GMP statement that validation is part of the complete life cycle (see below) means that the system will be developed in compliance with QA/QC norms, for example like the description in ISO 9000-3.

A system should be validated before use, as we are not supposed to use systems for regulatory purposes until they have been validated. However, quite often we have systems which have been in use for a long time without ever having been validated. These must undergo retrospective validation, which is described below.

Computer system life cycle

The computer system development life cycle (SDLC) and its requirements for QA and QC have been discussed by both McDowall (1991) and Segalstad (1995). SDLC means built-in quality from the very beginning, when planning a new system, to the very end when retiring the system. Buyers should include demands of quality in the requirement specification which is made before acquiring the new system. In this context, 'acquiring' means all nuances, from developing the whole system themselves to buying the complete system off the shelf.

However, we are often faced with being the owners of systems where this requirement was not included when we acquired the system. We might be using a system of uncertain, and possibly missing, built-in quality.

As owners we are responsible for knowing the state of quality of the system. We must be sure that the quality was built in from the beginning. This can be done by auditing the vendor or programmer. The liberty of doing so should be included in the requirement specification and/or the contract. Even if it were not included originally, it may be possible to have an audit, as most vendors welcome auditors.

A large part of the SDLC is the operation phase of the system. The quality of this can only be ensured by the users. As the chain is no stronger than its weakest link, the quality of the computer system is no better than the quality of the weakest part of the SDLC. The operation of the system should be well-described and documented, and is included in more detail below.

Handling computer systems of uncertain built-in quality.

When the pharmaceutical industry produces its drugs, the quality of the product is not determined by the end control only. We are required to apply QA procedures and prove that they have been followed all the way through the production of the drug. The end control does not replace the built-in quality. On the contrary, end control is virtually replaced by the procedures and is just a final check that the procedures were followed. Validating a computer system is equivalent to the end control, and does not replace built-in quality.

Whether we are sure or unsure of the built-in quality of the computer system, we must collect as much data as possible to show that the system is good enough to use in the pharmaceutical industry. If the vendors are still in operation, they might answer our letter with questions about the built-in quality of the system. We can also perform an audit if this is appropriate.

All available papers and documents regarding the system should be organized and stored in one accessible place. This includes all the documents created during the planning of a new system, letters to and from the vendor, log books for the system and SOPs. It may be possible to reconstruct some of the documents if they are not available, but they should be clearly marked with today's date, and not passed off as old originals. If SOPs have not been written, now is the time to do so.

Collecting the documentation which the organization feels is adequate for the purpose of validation is by far better than just telling the auditors that: 'This system has worked well for more than 6 years, so the quality must be good!' Having some documentation means that the auditor will have to prove that this is not enough, while having nothing will surely give rise to comment in the audit report.

Database validation

Most of the newer commercial database systems for G*x*P use have been built on databases regarded as industry standards. Oracle is probably the most widely used database, but others are also considered industry standards. The databases may run on VAX/VMS, UNIX and other computers or operating systems which may be regarded as industry standards. Some of the most used networking protocols fall into this category as well.

We do not need to validate the industry standards, because we can assume that they work the way they are supposed to. But our clinical system and our lab information system, built on the industrial standard tools, must be validated on site by us. There is no such thing as buying a validated database system, like some vendors like to advertise. The vendor can sell a quality system which has been built in conformance to, for example, ISO 9000-3 and tested, but it is not possible to sell a validated system. Even if the vendor sells the whole package of hardware and software, it still has to be validated in our environment, because every change, including moving the equipment, calls for change control with at least a minor revalidation or verification check. Also, the validation is not only the test, it is also the collection of the documents as described above. As users we must prove that our system works the way it is supposed to do in our environment, with our computer, our network and, not least, with our way of using the system.

When we buy the database program, what we are buying is a standard database with defined tables, columns, relations between the different tables and columns, and interfaces (screen pictures or forms) with the different column contents. Predefined keys for certain commands may also be included in the package for queries, updates or tables, moving around on screen, etc. The new database generally contains no data, and we must find out what kind of data we want to put where if there is a choice. We must also define the normal operating procedures for using the system, and document this in the SOP system we are required to have.

We have to validate our own use of the system. We do not need to validate parts of the system which we do not use, but we do have to explain in the protocol why we did not validate these parts. If we decide to use these parts later we must validate them before use.

Vendors can definitely help with their knowledge of the validation procedure, providing they also know the regulatory rules to which the customer has to comply. We might be able to get some suggestions from vendors on how to validate the system, but we should hesitate to use their validation diskette as our complete test suite. Usually their suggestion for validation does not reflect our use of the system. Then there is always a chance that they deliberately choose to omit a test which would show a bug or a deficiency in the program.

Validation protocol

A validation protocol must contain certain information briefly described below. For more details, refer to Segalstad (1994). Although this reference is targeting the LIMS system, it contains demands and suggests solutions for validating any type of computer system for GMP/GLP/GCP.

Well detailed SOPs (see Appendix 1) will automatically minimize the need for validating all aspects of the system. The validation can be limited to use according to the SOPs. It is therefore wise to write the SOPs before the protocol.

The content should include:

1 Descriptive chapters: describing what the system is, including details of version for hardware and software.
2 Responsibilities: who is responsible for what during the validation period.
3 Assumptions, exceptions and limitations: what not to include in the validation plan and why it is not included.
4 The validation plan: the plan must include all details for every step, so that it is possible to repeat the very same procedure later during revalidation.
5 Error handling plan: how to handle errors which may be found during the validation.
6 Acceptance criteria: set the frames for what errors may be acceptable, and what may not be acceptable for the use of the system.
7 Documents: list all the available documents for the system, as described earlier. The documents need not be in the protocol, but reference should be made to which documents exist and where they are located. Additionally, many new documents will be created during the validation.
8 Test plan: the test plan should include all aspects of how the system is handled in daily use. Follow a key object (study, sample, etc) through the system in all possible ways. The plan must be written in such detail that it is possible to follow it later for revalidation.
9 Post-validation: a validation report should be written, and the distribution list may also be included in the plan. The follow-up on errors found must be explained.

Protocols and reports should preferably be written by the application manager or other key person, but they must be authorized by QA. Good QA is to avoid testing being performed by the persons who wrote the protocol if possible, and definitely to avoid authorizing one's own work.

Retrospective validation

Retrospective validation is done when a system has been in use for some time. The same documents as mentioned above should be collected, but the test plan may be minimized or omitted provided we have other documentation to show that the system has operated properly during this time. Documents like that must be collected as well, and may include, but are not limited to:

1   Comparison: comparison between two systems, for example the old manual system and this system, or this system and an other comparable validated system.
2   Data collection: if the system has been in use for a long period, there may be data available which can show that the system has worked the way it should during the operational time.
3   Calibration and control data: if the system has been calibrated, controlled and checked directly or indirectly, records for this should be obtained.

Standard operation procedures needed

The extent of SOPs for any system depends on the complexity of each system. If there is more than one way to do something in the system, the standard way of doing it must be described if it makes a difference which way is chosen. A less complex system will have less need for SOPs as there are fewer things to explain. The SOPs must also reflect the organization where appropriate, for example when access, approvals and training are concerned.

There are no rules for how SOPs should be written, how long they should be, and how many topics each SOP should cover. The most important thing is that each system has an SOP or SOPs to cover all the necessary issues appropriate for the system. Many organizations generally keep the SOPs to a maximum of 10 pages, otherwise they are too troublesome to read, and thus to follow.

The art of SOP writing

Writing SOPs is an art. SOPs must be phrased so that it is possible to follow them, but at the same time not in such detail that they must be changed more often than once every year or two, at the most. It can save a lot of work writing them in an artistic way from the beginning. From our own experience we suggest that all the how-tos are referred to the manuals, but the whos, the whats, the whens, the whys, and the responsibilities must be explained in the SOPs. Refer to other SOPs instead of copying the content from one SOP to the other. If the content is copied, there are two or more SOPs to be updated every time there is a change. Try to avoid the use of personal names, but rather use titles which do not change as often as the names of the responsible person. Do not write: 'Jim Smith must do this', (if he is the application manager). Write instead 'The application manager is responsible for having this done'. The responsibility has been described, but the name of the person is not given, and he or she does not have to perform the job him- or herself. The job description for Jim Smith should state that it is his job to be the application manager, and thus the name of the application manager is given somewhere. If there is a new application manager later, the SOP does not need to be changed, as the new manager's job description will explain that this is his or her responsibility.

Our SOP for the use of our large LIMS system has only one page, which describes who can use the system, the training needs for the persons (reference to another SOP), access control (reference to another SOP) and the statement that the system should be used according to our own user handbook. In this way we do not have to update the SOP every time there is a change in the system. But we do have SOPs for change control, which comprises how and where to document changes in the system, including the user handbook.

References

Department of Health (1989) Good laboratory practice advisory leaflet number 1. *The Application of GLP Principles to Computer Systems.* United Kingdom GLP compliance programme. London: GLP Monitoring Authority.

Food and Drug Administration (1987).

GCP: EEC Note for Guidance (1990) *Good Clinical Practice for Trials on Medicinal Products in the European Community III/3976/88.*

ISO 9000-3 (1991) *Quality Management and Quality Assurance Standards – Part 3: Guidelines for the Application of ISO 9001 to the Development, Supply and Maintenance of Software.* Geneva: International Organization for Standardization.

McDowall, R. D. (1991) The systems development life cycle. *Chemometrics and Intelligent Laboratory Systems: Laboratory Information Management* **13:** 121–133.

OECD (1995) *Concepts Relating to Computerised Systems in a GLP Environment Monograph 10.*

PIC GMP (1991) *Pharmaceutical Inspection Convention Guide to Good Manufacturing Practice for Pharmaceutical Products. Annex 5, Document number PH5/92.*

Segalstad, S. H. (1994) A practical guide to validating LIMS. *Chemometrics and Intelligent Laboratory Systems: Laboratory Information Management* **26:** 1–12.

Segalstad, S. H. (1995) Quality assurance of computer systems. What is needed to comply with ISO 9000, GMP, GLP, and GCP? *Laboratory Automation and Information Management* **31:** 11–24.

Appendix

There are several issues in need of coverage in SOPs. Some issues are not applicable for some systems – access levels do not have to be described if there is only one level. The SOPs may be divided broadly into SOP issues needed for the end-user and SOP issues needed for the key persons if there is a need to divide the issues into more than one SOP. Again, the division is greatly dependent on the type of system.

1 Daily use of this system: What will it be used for? Who will be using it? Refer to user handbook or user manual if necessary.
2 Access to application: Who will have access to the system? If the system defines access levels, who will have access to what commands? How are additions and changes in access documented? Who will decide what access each user is to have? Who will perform changes?
3 Training: The extent of training for normal users and for expert users. Who is responsible for the training? What is the extent of the training in hours/days? What is training curriculum?
4 Responsibilities: Description of the roles for the system and their responsibilities.
5 Security: Security in and around the system. This may include access restrictions to the building, machine room and terminals, security for the machine, the operating system, the database and the application itself. It may also include a description of different types of access in the application.
6 System adaptation: How is the system to be constructed to suit our needs? (Describe in great detail.)
7 Standardization: Nomenclature for the fields in the screen, if this is not self-evident (the fields correspond to columns in the database), key definitions, upper or lower-case letters, language (important in multi-national companies), definitions.
8 System maintenance: Back-ups, periodic testing routines, maintenance. How and where are problem to be documented?

9   Change control hardware (machines, disks, network, peripheral equipment): What is to be done about desired changes and emergency changes? Documentation and procedures for change: Who will initiate the change? Who will approve the change to be done? Who will perform the change? Who will control what has been done and see if it had the correct effect? Who is to give final approval of the change? How is it documented?

10 Change control software (new versions of program, local changes in the system): What is to be done with desired changes and emergency changes? Documentation and procedures for change: Who will initiate the change? Who will approve the change to be done? Who will perform the change? Who will control what has been done and see that it had the correct effect? Who is to give final approval of the change? How is it documented?

11 Disaster recovery procedures: What is to be done when the system is not in operation? Definition of acceptable limits of down periods. How is the system to be set in operation?

Appendix I Animal health industries and GCP

Good Clinical Practice for the Conduct of Clinical Trials for Veterinary Medicinal Products (GCPV)

The EU note for guidance

This EU guideline on the *Good Clinical Practice for the Conduct of Clinical Trials for Veterinary Medicinal Products* (GCPV), takes its essence from the *Code of Practice for the Conduct of Clinical Trials on Veterinary Medicinal Products in the European Community* issued by FEDESA in 1993. Its content is therefore very similar to the FEDESA code. However, some modifications and improvements have been introduced by the Committee for Veterinary Medicinal Products (CVMP). The CVMP adopted the final text for this EU guideline in July 1994.

To avoid any confusion and to ease the implementation of the new requirements by companies, changes from the FEDESA Code are identified in this edition, with

| a single bar in the margin for minor changes (mostly wording)

‖ a double bar in the margin for major changes (i.e. changes of substance).

Where a point of the FEDESA Code has been <u>deleted</u> and not replaced, this is also signalled.

Contents

488   *Appendix I*

Chapter 5: Data verification

Chapter 6: Final trial report

Glossary

Foreword

The objective of this document is to provide a guidance for practice on the conduct of clinical trials on veterinary medicinal products in the European Community. It is directed to all those involved in the conduct of such trials and is intended to ensure that those trials are conducted and documented in accordance with Part 4, chapters II and III, and Parts 8 and 9 of the Annex to Directive 92/18/EEC.

Pre-established systematic written procedures for the organisation, conduct, data collection, documentation and verification of clinical trials are necessary to establish the validity of data and to improve the ethical, scientific and technical quality of trials.

The welfare of the trial animals is ultimately the responsibility of the investigator for all matters relating to the trial. All investigators must demonstrate the highest possible degree of professionalism in the observation of animals in the trials and the reporting of such observations. Independent assurance that the trial animals and the human food chain are protected should be provided by the authorization procedure of the competent authority and the procedure for informed consent of the owner of the animals.

Safety and pre-clinical trials, including pharmaco-kinetic studies, are not included in the scope of this document since guidelines are already in existence. However, in those Member States where it is required, data derived from such trials must be submitted to the relevant competent authority in order that the clinical trials or series of trials may be properly authorised prior to commencement.

In conducting clinical trials, due regard must be taken of the possible effects of the product on the environment, on residues in the produce of treated animals, and the eventual fate of animals used for food consumption.

Entry into force

All studies started **after 1 July 1995** should be carried out in accordance with this guideline

Chapter 1 – Responsibilities

Sponsor

1.1 Each sponsor will establish detailed Standard Operating Procedures (SOP) for the elements contained in the protocol.

1.2 With regard to trial protocols the recommendations contained in Chapter 2 of this guideline will be carefully followed during their construction.

1.3 Both the Sponsor and Investigator/Site Supervisor will sign the protocol as an agreement of the details of the clinical trial. Any amendments to the protocol must have the signed agreement of both Sponsor and Investigator/Site Supervisor.

1.4 Furthermore, the sponsor will:

a) select the Investigator/Site Supervisor, and assure his/her qualifications, assure his/her availability for the entire duration of the study, ensure that he/she agrees to undertake the study as laid down in the protocol, according to this note for guidance of practice, including the acceptance of verification procedures.

   (deleted): Point of FEDESA Code on the Suitability of Trial Site

b) inform the Investigator/Site Supervisor of the relevant chemical/pharmaceutical, toxicological and clinical details as a prerequisite in planning the trial.

c) submit notification/application to the relevant authorities where required.

d) provide the investigational medicinal product(s) in suitable packaging and labelling in conformity with the principle of GMP and in such a way that any existing blinding procedure is not invalidated. The labelling should include the words "For Veterinary Clinical Trial Only".

A sample of each batch should be kept for reference for one year after the end of the shelf-life.

Records of the quantities of the medicinal product(s) supplied should be maintained with batch/serial numbers. Certificates of delivery of the medicinal product(s) signed by the investigator must detail the method and place of storage to identify the exclusive use of the product(s) in the trial. It will subsequently be used to account for unused supplies.

Appropriate recommendations for disposal of unused supplies should be given.

e) appoint appropriately qualified and trained Monitor(s).

f) report all suspected Adverse Drug Reactions (ADR) in accordance with relevant requirements.

g) inform the Investigator/Site Supervisor of any critical information that becomes available during a trial and ensure that when required the relevant authority is notified.

h) ensure that a final trial report suitable for regulatory purposes is prepared whether or not the trial has been completed.

i) provide adequate indemnity for the Monitor and Investigator/Site Supervisor and compensation for animal owners in the event of injury or death of the animal or loss of productivity related to the trial.

Monitor

1.5 The Monitor will be the principal communication link between the sponsor and the Site Supervisor/Investigator and will:

a) help the Sponsor to select the Site Supervisor/Investigator.

b) work according to predetermined SOPs, visit the Investigator/Site Supervisor before, during and after the trial to control adherence to the protocol and ensure that all data are correctly and completely recorded and reported and that informed consent is being obtained and recorded from the owner(s) of trial animals prior to including his/her animals.

c) ensure that the trial site has adequate space, facilities, equipment, staff, and that an adequate number of trial animals is likely to be available for the duration of the trial.

d) ensure that trial staff have been adequately informed about the details of the trial.

e) be reasonably available to the Investigator/Site Supervisor for consultation, in person or via telephone, facsimile machine, telex, electronic mail etc.

f) check that the storage, dispensing and documentation for the supply of investigational medicinal product(s) are safe and appropriate, and ensure that any unused medication is returned by the owner(s) to the Sponsor or to an approved site.

g) submit a written report to the Sponsor at agreed intervals to include the reporting of all telephone calls, visits, letters and other contacts with the Investigator/Site Supervisor (audit paper trail concept). These reports will form part of the trial documentation.

(deleted): Point of FEDESA Code on Suspected ADR

Investigator/Site Supervisor

1.6 The Investigator/Site Supervisor will:

a) agree the protocol with the Sponsor via the Monitor and confirm in writing that he/she will work according to the protocol, and adhere to this note for guidance.

b) submit an up-to-date curriculum vitae and other credentials to the Sponsor.

c) obtain informed consent from the owners of trial animals The animal owner must receive written information from the Investigator/Site Supervisor in advance.

d) provide all relevant information to all staff members involved with the trial or with other elements of the management of the trial animals. This should include the local veterinary surgeon that normally attends the animals.

e) ensure that the investigational medicinal product(s) are correctly stored and safely handled. Ensure investigational medicinal products are dispensed to trial subjects in accordance with the protocol and to maintain a full inventory of receipt, usage and remaining stocks. At the end of the trial it must be possible to reconcile delivery records with those of usage and returns including accounting for any discrepancies.

f) manage any code procedure and documentation (e.g. randomisation envelopes), with due professional care, and ensure that any treatment code is only broken in accordance with the protocol and with the Sponsors/Monitor's knowledge and consent.

g) collect and record data in accordance with protocol requirements.

h) in the case of ADRs, immediately notify the Sponsor and Monitor and, where required, relevant authorities.

i) make all data available to the Sponsor/Monitor for the purposes of validation.

j) ensure the accuracy of any report drafted for him/her.

(deleted): Point of FEDESA Code on Confidentiality

k) forward signed Record Sheets to the Monitor. Collaborative Investigators and those responsible for the analyses (including statistical analyses) and the interpretation of the results should also sign the relevant Record Sheets. Where appropriate, all practice records will be clearly marked that the animal(s)/owner is participating in a clinical trial.

l) observe the following points particularly related to animal care:

the Investigator/Site Supervisor will be expected to give assurance that he/she has sufficient time to devote to the study, access to adequate staff and facilities for the conduct of the study, and that suitable equipment is immediately available in case of emergency.

the Investigator/Site Supervisor is responsible for animals under his/her care for the purpose of the trial and, where the Investigator/Site Supervisor is not a veterinary surgeon, will ensure that their care is maintained during and after the trial. The local veterinary surgeon should be kept informed.

Chapter 2 – Guide for the conduct of clinical trials

A well designed trial relies predominantly on a thoroughly considered, well structured and complete protocol which should be completed and approved by the Sponsor and Investigator/Site Supervisor before the trial is initiated.

The protocol will, where relevant, contain the information given in the following list of items, or this list should at least be considered, whenever a trial is contemplated and reasons for any omissions given.

2.1 General information

   a) Title of the study.

   b) Each study will be given an identifier unique to the Sponsor.

   c) The expected names and contact points of the Investigators responsible for the trial; the expected names of other possible participants and their professional background (e.g. veterinarian, biochemist, parasitologist, experimental animal attendant, statistician etc.) should also be made clear.

   d) The name and any contact point of the Sponsor.

   e) If known, the identity of the farm/department/group of veterinary practices where the trial will take place (affiliations, addresses).

2.2 Justification and objectives

   a) The objective in conducting the study must be clearly established.

   b) The essentials of the problem itself and its background, referring where appropriate to relevant literature.

2.3 Schedule

a) Description of the schedule of the trial, i.e. its expected date and time of commencement, investigation period, observation period and termination date where known.

b) Justification of the schedule, i.e. in the light of how far the safety of the medicinal product has been tested, the time course of the disease in question and expected duration of the treatment.

c) Justification of the withdrawal period before slaughter etc. Even if the post-medication period of observation of the live animal is in excess of this period, a withdrawal period must be proposed for all food producing animals in the trial.

2.4 Design

a) Specification of the type of trial, e.g. controlled study, pilot study.

b) Description of the randomisation method, including the procedures to be adopted and practical arrangements to be followed.

c) Description of the trial design (e.g. parallel groups, cross-over design) and the blinding technique selected.

d) Specification of other bias reducing factors to be implemented.

e) Description and justification of the experimental unit(s).

2.5 Animal selection

a) Specification of the type of animal to be used, including species, age, sex, breed, category, reproductive status, prognostic factors etc.

b) The housing and management of the animals.

2.6 Inclusion/exclusion criteria

a) Provision of a clear statement of diagnostic admission criteria.

b) Detailed listing of the criteria for inclusion and, if possible, pre-admission exclusions and post-admission withdrawals of animals from the trial.

2.7 Treatments

a) Clear, precise and detailed identification of the product(s) to be used. These should be fully formulated products likely to be proposed for marketing. There should be a justification of the doses to be used.

b) Description of treatment applied to control group(s) or for control period(s) (placebo, other products, vehicle only, no treatment, etc.).

c) Route of administration, dosing schedules, treatment period(s) for the test product(s) containing the active substance under investigation and for the comparative product(s).

d) Rules for the use of concomitant treatment.

e) Measures to be implemented to ensure the operator's safety whilst handling the test products prior to and during administration.

f) Measures to promote and control close adherence to the prescribed instructions/ordinances (compliance monitoring).

2.8 Assessment of efficacy

a) Definition of the effects to be achieved before efficacy can be claimed.

b) Description of how such effects are measured and recorded.

c) Times of, and periods between observations and concomitant recording of the effects.

d) Description of special analyses and/or tests to be carried out with times of sampling and interval before analysis/test.

2.9 Adverse events

a) Methods of recording and monitoring suspected adverse events.

b) Provisions for dealing with such events, e.g. treatment, changes to method of administration.

c) Information on where the trial code will be kept and how it can be broken in the event of an emergency.

d) Details for the reporting of suspected ADRs and all side effects, particularly the name of the individual designated to receive such reports.

2.10 Operational matters

a) A detailed plan should be drawn up of the various steps and procedures necessary to control and monitor the trial most effectively.

b) Definition of any instructions for anticipated deviations from the protocol.

c) The duties and responsibilities of the investigation team and their coordination.

d) Instructions to staff, including a trial description.

e) Addresses, telephone numbers, etc. enabling any staff member to contact responsible members of the investigation team at any hour.

(deleted): Points f), g) and h) of FEDESA Code on Confidentiality, instructions with regard to operator safety and sampling.

2.11 Handling of records

a) Procedures for handling and processing the records of various effects, including suspected ADRs, relating to the use of the product(s) under study should be defined.

b) Procedures for the maintenance of all the records for each individual (or test group) within the trial must be available. If animals are treated individually then the records must permit the identification of the individual concerned.

c) A copy of the test animal record sheet should be included.

2.12 Evaluation

a) Definition of the measure of test animals' response, e.g. a scoring system, and other measurements made in order to evaluate the clinical response.

b) Definition of the methods of computation and calculation of the effect of the medicinal product.

c) Description of how to deal with and report on animals withdrawn or otherwise removed from the trial.

2.13 Statistics

a) A thorough description of the statistical methods to be employed.

b) The planned number of animals to be included in the trial(s) and the reasoning for the choice of sample size, including reflections on (or calculation of) the power of the trial and the clinical justification, should be provided.

c) Description of the statistical unit/experimental unit.

d) The level of significance to be used.

2.14 Supplements

The protocol should compromise a comprehensive summary and relevant supplements (e.g. information to the owners of the animals, informed consent form, instructions to staff, description of special procedures).

2.15 References

A list of relevant literature, referred to in the protocol, must be included.

Chapter 3 – Data handling

3.1 *General*

a) The person recording an observation will sign and date it, or in the case of the supervisor, each page of observations.

b) Data should be recorded on pre-established durable recording sheets. Record Sheets should be diligently completed indelibly in ink or ball pen, with all the data points recorded as required in the protocol. However, when additional observations are considered necessary by the Investigator/Site Supervisor they should also be recorded on the record sheet together with a comment as to their perceived significance.

c) Units must always be stated, and transformation of units must always be indicated and documented.

d) All corrections on a record sheet and elsewhere in the raw data must be made by drawing one straight line through the erroneous values, which should still be legible. The correct data must be inserted with date and signature or initials, if possible with reasons for change. An alternative would be to use a correction form.

e) Laboratory values should always be recorded on a record sheet or attached to it. Values outside an accepted reference range must be certified by the Investigator. Normal reference values for the laboratory should be included.

f) If data are entered directly into a computer there will be adequate safeguards to ensure validation including a signed and dated print-out. In this case the electronic record or the print-out may be referred to as Raw Data.

g) If, for example, during (direct) data entry, data are transformed by coding, the transformation must be documented.

h) For electronic data processing only authorised persons should be able to enter or modify data in the computer and there should be a record of changes and deletions.

3.2 *Investigator*

The Investigator guarantees the correctness and completeness of the data with a signature and date on each record sheet.

3.3 *Sponsor*

a) The Sponsor will use properly documented and validated data entry handling and analytical systems/programmes.

b) The Sponsor will be able to identify each experimental unit (animal or group of animals) by unambiguous means.

c) SOPs will include systems for dealing with electronic data.

d) The Sponsor will ensure the greatest possible accuracy when converting data electronically. It should be possible to obtain a data print-out which can be compared with the raw data.

e) Computer data systems will be designed to allow correction after loading but the correction must be documented and traceable by date and identity of person making the correction.

f) The Sponsor will maintain a list of persons authorised to make corrections and protect the data by appropriate password systems.

3.4 *Archiving of data*

a) Wherever possible the investigational centre should forward all raw data to the Sponsor for archiving. Where this proves impractical, the investigational centre must ensure adequate archive facilities and forward copies to the Sponsor. The Sponsor must ensure that the Trial Master File contains a listing of all information which is available and where it can be found.

b) The Protocol, documentation (including data on Suspected Adverse Events), approvals and all other original documents related to the trial will be retained by the sponsor in the Trial Master File for a period of five years after the product is no longer authorised.

c) All data and documents will be made available for inspection if requested by relevant authorities.

Chapter 4 – Statistics

4.1 Access to biostatistical competence will be mandatory. Where and by whom the statistical analyses are carried out will be the responsibility of the Sponsor.

4.2 The type of statistical analysis to be used will be specified in the protocol and any subsequent deviations from the plan will be described and justified in the final trial report. Calculations and analyses will be confirmed by a named statistician.

4.3 The statisician and the Monitor will ensure that the data are of high quality at the point of collection and subsequent processing. The statistician will be expected to ensure the integrity of subsequent data processing by using proven and scientifically recognised statistical procedures. An account will be made of missing, unused and spurious data during statistical analysis. All exceptions will be documented for further review if required.

Chapter 5 – Data verification

5.1 Procedures for data verification will be applied to each stage of data collection, recording and processing.

5.2 The Sponsor/Monitor will be expected to perform the following functions before, during and after the study:

a) Monitor at the trial site to ensure that the investigational product(s) and record keeping are being handled correctly and that Adverse Events are properly recorded and reported.

b) Account for the supply and use of investigational and reference substances.

c) Monitor the Investigator's procedures and facilities in accordance with the Protocol and SOPs. Any deviations will be documented and justified.

d) Verify data through each processing procedure.

e) Account for all relevant trial documents and have them available for future audit if required.

f) Check all statistical methods, calculations and conclusions. Reference to validated statistical software will be acceptable.

g) Ensure that the Final Trial Report is in accordance with the methods used in the study, and the reported results and suspected Adverse Events reflect accurately the recorded data.

h) Report all discrepancies found during data verification.

i) Check data archives for ability to retrieve selected data.

j) Ensure that all the above elements are available for audit by an independent body, should this be required. Laboratory and other trial procedures may also be inspected.

Chapter 6 – Final trial report

As described in Chapter 1 of this document it is the responsibility of the Sponsor to prepare a Final Trial Report (FTR) for regulatory purposes whether or not the trial has been completed as planned. The FTR will form the primary record of clinical observations referred to in the Annex to Directive 92/18/EEC (Part 4, Chapter III, Section 2.1 and Part 9, Sections B and C). The structure of the FTR will follow the format of the trial protocol as defined in Chapter 2 of this document, and a copy of the trial protocol will be appended to the FTR.

6.1 In accordance with the above-mentioned Directive the FTR will include relevant information from the following list:

a) The names of all people involved in conducting the trial, including Investigator, Monitor, Site Supervisor, Technical Assistants, Statisticians and Veterinary Surgeons.

b) The address of the premises at which the trial was conducted (e.g. farm, institute or veterinary practice) and the name(s) of the owner(s) of the animals. In the case of a trial involving companion animals, it will only be necessary to use suitable practice reference codes on the Record Sheets to identify the animal owners.

c) Details of animal management including the composition of feed and the nature and quantity of any additives in the feed.

d) Disease history, relevant to the condition under investigation, especially in the case of specific disease problems associated with a farm unit.

e) Diagnosis of the disease being treated, including a description of the clinical signs according to conventional criteria. Reports from laboratory or post-mortem examinations used to identify the condition will be summarised in the FTR, and appended.

f) The precise identification of the clinical trial formulation used in the trial including lot or batch numbers.

g) The dosage of the medicinal product, methods, route, and frequency of administration and precautions, if any, taken during administration.

h) The duration of treatment and period of subsequent observation.

i) A full description of methods used and observations and measurements made.

j) A full description of animals involved in the trial, including numbers of each sex in each treatment group, and details of randomisation and blocking techniques used in the allocation of animals to treatment groups.

k) Full information on any animal withdrawn from the study.

l) Details of any other medicinal product(s) which was (were) administered during the trial, either prior to, during or after the test product, and details of any interactions observed.

m) A full description of the results of the trial whether favourable or unfavourable, including tables of all data recorded during the trial. Reports from laboratory or post-mortem examinations conducted during the trial will be appended to the FTR.

n) Details of any suspected Adverse Drug Reactions or other Adverse Events occurring during the trial and any measures taken as a consequence.

o) Any effects on animal performance (e.g. egg laying, milk production, or reproductive function).

p) A conclusion based on results from each individual case or treatment group as appropriate.

q) A summary of the trial including a statement of the objective, the materials and methods, the results, and the main conclusions that can be drawn from the results.

6.2 The FTR will be signed by the Sponsor and the trial Monitor indicating that it represents a complete and accurate record of the clinical trial.

Glossary

Adverse Drug Reaction (ADR)

A reaction which is harmful and unintended and which occurs at doses normally used in animals for the prophylaxis, diagnosis or treatment of disease or the modification of physiological function.

Adverse Event (AE)

Any undesirable experience occurring to a test animal during a clinical trial whether or not considered to be related to the investigational product.

Audit (of a trial)

A comparison of raw data and associated records with the interim or final report in order to determine whether the raw data have been accurately reported, whether testing was carried out in accordance with the trial protocol and standard operating procedures, to obtain additional information not provided in the final report, and to establish whether practices were employed in the development of data that would impair their validity. The audit must be conducted either through an internal facility at the Sponsor's, but independent of the units responsible for clinical research, or through an external contractor.

Clinical Study

A number of clinical trials conducted to a similar protocol.

Clinical Trials

Systematic studies in target species or in the particular categories of such animals, in order to establish the therapeutic effects which could include confirmation of the pharmacodynamics and/or to monitor any suspected adverse response from the use of veterinary medicinal products.

Documentation

All records in any form (including documents, magnetic and optical records) describing methods and conduct of the trial, factors affecting the trial, and the action taken. These include protocol, raw data, Investigator's reports, Monitor's reports, letters, biochemical reference ranges, final trial report, etc.

Final Trial Report

A complete and comprehensive description of the trial after its completion prepared by the Sponsor, Investigator or Monitor, including a description of material and methods, a presentation and evaluation of the results, statistical analyses and a critical clinical and statistical appraisal.

Informed Consent

The confirmation of an owner's willingness to participate in a particular trial. This confirmation should only be sought after information has been given about the owner's rights and responsibilities, about the risk and inconveniences related to the investigation and the objectives and benefits thereof. In the case of food producing animals, the owner shall be informed in writing of the consequences of participation in the trial, for the subsequent disposal of treated animals or for the taking of foodstuffs from treated animals. A copy of this notification countersigned and dated by the animal owner or the Investigator shall be included in the trial documentation.

Investigational Centre

A commercial or scientific body to which a Sponsor may transfer some tasks and obligations. Any such transfer shall be in writing and shall describe each of the obligations assumed by the Investigational Centre.

Investigational Product

Any active ingredient, medicinal product or placebo being tested or used as a reference in a clinical trial.

Investigator

The person responsible for the practical performance of a trial and for the health and welfare of the animals during the trial.

The investigator is:
- appropriately qualified
- experienced in the performance of clinical trials
- familiar with the background to and the requirements of the study.

Trained technical assistants may help in data collection and subsequent processing.

Monitor

A person appointed by the Sponsor or Investigational Centre to be responsible to the Sponsor or Investigational Centre for the monitoring and reporting on progress of the trial and for verification of data. The Monitor must have qualifications and experience to enable a knowledgeable supervision of the particular trial.

Protocol

A document which states the rationale and objectives of the trial with the conditions under which it is to be performed and managed. A list of items to be included in the protocol is given in Chapter 2 of this note for guidance.

Raw Data

The record of the original clinical and laboratory findings during a trial or certified copies of the same. Record Sheet: A record of the data and other information on each experimental unit as defined in the protocol. These shall be Individual Record Sheets in the case of individual treatments and Collective Record Sheets in the case of collective treatment. The data may be recorded by any means which ensures accurate input and presentation and allows verification.

Regulatory Authority

An independent or governmental body whose responsibility is to verify that the rights and integrity of trial animals and their owners are protected, and thereby provide public reassurance as to the welfare and well-being of the animals receiving Investigational Products, to determine the safety of products entering the food chain derived from trial animals, and to ensure safety to the operator and the environment from the use of Investigational Products.

Site Supervisors

Investigators responsible for an individual trial at a single location.

Sponsor

An individual or an organisation which takes responsibility for the initiation, management and financing of a clinical trial. When an Investigator independently initiates and assumes responsibility for a study that may subsequently become part of an application for a marketing authorization, the Investigator then also assumes the role of the Sponsor.

Standard Operating Procedures

Detailed written instructions describing the practical procedures, test methods and management operations to be performed or followed, precautions to be taken and measures to apply.

Trial Animal

A farm or companion animal, or groups of the same, included in a clinical trial.

Trial Master File

Document comprising protocol, raw data, original recordings from automated instruments, laboratory notes, records or telecons, documentation and final report.

Verification/Validation of Data

The process carried out to assure that the data contained in the final trial report match original observations. These procedures may apply to raw data, hard copy or electronic reports, computer print-outs and statistical analyses and tables.

Index